Dementia and Ethics Reconsidered

Reconsidering Dementia Series Editors: Dr Keith Oliver and Professor Dawn Brooker MBE

Dementia and Ethics Reconsidered

Julian C. Hughes

Open University Press

Open University Press
McGraw Hill
Unit 4,
Foundation Park
Roxborough Way
Maidenhead
SL6 3UD

email: emea_uk_ireland@mheducation.com
world wide web: www.openup.co.uk

First edition published 2023

Commissioning Editor: Sam Crowe
Editorial Assistant: Hannah Jones
Production Manager: Hannah Cartwright
Marketing Manager: Bryony Waters
Cover Design: Adam Renvoize
Cover Art: George Rook
Logo Design: Julia Heron

A catalogue record of this book is available from the British Library

ISBN-13: 9780335251001
ISBN-10: 0335251005
eISBN: 9780335251018

Library of Congress Cataloging-in-Publication Data
CIP data applied for

Typeset by Transforma Pvt. Ltd., Chennai, India

Praise Page

"Julian C. Hughes is to be wholly commended in producing this excellent new book in the Reconsidering Dementia series. He has made the complex field of ethics and moral philosophy accessible to everyone, whilst always keeping the experience of people living with dementia front and centre. I found his descriptions of everyday ethical dilemmas faced in practice illuminating and written with that rare mix of authority, humility and compassion. An essential read that both informs and delights at the turn of every page."
Professor John Keady, The University of Manchester,
UK/Greater Manchester Mental Health NHS Foundation Trust, UK

For me, as both a researcher and caregiver of people living with dementia, the most important work in dementia care is to see through the cognitive disorder no matter the severity of the condition and try to recognize and understand the person as the person he or she still is. This new book from Julian C. Hughes contributes hugely to this work highlighting the immensely important ethics of dementia care. Hughes cleverly shows how ethics run through all branches of life with dementia and why it is so important that we pay more attention to it in far more areas than we do today. In my view, this is where the book stands particularly strong as it helps to broaden the focus on ethics in dementia care to places often failed to be seen; that's what 'Dementia and Ethics Reconsidered' did to me!
Jesper Bøgmose Hansen, Associate Professor, Cand. Cur.,
Faculty of Health, University College Copenhagen, Denmark

"Julian C. Hughes is uniquely qualified to write about ethics and dementia. It's an area that requires insight into the clinical and lived reality of dementia, mastery of relevant philosophical ideas but perhaps most importantly, a sensitivity to what it all means. Dementia and Ethics Reconsidered not only explains the major approaches to ethics, but it also demonstrates the ways in which they are or are not applicable to thinking about dementia. This book skilfully brings together the threads of ethics and policy that are relevant to dementia and discusses them from a clinically nuanced perspective."
Professor John McMillan, Editor in Chief, Journal of Medical Ethics

"This book should be an essential read for all of us who support and navigate the ethical issues relating to people with dementia and their families. Sensitively and beautifully written, it offers a broad and

profound insight into the subject and provides a depth that is both contemporary and accessible. What we have here is a truly brilliant book that deserves so much credit. Read it."
Paul Edwards, Director of Clinical Services, Dementia UK

"Julian C. Hughes has made a significant contribution to the ethical dimension of dementia through his scholarly and comprehensive treatment of a range of pertinent issues, from the role of ethical theory to the moral dilemmas encountered in practice. He provides a balanced account of the diverse frameworks warranting attention, clarifying their strengths and limitations. His position on regarding people suffering from dementia as unique persons first and foremost but not at the expense of their human rights is presented impeccably."
Sidney Bloch, Emeritus Professor of Psychiatry,
University of Melbourne, Australia

"In this inspiring and important book Professor Hughes convinces us 'that ethics are all our business' but also that 'the questions to which thoughtful answers are required are not always asked'. Thankfully this book will help us do just that. This is a work of great depth but it is also accessible. The structure enables the reader to be eased into understanding ethical approaches and to consider these in a wide range of dilemmas in practice from sexuality and intimacy to death and dying. This is essential reading for anyone with a vested interest in the field of dementia."
Dr Simon Burrow, Division of Nursing,
Midwifery and Social Work, University of Manchester, UK

Titles in the series

Dementia and Psychotherapy Reconsidered Richard Cheston

Education and Training in Dementia Care: A Person-Centred Approach Claire Surr, Sarah Jane Smith and Isabelle Latham

Dementia and Ethics Reconsidered Julian C. Hughes

Forthcoming titles

Leisure and Everyday Life with Dementia Christopher Russell, Jane Twigg and Karen Gray (eds)

Reconsidering Neighbourhoods and Living with Dementia: Spaces, Places, and People John Keady (ed)

Talking with Dementia, Reconsidered Keith Oliver, Reinhard Guss and Ruth Bartlett

This book is dedicated to the memory of Tim Parry (1961–2017), an extraordinary nurse and an extraordinary human being.

Contents

List of boxes

List of figures

List of tables

About the author

Julian C. Hughes is honorary professor at Bristol University and visiting professor at Newcastle University in the UK. He was a consultant in old age psychiatry in the National Health Service (NHS) for over 20 years. He led both community and in-patient teams, with a focus on long-term and residential care.

Julian studied Philosophy, Politics and Economics (PPE) at the University of Oxford prior to studying Medicine at Bristol. He gained his PhD in Philosophy from the University of Warwick. He initially trained as a general practitioner (GP) in the Royal Air Force (RAF), where he also started his psychiatry training before moving for higher training to the Anglia & Oxford Regional Senior Registrar Training Scheme. His first consultant post was in Newcastle upon Tyne, but he then moved to North Tyneside General Hospital. From 2009 until 2016 he was honorary professor of philosophy of ageing at Newcastle University and was professor of old age psychiatry at the University of Bristol from 2016 to 2019.

As a researcher he has taken part, including as principal investigator, in numerous nationally-funded studies supported by bodies such as the Alzheimer's Society, the Medical Research Council, the Wellcome Trust and the National Institute for Health Research. He has also acted as principal investigator and national chief investigator on clinical drug trials. However, areas of particular interest have been palliative care and issues in connection with decision-making capacity and best interests. He has authored over 100 peer-reviewed journal papers and written 70 book chapters.

He was elected Fellow of the Royal College of Psychiatrists and of the Royal College of Physicians of Edinburgh. He has been an adviser to various national and international bodies, including Alzheimer Europe, the National Institute for Health and Care Excellence (NICE), the General Medical Council (GMC) and the Department of Health. He was the deputy chair of the Nuffield Council on Bioethics until March 2019, having served as a Member of the Council from February 2013 and as a member of their working party which produced *Dementia: Ethical Issues* in 2009.

Julian has written, co-written, edited or co-edited 12 books. His single author books are: *Thinking Through Dementia* (Oxford University Press, 2011); *Alzheimer's and Other Dementias: The Facts* (Oxford University Press, 2011); and *How We Think About Dementia* (Jessica Kingsley, 2014). He now concentrates on writing in the areas of ageing, dementia, ethics and the philosophy of psychiatry.

Apart from writing, Julian is a flautist (he is an Associate of the London College of Music and was for a time the flute teacher at Bristol Cathedral School) and enjoys walking and his family. He and his wife Anne have three children and currently four grandchildren.

The Reconsidering Dementia Series

The dementia field has developed rapidly in its scope and practice over the past 25 years. Many thousands of people are newly diagnosed each year. Worldwide, the trend is that people are being diagnosed at much earlier stages. In addition, families and friends increasingly provide support to those affected by dementia over a prolonged period. Many people, both those diagnosed with dementia and those who support them, have an appetite to understand their condition. Care professionals and civic society also need an in depth and nuanced understanding of how to support people living with dementia within their communities over the long term. The *Reconsidering Dementia* book series sets out to address this need. It takes its inspiration from the late Professor Tom Kitwood's seminal text *Dementia Reconsidered* published in 1997 which, at the time, revolutionised how dementia care was conceptualised.

The book series is jointly commissioned and edited by Professor Dawn Brooker MBE and by Dr Keith Oliver. Dawn has been active in the field of dementia care since the 1980's as a clinician and an academic. She draws on her experience and international networks to bring together a series of books on the most pertinent issues in the field. Keith is one of the foremost international advocates for those living with dementia. He also brings an insightful perspective of his own and others' experience of what it means to live with dementia gained since his diagnosis of Alzheimer's Disease in 2010.

Dawn and Keith have been professional colleagues for many years. They both worked together on the 2nd Edition of Kitwood's book entitled *Dementia Reconsidered Revisited: The person still comes first.* This 2019 publication was a reprint of the original text by Tom Kitwood alongside contemporary commentaries for each chapter written by current experts. Many topics in the field of dementia care, however, were simply unheard of in Kitwood's lifetime. When Open University Press approached Dawn and Keith with the idea of developing a book series dedicated to dementia, they were very pleased to accept. The subsequent titles in this series are cutting-edge scholarly texts that challenge and engage readers to think deeply. They draw on theoretical understandings, contemporary research and experience to critically reflect on their topic in great depth.

This does not mean, however, that they are not applicable to improving the care and support to those affected by dementia. As well as the scholarly text all books have a "So what?" thread that unpacks what this means for people living with dementia, their families, people working in dementia care, policy makers, professionals, community activists and so on. Too many books either focus on an academic audience OR a practitioner audience OR a student audience OR a lived experience audience. In this series, the aim is to try to address these perspectives in the round. The *Reconsidering Dementia* book series brings together the perspectives of professional practice, scholarship and the lived experience as they pertain to the key topics in the field of dementia studies. All the books aim to help us to think afresh, to reconsider our standpoint and to ultimately improve the experience of those affected by dementia for years to come.

Preface

Virtually every decision that is made in dementia care calls for an ethical framework. Deciding how to deliver a diagnosis (or not), whether to help someone eat their food, how to respond to someone's altered reality, how to help someone have medication and so on all require weighing up the pros and cons of different actions. The problem is that these are rarely made explicit and most people working in the field don't consider ethics as part of their professional development. Family carers and people living with dementia rarely see their decisions as having an ethical basis either. We mainly just do what we think is right at the time.

However, understanding and communicating clearly about ethical frameworks can make the tricky everyday choices much easier to navigate. It also makes it easier for us to challenge when we feel that people are getting a raw deal or when decisions feel wrong. We knew early on that we wanted someone to write a book on Ethics for our Reconsidering Dementia Series. We wanted a serious book but also one that spoke to everyday life. The one person we knew who would bring both the scholarship and practical insights honed over many years of clinical practice was Julian Hughes. We are delighted that this book is now part of our series and we hope that you will learn as much from it as we both have.

Series Editors: Dawn Brooker and Keith Oliver

Additional thoughts from Keith Oliver

When I first began to contribute to my various roles within the dementia world I had little or no understanding of what ethics in this domain entailed, and my early encounters did little to clarify this. What Julian does is to bring the subject alive in a very readable and scholarly way so that all who read it will take something useful from it. Whilst I wish this book had been available earlier its timing for me personally was most apt as when reading it for the first time my wife was in a geriatric ward in an acute hospital and many of the positives and negatives which Julian identifies were plain to be seen. My sincere wish was that those who could have influenced better care in that ward would be encouraged to read this book. If she is ever admitted again I will certainly signpost them to it!

Ever since accepting my joint voluntary roles as a NHS Dementia Envoy and an Alzheimer's Society Ambassador I have heard differing, often strongly held views about the term the medical model of dementia care. Whilst in my view, models are a bit like labels – helpful or not according to their application, what my knowledge of Julian based upon the eight years I have known him is that what both of us sincerely believe and is evidenced within this book is that the person affected by dementia should, and must always come first.

Finally, it was a genuine joy and privilege to play a part in supporting this book through to publication, and I am proud and honoured to stand alongside Dawn, Julian and the team in advocating for it. If read widely its positive impact will be significant, and the knowledge and wisdom professionals will derive from the book will be of great benefit to those like me who live with, and are affected by dementia.

Acknowledgements

I should like to thank the following:

Aileen Beatty, Charlotte Emmett and Jessica Kingsley Publishers for permission to quote from our 2021 book *Dementia, Law and Ethics*;

Dianne Gove and Alzheimer Europe for permission to quote from their 2021 report *Sex, Gender and Sexuality in the Context of Dementia*;

The Nuffield Council on Bioethics for permission to quote from the 2009 report *Dementia: Ethical Issues*, as well as from Prainsack, B. and Buyx, A. (2011) *Solidarity: Reflections on an Emerging Concept in Bioethics*;

Oxford University Press for permission to quote from the chapter co-authored with Chris Heginbotham (2013) on mental capacity and decision-making in the *Oxford Textbook of Old Age Psychiatry* (second edition); and

Russell Woodruff and SpringerNature for permission to quote from Woodruff's (2016) 'Aging and the Maintenance of Dignity' in *The Palgrave Handbook of the Philosophy of Aging*.

I would also like to thank Alan Howarth and Matthew Crooks who generously made helpful suggestions for Chapter 22. Aileen Beatty kindly read and commented on Chapter 27, for which I remain very grateful. Although mention of legal matters is deliberately sparse in this book, I must acknowledge (with thanks) that my knowledge of the law in relation to dementia owes considerably to Charlotte Emmett and John Horne. Hannah Zeilig has also been most helpful and inspirational when it comes to thinking about aesthetics and dementia. Dawn Brooker and Keith Oliver, the series editors, have been steadfastly supportive, encouraging, kind and assiduous in their comments on the book since its inception. In addition, I have benefited throughout from the careful and professional support of the editorial team at Open University Press: Sam Crowe, Beth Summers, Hannah Jones and their colleagues.

As I have gone over the drafts of this book, it has struck me how many of the authors I have cited have been colleagues, acquaintances and friends. This may just reflect a bias towards people I know. But it persuades me that I have been greatly privileged to have come across so many inspirational practitioners and thinkers to all of whom I owe considerable thanks. I acknowledge this and apologize that I cannot make my debts to them more specific.

Nevertheless, at the risk of being invidious, I must highlight three colleagues and friends who have inspired and guided me, especially in relation to clinical ethics and how we should think about people who live with dementia. They are Tony Hope, Stephen Louw and Steve Sabat. They will not agree with every word written in this book, but to them I owe considerable debts of gratitude alongside enduring affection. As always, I must thank Anne Hughes, my wife, for her ineffable support and impeccable proofreading. All the remaining errors and shortcomings of the book are mine.

The book is dedicated to a wonderful colleague who inspired me profoundly during my early career. I met Tim, who was working in a team of incredible nurses, at the old Radcliffe Infirmary in Oxford. The old age psychiatry unit then moved to the Cherwell Ward in the Fulbrook Centre at the Churchill Hospital. Tim, a philosophy graduate as well as a nurse, was a person of great compassion and wisdom. He later gave me two booklets about Saint Isaac the Syrian, who once wrote: 'There is no virtue which does not have continual struggle yoked to it' (Saint Isaac, 1997: §130, p. 16). Tim would have agreed with this and I think it remains relevant to our attempts to understand and care for the person living with dementia in a manner that is ethical and just. I am grateful to Pauline, his wife, and to Rosie, Isaac and Anna for allowing me the privilege of using Tim's name in this way.

Abbreviations

§	Paragraph
AD	Alzheimer's disease
ADHD	Attention deficit hyperactivity disorder
ADND	Acquired diffuse neurocognitive dysfunction
ADRT	Advance Decision to Refuse Treatment
AED	Advance euthanasia directive
AQT	A quick test of cognitive speed
BPSD	Behavioural and psychological symptoms of dementia
CJD	Creutzfeldt-Jakob disease
COVID-19	Coronavirus disease
CPR	Cardiopulmonary resuscitation
CRPD	*Convention on the Rights of Persons with Disabilities*
CSF	Cerebrospinal fluid
DLB	Dementia with Lewy bodies
DRSEIs	Dementia Research-Specific Ethical Issues
DVA	Driver and Vehicle Agency
DVLA	Driving and Vehicle Licensing Agency
DSM	*Diagnostic and Statistical Manual*
FTD	Frontotemporal dementia
GMC	General Medical Council
GP	General practitioner
HD	Huntington's disease
HIV	Human Immunodeficiency Virus
HMSO	His Majesty's Stationery Office
ICU	Intensive care unit
KNMG	Royal Dutch Medical Association
MCA	*Mental Capacity Act 2005*
MCI	Mild Cognitive Impairment
MHA	*Mental Health Act 1983*
NGT	Nasogastric tube
NHS	National Health Service
NICE	National Institute for Health and Care Excellence
NMC	Nursing and Midwifery Council
NPH	Normal Pressure Hydrocephalus
NVVA	Dutch Association of Nursing Home Physicians
p. (pp)	page (pages)
PDD	Parkinson's disease with dementia
PEG	Percutaneous endoscopic gastrostomy
PPE	Personal protective equipment
REC	Research Ethics Committee

REM	Rapid eye movement
SEA	Situated Embodied Agent
SOED	*Shorter Oxford English Dictionary*
UK	United Kingdom
UKCC	United Kingdom Central Council for Nursing, Midwifery and Health Visiting
USA	United States of America
VaD	Vascular dementia
VBM	Values-based medicine
VBP	Values-based practice
WMA	World Medical Association

Part 1

Theory and Everyday Life

1 Introduction: In anticipation – so what?

Ethical questions

Each month, the very helpful National Health Service (NHS) librarian in my local hospital kindly sends me a review of the latest academic literature on the topic of dementia. I decided to introduce this book by looking at the twelfth work cited in this month's literature review. You will have to believe that this was a random process! Prior to looking, I had no idea what the paper would be about. The point I wish to make is that it is inconceivable it would not raise ethical issues. Everything to do with health and social care, it seems to me, tends to raise ethical issues; and dementia raises particular issues.

The paper I found was called 'Reliability and validity of a quick test of cognitive speed (AQT) in screening for mild cognitive impairment and dementia' (Afshar et al. 2021). This is, of course, a perfectly proper topic for empirical research. In what sense, therefore, does it raise ethical issues? In Box 1.1, I have listed some questions which can be regarded as ethical in that they raise questions of right and wrong.

Box 1.1 Examples of ethical questions in connection with Afshar et al. 2021

Why do we need any further tests of cognitive function (we have enough)?
Why are we testing this particular test?
How were the participants recruited to the study?
Why do you want to screen for dementia (let alone mild cognitive impairment (MCI)) using a cognitive test at all, especially one that is so specific?
What are the likely consequences of such screening?
Would it be right to tell people that they have, or may have, dementia if they are not presenting with a problem?
What, in real terms, can be done to help them?
What is the point of screening for a condition (MCI), which is not dementia, but which might, or might not, become dementia?
Do the people in the study know they are being screened to see if they are eligible for research which will involve telling them that they may or may not have a condition, which they may or may not wish to know about, for which there is no specific treatment?

These are valid questions to do with the study. Some relate to the topic of research ethics, which I shall discuss in Chapter 14. The research was reviewed by the appropriate Research Ethics Committee (REC), which would have looked at its aims, objectives and methods very carefully. You might say it is not terribly surprising that research raises questions relevant to research ethics.

But we should stand back a bit. There are fundamental questions that can be raised about the point of doing this research at all, not just questions about the practicalities. For instance, is MCI even an illness? We shall return to this in Chapter 17. Of course, there are plausible answers to such questions which are more or less convincing. It might be said that an early diagnosis of MCI helps, for instance, in that you can do some advance care planning in anticipation of dementia. But, wait a second, you can do advance care planning even without a diagnosis and not everyone with MCI goes on to develop dementia. Furthermore, there are no treatments that work in MCI and the treatments for dementia are only marginally effective and do not treat the underlying condition. It could be said that an early diagnosis allows time to optimize the person's general condition. But why not do that anyway? If you are worried about raised blood pressure, screen for that! And so on.

All I want to establish is that there are lots of questions and they are ethical. They also, we should note, go beyond the normal remit of an REC (in the USA this would be an Institutional Review Board), because they start to question taken-for-granted positions, such as there being a diagnosis of MCI. Likewise, there are also lots of answers. To be candid, most researchers and clinicians accept that there is a condition called MCI and that early diagnosis is beneficial, so screening is a worthwhile thing. My aim is simply to point out that these fundamental assumptions can be questioned, and should be, because they are partly ethical assumptions. At the end of this book, it has been suggested that I should answer the question 'So what?'. In this chapter I am partly anticipating that question.

For now, I shall put the answer this way: sometimes asking questions – and seeing the ethical nature of the issues involved – is a step towards practical change for the better; but sometimes seeing something in a new light does not bring about immediate or obvious practical change. It may, however, change our attitude to something or someone. Coming to see, for instance, that the scientific inclination to measure things is not always the right approach to other human beings might induce a shift in terms of one's approach to others. This in itself might solve a particular problem. The link between a conceptual question (one which raises ethical concerns) and a practical attitude (one which de-escalates a tense situation) may not be overt. It may, however, be potent.

In any case, it can be added that asking relevant and profound questions is part of what it is to be a good human being: one who flourishes; one who uses the intellectual skills with which we are imbued to understand our situation; one who, in short, is alive to the moral uncertainties of our lives. It is a virtue to ask questions that should lead us to live our lives in as good a way as possible. Ethical questions are ethically imperative!

Dementia and its types

I shall now move on briefly to describe the dementias, or some of them. The aim is not to provide a compendious account or overview (see Ames et al. 2017 for the former and Hughes 2011a for the latter). I shall describe them in a manner that highlights how they might raise ethical issues. First, I shall cover some basic facts.

As illustrated in Figure 1.1, 'dementia' is an umbrella term. There are many different types of dementia, reflecting its many causes. Trauma (including heading heavy balls in football) can cause dementia; so can genetics. Biochemical abnormalities cause dementia; so do strokes. The list of causes is very long indeed. But they are all causes of dementia. There are, however, four more common types of dementia: Alzheimer's disease (AD), vascular dementia (VaD), dementia with Lewy bodies (DLB) and frontotemporal dementia (FTD).

What this means is that if you have Alzheimer's disease, you automatically have dementia; but if you have dementia, you do not automatically have Alzheimer's (you may have vascular or some other type of dementia).

The definition of dementia is that it is an acquired condition: it emerges later in life, albeit as early as in a person's thirties; it is not (unlike congenital conditions) present at birth. It is a global condition: it does not affect just one small

Figure 1.1 Types of dementia

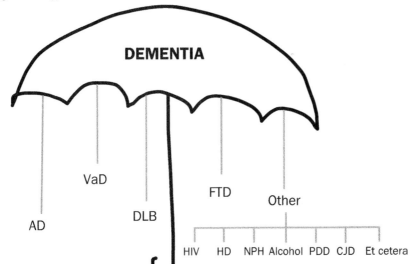

Key: AD = Alzheimer's disease; Alcohol = alcohol-related dementias; CJD = Creutzfeldt-Jakob disease; DLB = dementia with Lewy bodies; FTD = frontotemporal dementia; HD = Huntington's disease; HIV = human immune deficiency virus dementia; NPH = normal pressure hydrocephalus; PDD = Parkinson's disease with dementia; VaD = vascular dementia.

bit of the brain but affects different areas and therefore different functions of the brain. It tends to be progressive. It has psychosocial and behavioural components: it does not solely affect cognitive or so-called 'higher' brain functions; it affects how people behave, how they think and perceive things and it eventually affects activities of daily living. It will finally have physical effects too, although in some types these come early. All the many types of dementia will tend to have these main features.

But the different types of dementia will also have their own specific features. Table 1.1 gives some brief details about the four main types of dementia. Actually, it leaves out an important type, which is very common – that of mixed dementia. In this condition people will have a mixture of two or more types of dementia. Perhaps they have Alzheimer's disease, but they have also had strokes causing vascular dementia. They would then present as people with (what might seem like) an odd collection of symptoms and signs, until the nature of the mixed dementia is understood.

Further details of the specific types of dementia need not detain us. Its epidemiology is also complicated (see Lilford and Hughes 2020 for further details). Except we should note that, whilst most dementias start late in life, there is also young-onset dementia, where the dementia starts before the person is 65 years old.

To return to ethical issues, almost any issue might occur in any form of dementia. To anticipate, Table 1.1 also includes examples of typical ethical issues that might emerge in particular forms of dementia.

Before concluding, I should note that the literature which I review in this book can quite readily be seen as 'medical', so that it can become natural to speak of 'medical ethics'. I shall try to refrain from doing so on the grounds that ethical difficulties might arise for a great number of professionals, from care assistants in care homes to social workers in the community, from general nurses to psychiatrically trained nurses, from general physicians to old age psychiatrists, and so forth. Family carers of people living with a diagnosis of dementia also face ethical issues, as do other 'informal' (non-paid) carers, such as good neighbours or old friends. Moreover, people living with dementia themselves can face ethical dilemmas: when should they make advance decisions and, in doing so, how much burden do they place on their friends and family? Feelings of guilt are feelings about what is right or wrong. Policymakers, from those who run local organizations to national politicians, make decisions about the lives of people with dementia too. I hope the breadth of the ethical concerns that can arise in connection with dementia will be apparent throughout this book, even if there is a tendency to consider clinical issues. This tendency is because it is these issues that are mainly written about in the literature.

'Dementia' itself

To conclude, I want again to anticipate Chapter 17 by flagging an underlying ethical issue. I have described various types of dementia as if this is straightforward.

But now I want to ask whether it is even right to refer to 'dementia' itself. Dementia is not a thing; it is about a hundred things. When you are told that someone has dementia, you cannot presume you know what is mainly wrong with them: they might have problems recalling things; they might have movement or speech problems; or they might experience psychosis. Moreover, *de-mentia* means 'out of mind'. Is it good to be told you are out of your mind?

Table 1.1   Brief details of main types of dementia and examples of ethical issues

Type of dementia	Approximate prevalence (%)	Typical pathology	Description	Example of ethical issue that could occur (and chapter where such issues are discussed)
Alzheimer's disease (AD)	50	Amyloid plaques and neurofibrillary tangles in the brain	This is what many people might consider the archetypal dementia: gradually worsening memory lapses (of various types) broaden to disorientation and speech difficulties. Other cognitive problems emerge, to do with calculation, writing, perception and so forth. This all goes along with difficulties to do with activities of daily living: cooking, shopping, doing odd jobs around the house. Eventually there are also physical problems with eating, walking, swallowing; and the person becomes completely dependent on others.	Concerns about a person's decreasing ability to drive (see Chapter 18). When is it right or wrong to stop someone from driving?
Vascular dementia (VaD)	20	Strokes and small vessel disease in the brain	'Vascular' implies it is to do with the blood vessels. Depending on where and how extensive the blockages in or bleeding from the vessels has been, will determine the exact symptoms and their severity. Perhaps, as well as problems doing things (called 'dyspraxia'), there are also major speech problems. Or it might be much more gradual and look quite like Alzheimer's disease, except the deficits can be patchy – not quite what you would have expected, with one ability seeming good yet another very poor.	A person's irritability might be a sign of the extent to which insight can be maintained in VaD. How should this be approached in a manner that is good (see Chapter 21)?

(continued)

Table 1.1 (*Continued*)

Type of dementia	Approximate prevalence (%)	Typical pathology	Description	Example of ethical issue that could occur (and chapter where such issues are discussed)
Dementia with Lewy bodies (DLB)	20	Lewy bodies in the nerve cells of the brain	In this type of dementia, the cognitive (higher brain) problems might not present as forgetfulness, but are more likely to be signs of visuospatial problems: finding it difficult to copy or write when tested, or to sit down on a chair or perform certain daily tasks and so on. But DLB also typically involves very vivid visual hallucinations, often of small people or animals. There are associated sleep disturbances too (rapid eye movement (REM) sleep disturbance) and people develop some of the symptoms and signs of parkinsonism (for example, stiffness and slowness of movements).	The person with DLB, on account of hallucinations, might be very paranoid. Ought you to agree that there are people in the garden, or do you say it is all just a delusion (see Chapter 24)?
Frontotemporal dementia (FTD)	<10	Proteins called tau and ubiquitin in the brain	When this type of dementia – which is much commoner in people with young-onset dementia (where it starts below the age of 65 years), albeit AD still dominates – mainly affects the front of the brain, there can be behavioural disturbances. When it affects the temporal lobes there can be a variety of language problems. But like all the dementias, finally there is a general, global deterioration.	If there is sexual disinhibition as part of FTD, should the person be told off, or even arrested (see Chapter 25)? Would that be the right or wrong thing to do?

Is that a fair description of someone who has problems with recall, movement or speech? There are better ways to put it. It starts to look incredibly unkind. Should we change the terminology? It seems lazy not to and it is certainly something we should (ethically) reconsider! For in response to 'So what?' I am inclined to reply: for the sake of the standing of persons who live with the diagnosis we should not be lazy; our approaches to them – and to those who love and care for them – should be ethically and morally energetic.

2 The 'problem' of ethics

What are ethics and morals?

In Chapter 1, I was keen to establish that ethical and moral issues are common in dementia and that we must take them seriously. Perhaps we need to define these terms before we proceed. The words 'ethics' and 'morals' can almost be used interchangeably. They do, however, have different roots and can convey slightly different meanings. 'Ethics' comes from the Greek *ethikós* and, according to the *Shorter Oxford English Dictionary* (SOED), can imply a set of moral principles or the science of morals. We speak of nursing or medical ethics; nursing or medical morals would sound odd! Aristotle's famous *Ethics* (actually, he wrote more than one) could be described as presenting a system of moral thought. 'Morals' derives from the Latin *moralis* and it is here that the SOED speaks more obviously about good and bad, right and wrong, good and evil. Overall, these words – 'ethics' and 'morals' – suggest anything to do with questions of good and bad (or evil), right and wrong, whether this is to do with individual decisions, attitudes, dispositions, character and behaviour, people, practices, institutions or systems. In fact, the SOED suggests that *moralis* was the Latin rendering of *ethikós*, so using the words almost synonymously is excusable. There is, however, a slight tendency to regard morals as representing internal conceptions of right and wrong, good or bad, whereas ethics implies external restraints on our behaviour.

So, under extreme circumstances, we might argue that a clinician acted morally, even though the action conflicted with professional ethics. For instance, professional ethics codes (and the law) will typically say that a person must give consent before any treatment can be given. Still, we can imagine extreme circumstances (think of a young adult who has taken an overdose and is refusing treatment) where a doctor feels it is a moral obligation to treat even in the absence of consent. There would be consequences of such a decision – the doctor might be struck off – and the moral judgement may well be challenged. But such a case is enough to show that private morality and professional ethics do not always have to coincide.

What difference do ethics and moral philosophy make?

The title of this chapter suggests there is a problem with ethics. So, what is it? One problem is the gap between theory and practice. There will be times when an ethical theory will suggest a nice, clean decision or action, but in reality, in practice, it is hard to put into effect. Perhaps, for instance, an ethical theory suggests we should allow someone to die, but in practice this does not feel right. This might be one of those instances where external ethics and internal morals collide. Professional ethics might suggest it is reasonable to let the person die, but my internal moral compass is upset by this suggestion. One response to this might be to say that something needs to change: either the professional ethics advice is wrong, or my moral compass needs to be recalibrated. But how often can we change professional ethics or our moral compasses before things start to look rather random?

Another way of conceiving the problem is to point to the variety of ethical theories that might be brought to bear on any particular dilemma. Some of these theories may, indeed, conflict. So how do we decide between ethical theories or approaches? Is there some other meta-theory that tells us which theory is the most appropriate? There is a more worrying thought, which is that it does not really matter: as long as you can justify your actions according to some recognizable ethical principles, this should be good enough. This seems to make ethical arguments and debates rather redundant. You can seemingly choose anything that takes your fancy. As we shall see in Chapter 24, Immanuel Kant (1724–1804) says always tell the truth, whereas Utilitarians (see Chapter 3) might well say it is better to tell a lie to the person living with dementia. Take your pick!

This does not seem right because we often think of ethics as something we turn to when we want an answer. Hospitals in the USA have ethicists on their staff whom you can consult if you face a clinical dilemma. In the United Kingdom (UK), many NHS Trusts will have a clinical ethics committee or a clinical ethics advisory group ready to provide suitable advice. There is almost an expectation that these committees or groups will provide a definitive answer. The truth, however, is that clinical ethics advice is often not so clear-cut: alternatives are given but the relevant clinician still has to decide.

The problem is a general one to do with philosophy. Ethics in the sense we are talking of here amounts to moral philosophy. Professions (like medicine or nursing) will have their own codes of ethical conduct regulated in the UK by bodies such as the General Medical Council (GMC) or the Nursing and Midwifery Council (NMC). Other health and social care professions will also have their own regulatory bodies with codes of ethical conduct. This is largely true throughout the world. Similarly, there are well established ethical principles governing research (see Chapter 14). Important as all of these principles and codes undoubtedly are, the sort of ethics or moral philosophy I am considering at the moment may be considered to be more fundamental.

Moral philosophy deals with the theories and approaches which underpin the professional and research codes of ethical conduct. Such codes will, for instance, emphasize the importance of gaining valid consent, but underpinning this is thinking over centuries about personal liberties and autonomy, about duties and the nature of our personhood, about dignity and human rights, and so forth. All of that profound thinking will be summarized by a simply stated principle, such as this (taken from the *Code of Ethics* of the Royal College of

Psychiatrists): 'Psychiatrists shall seek valid consent from their patients before undertaking any procedure or treatment' (Royal College of Psychiatrists 2014: 11). A whole lot more thought is then required about what to do if the person lacks the capacity to give consent, but that is another story (see Chapter 11).

So, we are dealing with moral philosophy which should lead us to ask what philosophy itself is about. Bertrand Russell famously wrote that the point of philosophy was:

> ...not for the sake of any definite answers to its questions, ... but rather for the sake of the questions themselves; because these questions enlarge our conception of what is possible, enrich our intellectual imagination, and diminish the dogmatic assurance which closes the mind against speculation
>
> (Russell 1912: 93–94)

In a more straightforward statement Raphael (1981) suggested that the purpose of Western philosophy 'is the critical evaluation of assumptions and arguments' (p. 1); and that an essential part of philosophy is '[t]he clarification of concepts' (p. 5).

Critical evaluation does involve questioning, as Russell suggested, and such questioning may bring about clarity which enables a decision to be made and action to follow. But it may not. Rather than dictating a particular course of action, critical evaluation is more likely to rule out possibilities which come to seem untenable once what is being talked about and its implications have been clarified. Raphael put it bluntly: 'If you are faced with a dilemma on what is the right thing to do, moral philosophy will not find a decision for you. What it can do is remove some confusions and clarify some obscurities, so that the options stand out more plainly. But then the actual choice between them is something you must make yourself' (Raphael 1981: 10).

So, this is the problem: moral philosophy and ethics (as opposed to moral or ethical codes) do not in the end appear to help practically; rather, you have to make a choice. This seems like a slightly dismal view, because my inclination is to think that the process of arguing, questioning, evaluating and clarifying does have a practical effect. If we can see things more clearly, it is helpful. It can happen, however, that what we come to see is that the situation is more complicated – there are more things to consider – than we had at first assumed. But to reject this complexity would surely not be a manifestation of human flourishing, for it would amount to a failure of understanding – a refusal to see things as they are. This book will be full of arguments and if occasionally this makes the world look more complicated, then so be it: that is the way the world is!

But here is the problem the other way around, which is that ethics and moral philosophy will, in clinical practice, sometimes seem by the bye. Health professionals get on with treating people. They do not have to think about Kant or utilitarianism. They handle things in the manner to which they have grown accustomed. This may sound complacent. But perhaps we imbibe how to perform as health and social care professionals from our training and from familiarization with our codes of practice so that deeper reflection is not required except in exceptional circumstances. Mainly we know what we are doing and we do it well (clinically and ethically). Indeed, this is true for all of us: for family carers, for policymakers and for people living with dementia. And yet, we can always do better.

I think the worry about complacency and the need to do better and the possibility of exceptional circumstances means that we require moral and ethical reflection. More than this, we simply need to understand what we are doing. I shall leave this hanging until the end of the chapter.

Links with law and politics

Fairly briefly, I wish to consider how ethics fits in with law, but also with politics. The importance of law is straightforward, because often an ethical dilemma can be solved by looking at the relevant law. Obvious examples are matters to do with lack of capacity or competence. (In the UK we talk of capacity and incapacity, whereas in the USA they tend to speak of competence and incompetence.) Most countries have capacity legislation, so that when faced by a person who lacks the capacity to make a decision it is possible to find out what to do by consulting the legislation. A big warning needs to be inserted here because (as we shall see in Chapters 11 and 12) there is the danger that people will apply the law unthinkingly as if it were a tick box exercise. Thus, in an ethically dubious manner, it might be *presumed* that someone lacks capacity and that we should therefore act in their best interests. But these things may require much more thought. In particular, even if the law says act in the best interests of the person, what is best for someone often requires the wisdom of Solomon to judge. So, beyond the law, ethical judgement and moral thinking become essential.

For this reason, in this book I shall say relatively little about the law. In practice, as suggested above, the law will frequently be a necessary and vital constituent of decision-making in relation to someone living with a diagnosis of dementia. I am more concerned, however, with the underpinning ethical and philosophical issues. As shown in Figure 2.1, my presumption is that laws reflect moral thought. Unethical laws exist, but they are not good laws and they ought (where 'ought' is used in the sense that there is a moral imperative) to be changed. I shall say relatively little about specific laws, the main exception being capacity legislation. More detailed discussion of laws in relation to dementia can be found in Foster et al. (2014) and Hughes et al. (2021).

I have also included politics in Figure 2.1. Laws are made by the political institutions that exist in a country. Corrupt, unthinking or immoral politicians are likely to make bad laws. It is of note that Aristotle's ethics are regarded as leading directly to his politics: moral thought underpins political thought. Politics is ethics writ large. If morals are to do with something internal or personal, politics is the public expression of our private ethical beliefs. But politics (and its resultant legislation) has a different purview. It is not mainly about an individual's day-to-day decisions. It might be hoped that in democratic states it is

Figure 2.1 Connections and interconnections

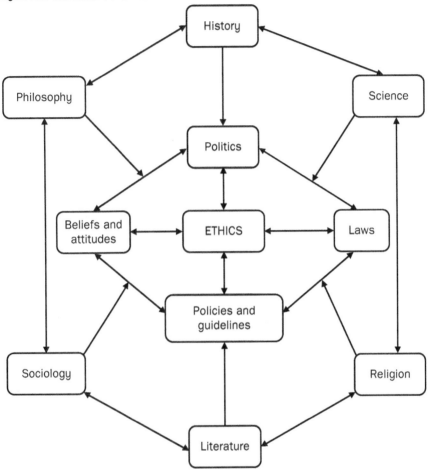

more to do with the common good. The question is about how we make things as good as they can be for everyone on a fair basis.

You might wonder how exactly this is relevant to ethics in relation to dementia. If someone faces a dilemma about what to do in connection with someone living with dementia, only occasionally will the answer be: write to your local politician! Yet, perhaps this ought to be a more frequent response. For one thing, as subsequent chapters will repeatedly show, the issue of human rights is ubiquitous when it comes to care of people living with dementia. So, too, stigma and resources (Chapter 7), dignity (Chapter 10) and worries about abuse (Chapter 22) are among some of the areas where background societal beliefs and attitudes, as well as guidelines, policies and legislation are potentially relevant. Societal beliefs and attitudes reflect underpinning ethical thinking; but also influence and are influenced by guidelines, policies and legislation.

Figure 2.1, therefore, suggests the complexity of the connections and inter-connections that make up the societies in which we live. In order to make this complexity more realistic, I have also included in Figure 2.1 some of the background disciplines that shape our world and which impinge on our politics, laws, beliefs and attitudes, as well as on our policies and guidelines. History, science, religion, sociology, literature and philosophy all influence our ethical understanding of the world. At the heart of this complexity, however, is an ethical core: an impetus to live well together as human beings.

Reconsidering ethics

The problem was that ethics could seem removed from everyday life. But what we have now seen is that it has a centrality to our complicated lives. I left hanging the thought that we simply need to understand what we are doing. One of the ways to reconsider ethics, therefore, is to see the richness of our lives as shot through by ethical and moral concerns. How we greet someone in the street is not irrelevant to how we might make a decision about ending a person's life-supporting treatment. Critical (ethical) reflection is, as Plato's quote suggests (see Box 2.1), quintessential for our lives as human beings.

Box 2.1 Socrates and the unexamined life

In Plato's description of the trial of Socrates he has him utter the now famous dictum:
    'the unexamined life is no life for a human being' (Plato 1970: 80).
    This is cited by Gillon (1986: 2) in his seminal work, *Philosophical Medical Ethics*, which continues to provide a useful and authoritative brief introduction to the whole field of clinical ethics.

A very obvious conclusion follows, which is that ethics is all of our business. It is the business of politicians and policymakers, of health and care professionals, of family and non-family carers and of people who live with dementia. Human beings are surrounded by ethics. Mostly we navigate this moral terrain without reflection. A crisis or dilemma, however, will give us pause to reflect and examine our lives. The content of this book takes a purchase at such moments.

3 Ethical theories: *Viva las virtudes!*

Introduction

In this chapter I shall present an overview of the four main ethical theories that are discussed in the literature, in clinical ethics committees and by ethicists: consequentialism, deontology, principlism and virtue ethics. Principlism may not be one of the main ethical theories discussed in general books of moral philosophy, but it is much discussed in the world of medical (or clinical) ethics.

I shall describe the main theories shortly but, in order to think more about their application, I have considered a particular case which we can look at from the varying perspectives of the different theories. The case is based on a real story which I first heard just over 20 years ago when, with colleagues from Oxford, we conducted research into the ethical issues that arose for family carers of people living with dementia (Hughes et al. 2002a). Incidentally, the family carers did not always think of the ethical difficulties they faced as overtly 'ethical', they were simply problems they had to overcome. But they were problems precisely because they raised issues of right and wrong, leaving the family carers worried about whether what they were doing made them good or bad. One interesting thing was that the breadth and nature of the ethical difficulties they faced seemed greater than the issues that emerged from the professional literature (Hughes et al. 2002b). The case I present below in Box 3.1 reflects some of this and also allows us to analyse the ethical theories we are discussing.

Box 3.1 The case of Mr and Mrs Carter

Mr and Mrs Carter had been happily married for over 40 years when he started to show symptoms of a dementia. He recognized this himself. For instance, he would become frustrated when he could not find the right word, which he felt was happening more frequently. He was not initially keen to see the doctor about the problem, but eventually went with Mrs Carter. She told the doctor that she was also concerned he sometimes did not seem to understand what she was asking him to do. For instance, he would make mistakes laying the table or doing the dishes. The doctor referred him to the local memory clinic and, after all the tests were done, he was told he had a vascular type of dementia. He was started on medication for raised cholesterol and his blood pressure tablets were modified. He was given advice about diet and exercise and was left with the impression that, with luck, his condition would stay fairly stable. He was pleased with the outcome and seemed quite positive about the future.

However, over the next several months Mrs Carter noticed that things are not as good as they could be and seemed to be getting worse. She was reluctant to bring these observations to her spouse's attention because he seemed to be happy, whereas he could become gloomy if there were hints that he was not doing so well. Mr Carter had always been very good at do-it-yourself and had always fixed things around the house himself.

After a particularly squally night, a part of their wooden garden fence blew down. Mr Carter set about fixing it immediately. The result was a complete mess, which was very uncharacteristic of Mr Carter. Mrs Carter suggested he needed to improve it, which he found very annoying. He attached some more bits of wood to the fence, scraps he had had lying around the garden for years. But there were still gaps in the fence and the whole structure remained wobbly. Their neighbour, with whom they had been on good terms for many years, offered to help and managed to sort matters out, but Mr Carter was quite annoyed that he had interfered and from then on complained about him.

A little while later, Mr and Mrs Carter agreed they needed to do something about the sealant in their bathroom shower and some of the adjacent plasterwork, which would then need to be repainted. Mr Carter set to work and within a day proudly told Mrs Carter that it was as good as new. In the old days, if he had said this it would undoubtedly have been true. When Mrs Carter went to look at it, however, she was shocked at what a mess he had made. It was actually considerably worse than before! She managed to stifle her expostulation when she realized that he had no idea how bad a job he had done. She arranged for someone to come in to put the thing right. Mr Carter was extremely annoyed when someone else turned up to do the job. Mrs Carter tried to pacify Mr Carter by saying that she had just fancied a bit of a change in the colour of the bathroom and asked the painter-decorator to paint the whole room. Having been very cross, Mr Carter then became quite morose and seemed to be depressed for the next few weeks.

Some months later it became apparent that the hinges to the sitting room door were coming off the wall. Mr Carter said he could fix it. But he attempted to do so in a bizarre manner using, amongst other things, Sellotape and Blu-Tack. Mrs Carter told him it looked great, but secretly arranged for someone to come in to rectify the situation whilst Mr Carter was out with an old friend (which she had also arranged secretly). She felt bad about this. Afterwards, Mr Carter was suspicious about the sitting room door, frequently quizzing his spouse about whether someone had done something to it. She would gently remind him that he had fixed it.

Mrs Carter next noticed that a shelf in the kitchen was coming away from the wall. Mr Carter had not yet noticed it. She decided that the best thing was to get someone in to fix it before it became any worse. Again, this would involve a degree of deceit, because she would need to get Mr Carter out of the house while the shelf was being fixed. She felt guilty about the deceit, about her inability to be honest with him and about the mere fact that she was keeping these tasks from him, which she knew he would have loved to be able to pursue himself. She felt bad about herself and questioned whether she was doing the right thing taking even small jobs from him in order to avoid the hassle.

For Mrs Carter, this whole business of keeping tasks from her spouse was the most difficult issue she faced. She saw it as a practical issue. There were jobs to be done; quite simply, how was she to arrange things to make sure they got done without upset to Mr Carter? In other words, she did not see this primarily as an ethical issue, although she readily agreed that her concern was whether she was doing the right or wrong thing. She felt she might be a bad person concealing matters from her spouse with whom she had always enjoyed an open and honest relationship and she felt guilty upsetting him.

In the unlikely event that she had consulted a book on ethics, what help might the four main theories have offered Mrs Carter? Table 3.1 presents an overview of the four theories which we shall be considering.

Let us now apply these theories to the case of the Carters. We should keep in mind that, for carers such as Mrs Carter living with her spouse, there is plenty of evidence of carer burden and poorer psychological wellbeing (Brini et al. 2021). The problem Mrs Carter faces, therefore, is a serious practical one with important implications (for example, if Mrs Carter felt she could no longer cope, or if Mr Carter became annoyed and aggressive), as well as being ethical in nature.

Table 3.1 Four main ethical theories

Theory	Classical proponent	Description	Background references
Consequentialism	Jeremy Bentham (1748–1832) and John Stuart Mill (1806–1873)	Consequentialist theorists look at the consequences of an action in order to decide whether or not it is a right action. Bentham is famous for saying that the right action is the one that brings about the greatest happiness for the greatest number. His godson, Mill, in *Utilitarianism*, then defined 'happiness' in terms of pleasure or the absence of pain. The main thing in consequentialist thinking (of which utilitarianism is the best known variety) is that the rightness or wrongness of an action is decided by the degree to which it does or does not maximize some good, such as happiness, pleasure, utility welfare or health. There are act utilitarians and rule utilitarians. Act utilitarians hold that we should look at each particular act and ask whether it maximizes pleasure or not. Rule utilitarians consider the important thing is to consider whether, if it were to be made into a general rule that this action should be done, it would be a rule that would maximize pleasure.	Bentham (1789) Mill (1861) Smart and Williams (1973)

(continued)

Table 3.1 (Continued)

Theory	Classical proponent	Description	Background references
Deontology	Immanuel Kant	The Greek word Deon suggests a duty, something that is right, proper and necessary. Deontology, therefore, suggests any theory that depends on a sense of duty (more or less whatever the consequences). In Kant's hands the theory was that certain actions would be such that all rational people would wish to pursue them: they would be categorical imperatives. For instance, he said all people would rationally wish to be treated as ends in themselves and not simply as means to an end. Hence, as a matter of duty, we should treat all humanity similarly. Any maxim or law you might make should be such that it could be applied universally, including to yourself. This sort of idea was picked up much later by John Rawls (1971) when he developed his idea of 'justice as fairness'. His idea (roughly) was that we should imagine ourselves making laws from behind a 'veil of ignorance', so that we do not know what our position will be in the kingdom that results. Rationally we would then make laws that were fair to everyone (irrespective of class, race, colour, intellect, position and so forth) in case we ended up in a worse position than others.	Kant (1785) Rawls (1971)
Principlism	Tom Beauchamp and James Childress	Beauchamp and Childress (2001) have made famous the 'four principles of medical ethics', which are autonomy, beneficence, non-maleficence and justice. They have derived these principles from a variety of other thinkers such as Mill and Kant. The principles provide a language with which clinicians can examine the ethical nature of their decisions and actions. Will the action promote respect for the person's autonomy? In other words, has the person been listened to? Do we really understand what the person wants? Does the action promote the person's good (beneficence) and avoid harming them (non-maleficence)? Finally, as a matter of justice, when the action is pursued, will resources be used appropriately and fairly? Of course, there is some weighing up to be done when the principles conflict, but at least our thoughts, guided by the principles, will be relevant.	Beauchamp and Childress (2001) Gillon (1986) Gillon (1994)

Table 3.1 (*Continued*)

Theory	Classical proponent	Description	Background references
Virtue ethics	Aristotle (384–322 BC), St Thomas Aquinas (c.1225–1274) and Elizabeth Anscombe (1919–2001)	Aristotle emphasized the importance of acting virtuously. This is how we flourish as human beings: we become the best type of people we can be if we are brave, true, caring and compassionate, steadfast, just, honest, wise and prudent, show temperance or self-restraint, and so on. A good action is one that is in accord with what the virtuous person would do; in other words, it demonstrates the virtues. Aquinas took Aristotle's teaching on ethics and incorporated them within Christian (and Western) beliefs. But for many years virtue theory all but disappeared (utilitarian thinking and deontology ruled the ethical roost). Anscombe is credited with revitalizing interest in the virtues and subsequently there has been considerable interest in this approach to ethics.	Aristotle (1980) Aquinas (1990) Anscombe (1958) MacIntyre (1985) May (1994) Hursthouse (1999) Foot (2001)

Consequentialism

A very quick assessment, by an act utilitarian, might be that Mrs Carter should simply go ahead and get in workers whenever she needs them, without any worries about deceiving her spouse. After all, the job would then be done, Mr Carter would not need to be bothered and would forget anyway if he were to notice that something had changed. The only thing against this, the act utilitarian might say, would be if Mr Carter were to get very upset, perhaps even aggressive, about any changes that he noticed. Also, if it were very difficult to get him out of the way when the work was being done, this too might weigh against it being the best option.

Raising these caveats to the quick assessment, however, starts to make it seem that perhaps it was too quick. Perhaps the stress and upset it causes Mrs Carter to deceive Mr Carter, by planning that he should be taken out and by having to concoct stories about why something might have changed, will all be too much. Perhaps Mr Carter will sense Mrs Carter's unease and will, in any case, notice things are different around the house. Worst of all, perhaps he will one day be brought home early or discover someone else's tools inadvertently left lying around. Perhaps he will develop the idea that his spouse is having an affair. This may then be called a delusion and he might be put on medication to 'calm him down', but there might be untoward effects from the medication.

All of this highlights a major problem with consequentialism, which is that we can hardly ever know what the full consequences of an action might be.

Perhaps the Carters have a daughter who disagrees with her mother's approach. If mother and daughter fall out over this, or even if the daughter simply harbours resentment, what will the short- or long-term consequences be? A slightly different act utilitarian assessment, therefore, might be that getting people in to do the work is too fraught with potential problems and it might be better to put up with some deficiencies in the house. Mrs Carter could simply stop using the kitchen shelf that is coming away from the wall. Or perhaps it is better to confront the situation and tell Mr Carter what is going on. But would he remember anyway? Meanwhile, the rule utilitarian might reason that to establish a rule that it was right for spouses to deceive each other (under certain circumstances) would not be good. They may say honesty is the best policy.

Deontology

In this, the rule utilitarian would probably be in accord with the deontologist. Certainly, Kant was absolutely against lying. He saw it as a duty always to be truthful, because it could not rationally become an ethical law that people should deceive each other. This sort of stance sometimes gets called absolutism, because no other approach would be countenanced. But you could argue, deontologically, that Mrs Carter also has a duty to look after herself, including her mental health. You could even argue that she has a duty to look after her house and environment. Further, she might be considered to have a duty to ensure her spouse stays safe and, given his increasing dyspraxia, this might involve keeping him away from hazardous tools.

The good thing about these ethical theories, therefore, is that they get us thinking in suitably sensible ethical ways, either about different consequences or about different duties. However, no definitive answer emerges: either stance might be correct and suggest the right thing to do, but neither is definitive.

Principlism

The benefit of the four principles is that they also get us thinking about ethically relevant matters. Respect for autonomy suggests that we should try to discover Mr Carter's views. Talking to him to find out what his current views are, if not about specific matters (like the kitchen shelf) then about the general issue of what should be done if he were not able to do jobs himself, would seem like the right thing to do if at all possible. If not possible, then finding out about or considering his previous wishes or beliefs would be helpful as a guide to what might be the right thing to do from his perspective. At any rate, it would seem right to aim at doing some good (by getting the job done) whilst avoiding doing harm (by taking him out whilst the work is being done). Justice seems less relevant if we are thinking of resources, although using up the good will of friends who might need to take him out is a consideration. If he had to be given medication to calm him down, this would also use resources, especially if there were the risk of side effects. Principlism, therefore, gives us a lot more to think about in deciding what is right or wrong in this situation.

Virtue ethics

One thing about the virtues is that they change the conversation. The focus becomes the person's character. If Mrs Carter wishes to do the right thing and be a good person, she should do what the virtuous person would do; in other words, she should demonstrate the virtues in what she does. How does she show compassion and charity towards her spouse? How does she remain as honest with him as possible and demonstrate her fidelity? Can she summon up the courage to deal with the situation? Does she have the requisite fortitude? There is also the virtue of justice again: how can she be fair to her spouse? What about practical wisdom, sometimes called prudence, which is regarded as the ability to see how to achieve the good that is being aimed at? The aim is to keep managing the house without belittling or upsetting Mr Carter. We could describe this as a matter of friendship or sociability, which can be regarded as basic human goods worth aiming at (Finnis 2011: 88). The virtue that helps us to achieve this end is practical wisdom (or, in Greek, *phronesis*). It might involve Mrs Carter in a good deal of explanation and negotiation with Mr Carter. Perhaps, the person who comes in to help would be patient enough to involve Mr Carter in the repair so that he does not feel useless or undermined.

In any event, virtue ethics is about our inner dispositions, instilled in us by temperament, by upbringing, by education. It recognizes that what we do affects what we become, because putting the virtues into effect makes us into virtuous people; by being compassionate and honest we become the sort of people who are compassionate and honest.

Virtue ethics also allows that we can feel regret for whatever it is that we feel we have to do. In this it differs somewhat from consequentialism and deontology, which both seem to tell us what the right thing to do is in a manner that elides this with what the good thing to do might be. Virtue ethics recognizes that sometimes we are presented with choices where no choice makes us feel comfortable, no choice seems like a good one. But, nevertheless, one of them must be the right thing to do, however bad it makes us feel. Mrs Carter may just have to accept that she will feel guilty about her decision to hide from Mr Carter the repairs that are being done. Practical wisdom might suggest that this is the only way. She can still consider how she will be compassionate and honest with him.

Conclusion

It may be apparent that I prefer virtue ethics to the other theories. You might decide to disagree with this, but it explains my sub-heading: *Viva las virtudes!* I am not sure where I got this exclamation from originally, but there is an element of humour in it because it mimics the name of a 1964 film, starring Elvis Presley (1935–1977) and Ann-Margret, *Viva Las Vegas!*

There is a certain richness to virtue ethics. It seems a nuanced approach. How things are done is as important as what is done. It also allows that ratiocination is not the main thing. Mrs Carter just is honest with Mr Carter. She does not have to rationalize this in terms of consequences or in terms of duties that emerge as categorical imperatives. This is simply the way that she is as a virtuous person, without even knowing it. If her immediate reaction is to lie and, furthermore, she feels no sense of guilt about doing so, then she is a different sort of person. She may have other virtues, but she is certainly lacking the virtue of honesty and perhaps integrity. So, I would be inclined to plump for virtue ethics as the main ethical theory to be pursued because of its nuance about the reality of our moral lives.

We should still note that virtue ethics, like the other main theories discussed here, does not give us slam dunk answers to our ethical problems. On the other hand, together they provide us with a moral vocabulary, and they offer challenges and questions which should help us all – whether we are health and social care professionals, family or non-family carers, politicians or policy advisers working for charities, or even people living with a diagnosis of dementia – to think more clearly and more broadly when faced with moral difficulties.

4   Ethical approaches

Introduction

Having introduced what might be considered the big ethical theories, in this chapter I highlight different ethical approaches. They are approaches which have emerged (roughly) in the last 50 years. There are two reasons I like them: first, they are engaging – they engage with reality; they make sense in the real world. Secondly, one way or another, they all stress relationships and communication. This seems very sensible to me. Apart from anything else, relationships and communication are highly prized by people living with dementia (Reilly et al. 2020). I am sure that many ethical difficulties would be solved on the basis of good relationships aided by good communication. Some of these approaches (and much more besides) are discussed in more detail in the authoritative *Principles of Health Care Ethics* (Ashcroft et al. 2007).

Once again, we can apply our different ethical approaches to the fictional case of the Carters (see Chapter 3). In Table 4.1, I have sketched the sort of questions that these approaches raise for the Carters. I shall then say something further about each of the approaches.

Feminist and care ethics

Strictly, it is probably wrong to lump together feminist ethics and the ethics of care, but they are entwined. Indeed, it is probably inaccurate to talk as if feminist ethics is only one thing. For a start, some might wish to make a distinction between 'feminist' and 'feminine' ethics. Nevertheless, it is more straightforward to point to threads that link these various approaches together.

In this spirit, it is possible to highlight the work of Carol Gilligan as kick-starting a movement which pointed out that there were different approaches to ethical dilemmas and problems in terms of the ways in which they were conceptualized (Gilligan 1982). Gilligan's work suggested men approached ethical problems in a more abstract manner, with an emphasis on rules and concepts such as justice. A more feminine (or feminist) way to look at things was from the perspective of relationships, where context and, therefore, the particularities of the case were important. It was not being suggested that there was a strict gender difference, but nevertheless different themes and approaches seemed apparent.

Gilligan's book was quickly followed by Nel Noddings's writing, again from a feminist perspective, about care and caring (Noddings 1984). She emphasized the way true care required the carer to be engrossed in the person being cared for.

Table 4.1 Questions raised by four ethical approaches

Ethical approach	Possible questions raised by the approaches	Indicative references
Feminist and care ethics	What has the relationship between Mr and Mrs Carter been like (over the years and now)? How have they cared for each other? How have responsibilities shifted over time (if at all)? Are they able to speak about their relationship and how it might be changing or likely to change? Has their relationship been one of genuine trust? Is this something they can use in the current situation? How are they supported by others? What are their relationships like with the people who can help them?	Sherwin (2007)
Narrative ethics	Who are the protagonists in this story? Who are the people with supporting roles and how do the Carters get on with them? How do the Carters see themselves and their relationships? How would they like the story of their lives to go? Do they feel they have control over this? How does Mrs Carter now see her life's narrative? How would Mr Carter tell his story? Is there a way of interacting with Mr Carter that would be more or less helpful? Would it be possible (in a helpful way) to see the current problems as part of a bigger narrative or story?	Brody (2007)
Hermeneutic ethics	From the perspective of each of the Carters, what is the meaning of their respective behaviours? How do they each interpret what the other is doing? What is the explanation that they give as to what they are doing? Would they be willing to accept a different interpretation of their own or the other's behaviour and reactions? What potentially helps them to understand the other's behaviour and reactions? Do their background beliefs help or hinder their interpretation or understandings of the current situation?	Widdershoven and Abma (2007)
Communicative (discourse) ethics	How are Mr and Mrs Carter communicating? Haver they always communicated in this way? Could they change the way they discuss things? Is there anyone else involved who might be able to help with communication? Are there better or worse times of the day to discuss matters? Might it be good to write some things down to aid recall of what they have agreed? Do they have enough time together to allow normal (non-controversial) communication?	Moody (1992a) Also see Habermas (1990) – especially the chapter 'Discourse ethics – notes on a program of philosophical justification'

In other words, the carer had to be able to put themselves thoroughly in the position of the other. Care is not providing someone with what you think the other needs; it is providing the care that they want and actually require. At an authentic level, the carer must really think about the person they are caring for. This will often reflect a tendency to nurture, not to control.

In a further development of the feminist-care ethics theme, Annette Baier (1929–2012) was interested in, amongst many other things, the theme of trust (Baier 1986). Again, it makes sense to think in terms of authentic trust. For as Baier pointed out, some trusting may be out of necessity because of powerlessness. The importance of power relations thus emerges from this feminist critique. It will almost always be a potential issue in relationships with people living with dementia. Consciousness of this tendency can be seen as a potent impetus to the development of the notion of 'social citizenship' for people with dementia (see Chapter 13), with all that this implies in terms of agency and social identity (Bartlett and O'Connor 2010).

Narrative ethics

It has to be said that not everyone agrees that our lives can or should be thought of as narratives (Strawson 2004). Even so, people will sometimes tell the story of their lives. They may feel their lives have some sort of direction; or that they have changed direction. There are at least three aspects to the idea that we live narrated lives which can be helpful in our thinking about ethical problems of the sort faced by the Carters.

First, there is the idea that we are the narrators of our stories. This can be helpful. It can simply be therapeutic to tell your story. It can be therapeutic in another sense, because realizing that it is *your* story may give you a sense of permission and the power to act to change things in some way. This might be relevant for a family carer such as Mrs Carter. But it might also be relevant to people living with dementia. Hydén (2013) argued, using case vignettes, that it is not always the textual aspects of the narrative that count (where a person living with dementia may have difficulties), but the performative and embodied aspects of storytelling. Hence, storytelling can become a collaborative affair. And when a person's story is told, understanding is likely to increase. An impressive example of this is seen in the book by Steve Sabat (2001), *The Experience of Alzheimer's Disease*, where (in effect) the careful telling of stories using extensive verbatim quotes greatly increases our understanding of the lives of the people concerned and the conceptual issues that need to be considered.

A link has also been made to personal identity, in that, if we can tell our stories, we present and confirm *what* we are and *who* we are as persons with narratives. Ryan et al. (2009) have looked at how people living with dementia who write can maintain their social identity by the meanings they create through dialogue with their readers. Baldwin (2010) spoke of:

- narrative agency – 'having the ability and opportunity to author one's own story' (p. 247)
- narrative webs – 'made up of stories of individuals, stories of others, ... meta-stories (stories that seek to provide a framework for other stories...)' (p. 249)
- narrative resources – having a stock of stories sufficient 'to hold a person with dementia within a web of meaningful stories'; that is, to maintain identity partly by acknowledging 'retained abilities' and 'meaningful inter-actions' (p. 250).

Secondly, there is the idea that our stories interconnect with the stories of others (Baldwin's 'narrative webs'). We are not the sole authors of our narra-tives. The narratives of spouses will be intimate. But anyone who comes into the house will also be entering the ongoing stories. The painter-decorator, for example, if suitably attuned, might be able to alter the story in a positive way. Equally, the painter-decorator might misunderstand the situation and make matters worse.

Thirdly, there is the idea that our narratives have meaning or give us mean-ing. This is so even when stories are told by others. Meanings have to be understood. This in itself is an ethical matter for people living with dementia. They remain semiotic subjects because of the accounts they can give, the sto-ries they can tell (Sabat and Harré 1994). Whatever detractors might suggest, there is a richness to the notion of narrative (Bitenc 2020) that is helpful in discussing ethical problems.

Hermeneutic ethics

The relevance and importance of meaning for the person living with dementia continue in the approach of hermeneutic ethics. A hermeneut is an interpreter. Hermeneutics is about interpretation, about conveying the meaning of a text for instance. There is the notion in philosophy of a hermeneutic circle, which: 'Has to do with the inherent circularity of all understanding, or the fact that comprehension can only come about through a tacit foreknowledge that alerts us to salient features of the text which would otherwise escape notice' (Norris 1995: 353).

We know things even before we read a text, but the interpretation of the text gives us further insight which in turn can be useful in how we deal with the world to which we return from the text. But the world also instructs us – anew having read the text – so that when we return to the text, novel insights, new interpretations arise and so on. Through experience and education, we become more astute in our interpretations.

All of this can be transposed into thinking about dementia. The person living with dementia can be thought of as the text, whom we come to understand. Widdershoven and Berghmans (2006) have shown how a hermeneutic perspec-tive is relevant to dementia, especially where there is some sort of breakdown in terms of understanding. We can become proficient at interpreting or understanding the person living with dementia. Elsewhere they have written: 'Instead of waving away the perspective of the person with dementia as irrelevant ..., or of treating it as the only relevant point of view ..., the hermeneutic approach claims that the confrontation of perspectives may lead to a new and better (shared) perspective' (Widdershoven and Widdershoven-Heerding 2003: 106). Perhaps this approach would be useful for the Carters. Having discussed matters, there could be some sort of negotiation, for instance, with the painter-decorator, which might allow progress to be made.

Communicative (discourse) ethics

Dialogue can be key to the hermeneutic approach, but it is central to communicative or discourse ethics. Put simply, we might say that actions are ethically right when the communication is right. If we get the communication correct, it is more likely that we shall do the ethically correct thing. This will be precisely because we have listened to and understood the different perspectives. More than this, we should try to reach a consensus if there are disputes (we shall see the importance of this in the next chapter when we discuss values-based practice). This will not always be possible. But at least if we have really listened, and the person concerned feels listened to, there may be understanding about the decision that has been taken. Attentive, genuine discourse is likely to engender trust, of which we have seen the importance in feminist and care ethics.

Harry Moody, a geriatrician, pursued the idea of communicative ethics in his important book *Ethics in an Aging Society* (Moody 1992a). Elsewhere he has written: '... in place of an abstract ethics of rules or principles, we need a communicative ethics grounded in practice and in lived experience' (Moody 1992b: 93). Apart from the importance of right discourse between individuals, Moody (1992a) helps to emphasize that much of this will be to do with communication within institutions and how this is encouraged or inhibited. A care agency sending care workers out to attend to older people living with dementia, but only giving them the minimum time to carry out basic tasks, is not affording them the opportunity to engage in helpful and meaningful dialogue with the people they serve. Before we heap all of the blame on to the care agency, however, we should consider how they are funded. Who are the people making funding decisions at the local and national level? Should voters have voted for a tax-increasing government to ensure that funding for those who look after people living with dementia is adequate? Or should money be moved from the defence budget to the care budget? Communicative ethics is pertinent to the individual, but also has political ramifications (which takes us back to the discussion of ethics and politics in Chapter 2).

As suggested in Table 4.1, communicative ethics owes much to the work of philosophers such as Jürgen Habermas. Moody (1992a) sums up matters this way, saying that Habermas favours:

... a 'communicative ethics' based on shared discourse among persons who respect the position of others in the communication process itself. According to this perspective, finding the 'correct answer' to an ethical dilemma may be less a matter of agreeing on an abstract set of principles than it is a matter of sharing a commitment to free and open communication and working on behalf of institutional structures that support such communication.

(p. 38)

Well, 'free and open communication' is not a bad place to start when ethical dilemmas emerge.

Conclusion

It is not that the ethical approaches sketched in this chapter will solve all the ethical dilemmas we may encounter. But they do get us closer to the reality of everyday lives. They encourage us all to look at the details of any ethical dilemmas and difficulties that might face us. The vocabulary, which they encourage us to use, provides us with the possibility of nuance and subtlety in our approach: contexts, relationships, nurturing, caring, trust, identity, stories and narratives, collaboration, understanding and meaning, meaningful interactions, interpretation, alternative perspectives, negotiation, free and open communication, dialogue and discourse. The impetus, then, is not to seek quick fixes via abstract theories and principles, but to think broadly and to interact showing authentic solicitude.

5 Practical approaches: casuistry and values-based practice

Introduction

The big ethical theories are useful. They give us a framework. But as we saw, they still leave us having to make decisions even if they suggest the direction we should take. The ethical approaches add nuance and deepen our thoughts about the particularities of the case. On the basis of these theories and approaches we may well be able to make a good decision about what to do. In this chapter, I shall present two further approaches to moral reasoning which suggest practical ways to deal with ethical dilemmas.

Values-based practice

Some years ago, Bill Fulford (the doyen of philosophy of psychiatry) set out ten principles of what at the time was referred to as values-based medicine and in doing so he provided a useful definition: 'Values-based Medicine (VBM) is the theory and practice of effective health-care decision making for situations in which legitimately different (and hence potentially conflicting) value perspectives are in play' (Fulford 2004: 205). Subsequently, the name has broadened beyond medicine, to be designated 'values-based practice' (VBP); and the ten principles have been slightly modified. But the foundations have remained the same: that values – which are important in our lives and which guide our actions – are pervasive in practice, need to be seen and understood, and can cause difficulties when they conflict. It also remains true that VBP relies on both principles and skills.

A more up-to-date presentation of the ten-part process of VBP is shown in Table 5.1. Further details can be found in Fulford et al. (2012). A key feature of VBP is that it 'aims to support *balanced decision making of shared values* (the main *point* of VBP), based upon *mutual respect for differences of values* (the main *premise* of VBP) within a given situation' (Hughes and Williamson 2019: 14). Of course, VBP is aimed at practitioners, but it is not irrelevant to others such as policymakers, family carers and people living with dementia. The right-hand column in Table 5.1 gives examples of how the elements of VBP might be relevant to people other than professional health and social care workers.

Table 5.1 Ten-part process of values-based practice

Areas	Key elements	Description	Relevance to dementia care
Clinical skills	1. Awareness of values	The first clinical skill is simply that values must be recognized. This is not always so simple! Sometimes values will be taken for granted and may not be noticed as a consequence. Sometimes values may be obscure if, for instance, they reflect particular cultural beliefs of which practitioners are not overtly aware. They can be brought into conscious awareness by paying close attention to the language people use. The values of everyone involved in decision making need to be considered.	Staff must be aware of values. Policymakers, too, should consider the values that their policies suggest. Closing services, for instance, might simply show that people living with dementia and their families are not valued, unless such closures enable something good to emerge elsewhere. People living with dementia might wish to reflect on their values and note them down for future reference. Family carers should ask themselves to what extent they know the values of the person for whom they care.
	2. Reasoning about values	Having recognized that people's value judgements are relevant, the next skill is to be able to reason about them. This may require some knowledge of moral theories such as consequentialism or deontology. But also, where do the values come from? What do they imply? Are we dealing with compatible values and value systems?	People other than professionals might have knowledge of ethical theories and approaches. They should feel able to use their knowledge to contribute to discussions about dilemmas. When family carers and people living with dementia are faced with ethical dilemmas it would be useful for them to be aware of what is important to them and why. Are there some values (e.g. religious values) held within the family that cannot be compromised?
	3. Knowledge of values (and facts)	In turn, this implies that professionals know about values and, in particular, that they can see the values relevant to the specific circumstances they face. But it is not just values. There will also be relevant facts that have to be known. One problem is where people latch on to the facts and ignore the values. But another is that too much attention is paid to values without acknowledging the facts.	A clinician might be focused on the fact that the house of the person living with dementia is not clean, whereas the family might be able to confirm that the person with dementia never valued cleanliness. Someone living with dementia might assert how much they value their freedom to drive, but the family might emphasize the fact that they have already been involved in several small accidents.
	4. Communication skills	Practitioners have to be able to elicit the different values that people hold, but then they need to use their communication skills in order to come up with balanced decisions where the values of as many participants as possible are taken into account and differences are resolved.	People living with dementia and families and their supporters should be able to expect that professionals will communicate with them clearly and with care.

(continued)

Table 5.1 (*Continued*)

Areas	Key elements	Description	Relevance to dementia care
Relationships	5. Person-centred practice	Essentially, the person at the centre of the decision or dilemma must come first. So, for example, it is essential that practitioners know or learn of the values important to the person living with dementia. This does not mean that this person's values will eclipse all the values of everyone else. But the main person's values must be centre stage. They are given priority in terms of acknowledgement.	The person living with dementia may be determined to stay living at home – this is of great value – and everyone involved should do all they can to make this possible. If there are real reasons – facts – why it is not possible, these will need to be conveyed to the person clearly and with care. It may be that some form of residential care becomes inevitable, but this should not be presumed when it is not what the person wants.
	6. Multidisciplinary teamwork	One of the reasons for having multidisciplinary teams is to allow and encourage diverse values and perspectives. This allows that, potentially, we get to hear the anomalous view, representing idiosyncratic values, which might make people stop and think. The different perspectives, in any case, may facilitate thinking about how to bring diverse values to a consensus.	It is useful for family members and the person living with dementia to know who all the members of the team are and what their contributions will be to decision-making.

(continued)

Table 5.1 (Continued)

Areas	Key elements	Description	Relevance to dementia care
Principles linking evidence and values	7. 'Two-feet' principle	This principle restates the point that we shall always need to consider facts and values. Good decision-making will stand on both of these feet.	People living with dementia and their family carers should know that what they value is important, just as facts are. Early on, whilst still able, they may wish to prepare a values statement listing the things that make their lives worthwhile. Advance care planning is better done early before incapacity makes it more difficult.
	8. 'Squeaky-wheel' principle	In many instances people will have underlying values which cohere, so there is no problem. When there is a problem, when the wheel squeaks, this can be a sign of conflicting values and values diversity. Then we need to pay more attention to what is going on at the level of values.	If families have different views about what is important, they should discuss these differences and decide, if they can, how they will handle them. It is better that differences in values should be out in the open.
	9. Science-driven principle	We need to note that advances in science lead to greater chances that there will be values diversity. Science provides answers, but it also creates ethical debates partly because opportunities have changed or been created. Along with such changes come varying value judgements, which might conflict.	Families and people living with dementia need to be made aware of new technological or pharmacological options so that they can form views about them and work out the extent to which they may or may not feel the innovation is of value to them.
Partnerships	10. Consensus or dissensus	If all goes well, there can be consensus – not as a matter of luck, but because the process has been handled skilfully and with attention to the values that have been pertinent to a particular decision. But it may not always be possible to balance all the values in a way that leads to consensus. The notion of 'dissensus' makes the point that, where there are differences of opinion, we should not simply dismiss the dissenting voices. They remain in play and might yet become relevant. Diverse values are never entirely off the table.	Even if a person living with dementia or a family member finds that a decision has been made with which they disagree, they should not feel that they have been ignored; and if circumstances were to change so that what they thought was important could be pursued, it should be.

A further example, to help with understanding the relevance to dementia of VBP, is to consider the end of life (of which more will be said in Chapter 31).

Those involved with someone who is dying need to be aware of the values of that person, but also open to the possibility that others, in the family or in the care team, might have different values. Let us take it that there is a decision to be made about whether to use artificial feeding to keep someone with dementia alive (this is discussed further in Chapter 28). There might well be a variety of views. The person who has to make the decision will need to be alert to the possibility of conflicting values. If different opinions are expressed, some sort of weighing up and discussion of them will be needed, which itself requires appropriate reasoning skills. The facts must also be known, along with concomitant values. The person leading the discussions about the decision will need good communication skills in order to elicit people's concerns and the values that might be hidden, as well as to ensure that all involved, insofar as possible, listen attentively to the views of others. At the centre of all of this must be the views of the person with dementia who is dying. Do we know about this person's values, wishes and preferences? Perhaps there is some form of advance care plan, or perhaps someone has been appointed with the relevant power of attorney. What do members of the multidisciplinary team think? Have they, from their different perspectives, been able to find out anything else from the family that might be relevant? There clearly are both facts and values to be considered. It might also be clear that two members of the family do not agree with the decision, say, not to use tube feeding. It is important that their views should be heard and their values understood. We know that the increased possibilities, brought about by advances in science and technology, such as providing nutrition through percutaneous endoscopic gastrostomies (PEGs), means there are more choices, but also more room for dissenting voices reflecting different values. If there is no consensus a decision still has to be made; but if so, it should be made plain that the conflicting values are not being dismissed irrevocably. If not using a PEG tube leads to obvious distress, because of choking, the decision can be reconsidered.

VBP shows us the skills that are required for such difficult decisions, but also highlights an inclusive process of good communication, fact-gathering, awareness of values, with the person concerned at the centre and the aim being to develop a consensus; or, if this is not possible, at least the aim should be an open process where everyone's values are acknowledged and kept on the table. A more detailed discussion of how VBP is relevant to dementia care can be found in Hughes and Williamson (2019). One thing VBP highlights is the importance of values being known if they are likely to be salient to future decisions. Hence the importance of advance care plans and statements of values which people living with dementia might wish and could be encouraged to draw up.

Casuistry

Of course, if we were really discussing the end-of-life scenario above, we should need to think in much more detail about the particularities of the case. This is true in VBP. But it is of the essence in casuistry.

The word comes from the Latin *casus*, meaning case. It can be thought of as case-based deliberation. It involves arguing case by case, in the light of basic moral instincts, but with regard to the particularities of and important differences between cases. Casuistry has a long and interesting history (Jonsen and Toulmin 1988). Indeed, it places an emphasis on history, or at least on tradition. Murray (1994) wrote: 'The professions are one place where the genuine vitality of moral traditions may be especially apparent' (p. 94). Then, in discussing casuistry, he talked of 'the 'data' of ethics – considered moral judgements and moral maxims developed out of the experience of a moral tradition' (p. 100).

These arguments are relevant to the four points that can be used to summarize the approach of casuistry:

- It is an *inductive* process, arguing from the details of individual cases to general principles.
- It requires *immersion* in the particularities, perspectives and contexts of the case (Murray 1994: 96–99).
- There must be *interpretation* of the moral relevance and meaning of cases (Murray 1994: 96–99).
- The conclusions of such reasoning are *presumptive* and revisable (Louw and Hughes 2005).

When we think of logical reasoning, we think in a deductive way. We apply principles to particular instances. The law of the excluded middle, for instance, states that for any proposition (*p*), either it is true or its negation (*not-p*) is true: in other words, either *p* or *not-p* is true. This overarching rule can then be put into effect in particular instances. Thus, it cannot be true for a particular case both that 'resuscitation is appropriate' and that 'resuscitation is inappropriate'. Similarly, if we are committed utilitarians, the presumption might be that utilitarian principles can be applied to any and every ethical dilemma we come across, whatever the particularities of the case.

Contrariwise, inductive thinking – as in casuistry – does the opposite. It starts with the particularities of the case: the relevant facts in which we must be immersed. It is a bottom-up and not top-down process. Immersion means really understanding the details of the case. 'Details', however, implies the broad context. One detail might be a biomedical fact (that the person's potassium is low) and another detail might be a social fact (that one half of the family live in Australia and the other half in England). This immersion is also in terms of perspectives, so that much of what was said above in connection with VBP is also relevant: it will always be facts *and* values.

Interpretation follows. Having been immersed in the details, moral judgements and moral maxims are then applied. Comparison can be made with previous precedent cases, where the moral judgements have already been established. The application of judgements and maxims, however, must be appropriate to the current case and its particularities. We should not be, as it were, simply taking off the shelf whichever moral tools are handy to us. Which are the right tools for this case? Is it relevant to think in terms of maximizing welfare, or would it be more useful to consider the appropriate virtues?

In all of this, casuistry is little different from law or medical practice. In law, a case is decided by looking in detail at the circumstances. If it is the same in all its particularities as a clear-cut precedent (or sentinel) case, it can be judged similarly. But if there are important differences it must be judged differently. Thus, one case is murder and another is manslaughter.

Likewise in medicine, if a person presents with the classic symptoms and signs of left heart failure, it is sensible to treat them for this condition. This may not require much thought because this case is such a classic presentation. We certainly do not need to go back to the principles of cardiac pathophysiology to figure it out. If, however, there is something that does not quite fit – an abnormal symptom (significant pain) or sign (a discrete opacity on the chest X-ray) – then our interpretation must be different. We cannot regard this simply as heart failure; it needs more thought, different tests and a different approach.

Hence, the last feature of casuistry is that judgements are presumptive and revisable. The law case can be appealed; a medical diagnosis can be changed in the light of new findings. New details in an ethical dilemma can also change our opinion. We might think it is wrong for the person living with dementia to drive (see Chapter 18). But when the report arrives from the driving assessment centre to say they passed their test with flying colours, we should revise our judgement.

Conclusion

In the end, a judgement is always required. There are, however, different (even if connected) ways of reaching moral judgements. VBP and casuistry indicate processes which might be helpful. Awareness of VBP and casuistry could be as relevant for the person living with dementia, for family carers and for policy-makers as it is for practitioners of any type. As in communicative ethics, active listening is a requirement. As in hermeneutics, interpretation is inevitable. The details of the narratives are crucial. Indeed, many years ago Aumann and Cole (1991) commended the idea that we 'need to attend more closely to *interpreting the particularities* of cases as stories', thus bringing together the approaches of hermeneutics, narrative ethics and casuistry. In any case, those involved must show great care. We must all (whether we are professional practitioners, family members or people living with a diagnosis) start with facts and values from which our moral judgements (reflecting our virtuous dispositions or otherwise) will emerge.

6 An idea: patterns of practice

Introduction

One of the strange things about practice of any sort, but here we are thinking about dementia care, is that mostly we do not notice it involves ethical judgements. Yet, all judgements in dementia care are, at one and the same time, ethical. Prescribing a drug, providing personal care or going to the daycare centre, these activities all invite ethical questions. Is this the right thing to do at the moment? Are we doing it in the correct manner? Will it bring about good? Mostly, however, the inherently ethical nature of what we do passes us by: we simply get on with the job. We do not consciously think about consequentialism or deontology. We do not even remark that we are now part of someone's narrative or notice the ethical interpretations we are making. And building relationships or good communication are seen as care skills, not as moral acts.

I suggest that patterns of practice might be helpful in understanding this aspect of our work in health and social care (Hughes 2006; Hughes 2009). Patterns of practice might also be helpful when we are actually making decisions. This chapter will expound these ideas.

Our patterned lives

To say that our lives are patterned seems mundane. It is obvious that we mostly live regular lives. We mostly sleep at night. We eat in a more or less set way: certain foods at certain times, in a certain fashion. We travel to work by more or less the same route and have the same routine when we get to our places of work. Even if we are lucky enough to have work that varies, we tend to perform the varied aspects of our work in a patterned way. Doctors tend to examine people from their right side, and if this is not possible, it can be disconcerting. Nurses have routines associated with drug rounds. The spouse of someone living with dementia will tend to have particular routines for providing care. Social workers will carry out assessments of a person's needs in set ways that ensure, as far as possible, all particulars are recorded. To have those routines interrupted can be annoying and might be in some cases be dangerous, for example if the nurse's concentration were to be disturbed during the drug round.

If these things seem mundane, we should note that our patterned behaviours and responses run deep. At a psychological level, it might be that certain circumstances induce a pattern of anxious behaviour which reflects something deep in our makeup – insecure attachments when young, perhaps. Biologically, we have circadian rhythms, which regulate the sleep–wake cycle, but which in turn are connected to the release of hormones in a patterned manner. There is a diurnal cycle of cortisol release, for instance, which has a profound effect on metabolic and inflammatory processes. Sociologically, you only have to think of crowd behaviours, for example at a football match, to recognize that there are shared patterns of practice, with seemingly instantaneous similar reactions from thousands of people to specific stimuli.

Importantly, we should also notice that our use of language is a matter of patterns of practice. This is not necessarily immediately intuitive. You could think of words as signifying objects in the world, so that learning a language is a matter of learning which thing corresponds to which word. But this can be tricky for a variety of reasons: think of words that connote abstract things ('time' might be an example), or of words with multiple meanings ('game' is an example) or many non-nouns (such as the adverb 'quickly'). What do we point to when we come across such words in order to convey their meanings?

To cut a long story short, Ludwig Wittgenstein (see Box 6.1) established that, rather than any correspondence theory of meaning (*this* word corresponds to *that* object), it makes more sense to say: 'the meaning of a word is its use in the language' (Wittgenstein 1967: §43). It is truer to say, therefore, that we understand a word (we know what it means) when we understand a whole sentence. This is not because we understand how each word represents something, but because we have grasped the use of the whole. More than this, it is not that we (as it were) stand aside from language in order to learn and use it. Rather, we are enmeshed in the practice that constitutes the language. As Wittgenstein also says: '... to imagine a language means to imagine a form of life' (Wittgenstein 1967: §19). Commenting on this (in a rather brilliant if philosophically challenging essay entitled 'Theories of Meaning'), Charles Taylor wrote: '... it is plainly impossible to learn a language as a detached observer. To understand a language, you need to understand the social life and outlook of those who speak it' (Taylor 1985: 281).

The point I wish to make is that a language is a pattern of practice. We do not just learn words, we buy into a practice, or what Wittgenstein calls a 'form of life' (see Box 6.1).

Box 6.1 Wittgenstein, language and forms of life

Ludwig Wittgenstein (1889–1951) was perhaps the most brilliant philosopher of the twentieth century. He was Austrian but spent much of his working life in England and was for a while Professor of Philosophy at Cambridge. In *Philosophical Investigations* he wrote: '...to imagine a language means to imagine a form of life' (§19) and '... the term 'language-*game* is meant to bring into prominence the fact that the *speaking* of language is part of an activity, or of a form of life' (§23).

Our lives, therefore, are patterned in profound ways. To be a human being, to be part of this complex language community, is to be situated in a form of life that is deeply patterned. Hence, I want to suggest that our ethical responses – our immediate non-rationalized reactions – are part of this patterning. Normally, in most cases, we do not have to ask, for example, 'What would the virtue ethicist do under these circumstances?' because our responses form part of a pattern of practice in which those responses are taken for granted.

How do patterns of practice help?

This is all very well, you may say, but how does it help? I think the notion of patterns of practice helps in two ways, which I hinted at in the introduction to this chapter. First, it gives an explanation to our experience of dementia care and the way this can also be, at one and the same time, covertly ethical. Secondly, once we see what is going on, we can use it to guide what we do in a more conscious or overt manner. So the notion of patterns of practice has both explanatory and determinative functions.

The explanatory force of the notion can be seen when we consider an everyday aspect of care such as showering someone. For the practice to make sense I must engage in it. There must be (at least potentially) such a thing as showering someone (such an activity must potentially exist) for there to be such a concept as 'showering someone'. The word 'potentially' is used to cope with the unlikely possibility that everyone stops showering – or never starts; even so, such an activity must be potentially possible for the concept to exist in a meaningful way. This is not to lapse back into thinking that words correspond to things. It is rather that the words only come alive in the context of a meaningful practice – one that makes sense. We can start to see how our actions are patterned through and through.

Two thoughts follow. The first is that the notion of patterns of practice, when considered in the way I am suggesting, reveals to us how our lives – which involve showering – are meaningful. Any human activity, *as* a human activity, shows our humanity. This is not a tautology. It says that our activities show (and are part of or constitute) our humanity. A human activity reveals the nature of our humanity. We are the sort of creatures that shower ourselves and help others to shower if they are unable to do this for themselves. Our activities, then, are replete with meaning and significance. They have significance for us *qua* human beings.

The second thought follows on from the first. This deep patterning of our lives (through and through) will inevitably involve an ethical dimension. 'Inevitably' because ethics and morality are about how we live our lives and the sort of people we are. So I am going to help someone to shower, but I can do this well or badly. I can be rough and gruff, impatient and insensitive; or I can be the opposite. Patterns of practice provide an explanation for how it is that actions are, at one and the same time, ethical.

What is true of showering someone is true of all our activities – from dressing the person to putting up an intravenous infusion of saline, from helping someone with their finances to providing them with a meal – these are all, at one and the same time, a matter of ethics and morality. We can do such things without the word 'moral' entering our heads and without any thought of the ethics committee. They are morally unproblematic. The lack of moral reflection should seem remarkable. And the reason is that such activities form patterns of practice within which we are situated. Inculturation has occurred. We have acquired these habits of performance. The nurse puts up an infusion without obvious concern and, similarly, an adult helps their parent wash or a care worker gives someone a shower. This is simply what we do. It is our way of life. It is how we practise. The notion of patterns of practice alerts us to the profound nature of what we do and how we live. This is its explanatory function.

I also said that thinking about patterns of practice has a determinative function in that it can be useful as a guide to ethical practice. Simply seeing that our actions are practices which fall into patterns can in itself be helpful. I realize that I am about to do something to a person living with dementia for which, if I were doing it to someone without a diagnosis of dementia, I would normally seek consent. Seeking consent is my normal pattern of practice. So the question arises, why would I not seek consent from the person living with dementia? Obviously, I may presume that they lack the requisite decision-making capacity. But have I tested this? Perhaps I ascertain for sure that the person does lack the capacity to make this particular decision. Now what am I to do? We shall discuss answers to this question in Chapters 11 and 12. The point here is simply that recognizing a pattern of practice raises questions and can help us to do the right thing.

Internal coherence

But there is a deeper sense in which thinking about patterns of practice can be determinative and guide our actions. For there needs to be some sort of coherence to our practices. This is a matter of rationality. A practice has to have a certain coherence in order to be the practice that it is. As shown in Box 6.2, coherence can be spoken of as internal and external; and internal coherence is of two kinds: intra-practice and intra-personal.

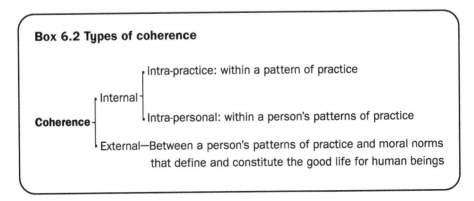

Box 6.2 Types of coherence

Coherence
- Internal
  - Intra-practice: within a pattern of practice
  - Intra-personal: within a person's patterns of practice
- External—Between a person's patterns of practice and moral norms that define and constitute the good life for human beings

The demand for coherence is not a demand that everything must be done in a uniform and dull manner. We can help someone to shower whilst wearing a red nose. But it normally makes no sense to go to try to shower someone with their clothes on. Similarly, routine operations on the abdomen might be performed in a variety of ways – there are patterns of practice associated with such procedures – but they do not require burr holes in the skull. We can call such coherence *intra-practice* coherence. Within themselves practices need to cohere. I do not think this is controversial.

By internal coherence I also mean that one person's practices should all cohere – not necessarily absolutely, but largely. Just because I can claim that a particular practice shows intra-practice coherence, this should not mean that I can do whatever I want. The doctor who is a serial killer cannot simply say, 'Well this is my coherent pattern of practice, so that is okay'! In the UK, we think of Dr Harold Shipman (1946–2004) who was found guilty of murdering 15 people, but who may have killed up to 250 individuals. The thought that such evil could be excused by regarding it as having intra-practice coherence is execrable.

No, there has to be coherence with the rest of the patterns of practice exhibited by the person; that is, intra-personal coherence. Presumably, during his professional career and in his family life Shipman showed compassion towards some people. He did not aim at the death of all his patients. In which case, there was large-scale incoherence in terms of how he practised. To show compassion to one person whilst callously killing another is not compatible behaviour. There are patterns of practice here that seem incompatible.

In a less dramatic fashion, we might consider a community nurse visiting an older person living with advanced dementia. Say the nurse finds that the person has an incipient leg ulcer, preventative measures would seem to be required. Not to give such treatment in this case would be incoherent if usual practice were to do so. We wish to see intra-personal coherence between practices in connection with looking after people living with advanced dementia. This is not to say that another course of action is impossible. If, for instance, the nurse felt sure that this person was likely to remove any covering put on the suspicious site and that, in fact, highlighting it might make it worse if the person were to start scratching and picking at it, then there might be reasons to leave the lesion for now and simply keep a watchful eye. A pattern of practice around watchful waiting, to see if the ulcer actually materializes, might not be incompatible with the nurse's other practices. There is, then, evidence of intra-personal coherence here because treating (on the one hand) and watchful waiting (on the other) are not incompatible approaches.

External coherence

In Box 6.2, I have described external coherence as being between a person's patterns of practice and moral norms that define and constitute the good life for human beings. What I mean is that, as well as internal coherence, we should also seek coherence between a pattern of practice and something external to the person, something with normative authority because it is a description of how we should humanly flourish. We could take as an example the two patterns of behaviour we just highlighted in the practice of the nurse who will either treat the incipient ulcer or will watchfully wait. These patterns of practice seemed to have internal coherence (in both senses), but what we can say in addition is that the two patterns also cohere under the rubric of good care. This is not something we can say about the evil activities of Shipman. I cannot think of accepted moral norms that define and constitute the good life which cohere with aiming at an innocent person's death. This is complicated, of course, because you might think that your aim could be to alleviate suffering. But then you would have to look in detail at what Shipman actually did: were the drugs and dosages he used of a kind to relieve suffering in the older people he was treating, or were they of a kind to kill them? Shipman's aim was to kill them, which does not cohere with good medical practice. The complication here is to do with what is intended by an action, which we shall come back to in Chapter 31.

There is obviously more to be said and clarified about all of this! Let me just add two things. First, we are looking for a degree of coherence. It is not anticipated that there must be complete coherence of every type. Can this be defined further? Well, patterns of practice cannot be completely contradictory. This would be for them to fail a test of rationality. They must largely hang together. The important thing is that we, as human beings, should be striving for coherence. It is the natural thing to do, otherwise we are left with an uncomfortable feeling: a guilty conscience, perhaps. I know I should have called so-and-so to reassure them. Not to have done so does not cohere with my normal practice, which I know to be good practice because it coheres with norms that define what it is to flourish or live the good life for human beings. We are not perfect, but the mindset I am describing grasps the inclination to seek perfection.

The second thing I wish to suggest is that intra-personal internal coherence is akin in my mind to features of casuistry. We compare our patterns of practice to each other, looking for morally significant similarities or differences. Meanwhile, external coherence is nothing other than virtue ethics, which provides us with a description in the virtue words of what it is to flourish as a human being. Patterns of practice are determinative, therefore, if we ask ourselves, first, in this case have I acted coherently (intra-practice coherence)? Secondly, does this practice show coherence in comparison with my other ways of doing things (intra-personal coherence)? And, finally, is what I am doing in keeping with the life of virtue: the good life (external coherence)?

Conclusion

The notion of patterns of practice is, I suggest, helpful in making the point that even in the mundane details of our lives there are ethical and moral concerns, chiefly the concern for coherence. This applies to practitioners, clinical and non-clinical, but also to policymakers, family and non-family carers and to people living with a diagnosis of dementia. We can all ask: are my actions coherent within themselves, together and with respect to the precepts of a life that is good?

Having introduced the notion of patterns of practice and described its explanatory function along with the internal and external coherence required for its determinative function, I shall now park the idea until Part 4 of this book, where I shall use it in my discussions of dilemmas in practice. Meanwhile, in Part 2, I shall review a range of concepts relevant to ethics and dementia.

Part 2

Notions of Note

7 Stigma

Introduction

The word 'stigma' derives from the Greek word meaning 'to prick': it conveys the idea of being marked or labelled. People living with dementia are labelled in various ways. In this chapter, we shall look at a variety of stigmatizing representations of people living with dementia. Stigmatization is not a new thing and seems well embedded in our culture. In an essay in 1990, Kitwood defined it as an aspect of labelling, 'but it also carries connotations of exclusion. The dementia sufferer becomes strange, alien, a diseased object, an outcast' (Kitwood 1990: 183). A mild irony is that Kitwood, whose work was and is so inspiring (Kitwood 2019), uses language in this definition that would now be considered stigmatizing. These days to describe people living with dementia as 'sufferers' would be frowned upon. But let us put the use of language to one side for a moment. Stigma is very real and it has real consequences. It links to ageism, with which I shall start.

Ageism and components of stigma

Sexism and racism are where we impose stereotypes on those from a certain gender or race in a systematic way and discriminate against them *because of* their gender or race. Ageism has the same characteristics (Nelson 2004). We lump all older people into one box – for instance, we think of them all as slow-witted and frail – and we then discriminate against all older people on the grounds that they are all slow-witted and frail. Ableism is closely related: it is discrimination against people with disabilities precisely because they are disabled. Or, the other way around, it is discrimination in favour of able-bodied people.

There are (at least) two things that are wrong with these '-isms': first, they are stereotyping; secondly, they are discriminatory on the basis of the systematic stereotyping. Ageism can be obvious, for instance in connection with employment. But it can also be more subtle. Direct discrimination is where a person is treated unfavourably because of their particular characteristics (for example, being old). Indirect discrimination is where practices, policies or procedures lead to discrimination because of a characteristic. An example of direct ageist discrimination would be if an advert for a job vacancy stipulated that people must be under 65 years of age. Indirect discrimination would be if a type of surgery were only going to be provided to people who could run fast. Although not stating that older people are excluded from such surgery, in effect this exclusion criterion would exclude most older people. In Great Britain, the *Equality Act 2010* affords older people protection against discrimination on the grounds of age – one of its 'protected characteristics'; the others are: disability, gender reassignment, marriage and civil partnership, pregnancy and maternity, race, religion or belief, sex or sexual orientation. 'The person, however vulnerable, infirm or 'different', is to be accorded respect and dignity under the law' (Hughes et al. 2021a: 60).

The link between ageism and the stigma of dementia is fairly obvious. Older people, just on account of their age, may be regarded as cognitively impaired in some way. It is their age that leads to the stereotype of 'incapable', which amounts to ageism on account of dementia. At the same time, since most people with dementia are older, the impression that they are incapable is reinforced. Both age and dementia are stereotyped as suggesting incapability. People living with young-onset dementia might also be regarded as incapable simply because of the label of dementia. Moreover, anyone living with dementia also has to put up with a different stereotype: that of having a mental illness. So, it soon becomes apparent there are three types of stigma people living with dementia might experience: not only the stigma associated with dementia itself, but also the stigma associated with ageing and mental illness. Since we can regard dementia as a disability, we might as well add the stigma of disability too.

But now I shall try to be more specific about what stigmatization amounts to in the context of dementia. Goffman (1963) famously described stigma in terms of groups who become discredited or spoiled because of their attributes, which often include deformity or perceived deviation from societal norms. Nguyen and Li (2020) highlighted the difference between public stigma and private (or self-) stigma, which can then be analysed in terms of:

- stereotype – a negative belief about the group or individual
- prejudice – emotional agreement with the belief
- discrimination – a behavioural manifestation of (in the case of public stigma) or a behavioural response to (in private self-stigma) prejudice (Corrigan et al. 2005; Corrigan and Watson 2002).

In terms of public stigma, in a systematic review of the global literature, Nguyen and Li (2020) demonstrated emotions ranging 'from negative (fear, anxiety, disgust), to neutral (pity), and positive (sympathy, empathy)' (p. 175). But they confirmed that negative emotions were reported more frequently. About self-stigma, they found: 'Fear, frustration, anger, grief, loss of confidence, and depression were the common emotions among people with dementia, whilst negative beliefs, fear, guilt, hurt, embarrassment, and shame were the common themes found among family caregivers' (Nguyen and Li 2020: 175).

Drawing on the work of Link and Phelan (2001 and 2006), Gove et al. (2016) listed the components of stigma as: labelling, stereotyping, separating us from them, status loss and discrimination, the exercise of power and emotional reactions. In their interviews with general practitioners (GPs), an example of the sort of negative belief that may then lead to prejudice and discrimination was this:

'You know the advanced dementia case becomes a non-person so there is very much a separation in that sense' (Gove et al. 2016: 395).

Another GP made a similar point:

'It's still them but their brain's so scrambled that mentally ... mentally it's not them ... But the mind, the mind isn't there' (Gove et al. 2016: 395).

Gove et al. (2016) concluded that there were specific aspects to the stigma attached to dementia in comparison with other conditions, which they characterized as 'existential anxiety and perceived similarity'. Because GPs could see themselves in the people living with dementia, arguably they were fearful about their own morbidity and mortality. This might have contributed to slower referrals, because GPs at some level might have been trying to protect people from a much-feared diagnosis.

Media and metaphor

I want to return to the use of language because what we say shapes the world. How we describe people influences how we think of them. The verbatim quotes from GPs given above from Gove et al. (2016) provide good examples of this. If we think the mind 'isn't there' because it is 'scrambled' and that the person is now a 'non-person' (we shall come back to this in more detail in Chapter 13) it must be the case that we look on the 'non-person' living with dementia in a particular way. It need not be that we despise them; we may simply feel immense pity for them. But they are stigmatized as different and separate from us and the inclination will be to treat them differently by, for instance, not regarding their possible or actual wishes and preferences with as much importance as we would if they were 'normal' people.

The media is a good place to observe how people living with dementia are talked about and therefore considered. Bailey et al. (2021) looked at articles in the British press between 2012 and 2017. The language used was analysed and the authors found that 'The most salient discourse ... was the portrayal of dementia in biomedical terms, with a particular focus on the pathological processes of dementia, and pharmaceutical treatments and research' (Bailey et al. 2021: 362). They found that the most popular metaphors (where words are applied to something to which they are not literally applicable) to describe dementia included talk of '...a zombie apocalypse ..., a military battle ... and an epidemic'; and they found '...the language of machinery, warfare, waste disposal and infection' were used to convey the neurological processes involved in dementia' (Bailey et al. 2021: 369).

We might be inclined to ask if all this matters terribly. If it helps people to understand what is going on, then all well and good. The trouble is that it presents only a limited view of what it is to live with dementia. It leaves out agency and the positive social aspects of life as opposed to the negative image of the victim. Bailey et al. (2021) went on to say: 'The absence of other named social actors gives the impression that the *patients* and *sufferers* are at the mercy of anonymous medical authorities, continuously being acted upon rather than acting for themselves with regards to their care and treatment' (Bailey et al. 2021: 371). These researchers pointed out that we tend not to hear anything from people living with dementia themselves in the media (at least between 2012 and 2017). Bailey et al. (2021) concluded: 'Such metaphors tend to obscure the agency of the person with the syndrome and perpetuate fear and anxiety, such as in the metaphor of dementia as a zombie apocalypse, which insinuates a global epidemic and promotes the belief that death is preferable' (p. 372).

Indeed, in a review of the literature, Johnstone (2011) had already spotted how there was an 'Alzheimerization' of the social debates around euthanasia and physician-assisted suicide. Although metaphors can help us to understand and make fresh meanings, they can 'also mesmerize and mislead people into thinking and behaving in problematic, wrong or morally risky ways' (Johnstone 2011: 387). Hence, Johnstone (2011) suggested: '… there is a need to examine critically how Alzheimer's disease and other dementias are portrayed in the public media and used as linguistic framing devices to influence public opinion on the permissibility of euthanasia/physician-assisted suicide as a bona fide medical regimen' (p. 390).

The heroes and heroines of the story as presented in the media are the medical people, the scientists and the drug companies who heroically fight back against the onslaught of dementia. Drawing out a critical point to emerge from their research, Bailey et al. (2021) went on to say:

> Notably, the reliance on the biomedical discourse conceals alternative discourses and ideologies, such as a discourse of political and social action which would reinforce dementia as a global issue requiring collective responses … Moreover, there is little evidence in the biomedical discourse that people with the condition may live full, active lives, despite the fact that it is very possible to continue to live well after a diagnosis of dementia with the right support …
>
> (p. 373).

Looking at two newspapers, one American (*The New York Times*) and one British (*The Guardian*), during a slightly later time frame (2014–2019), sm-Rahman et al. (2021) were able to report less negativity over time; yet the overwhelming picture was still negative and, again, the dialogue was mostly about scientists and drug companies and their potential cures (albeit none actually emerged). They referred to this as 'biomedical colonization' which 'perpetuates dehumanized healthcare … through the practice of infantilization, intimidation, stigmatization, and objectification' (sm-Rahman et al. 2021). They suggested that the typically negative picture in the news media will encourage stigma and distancing and a stereotypical image that people living with dementia '... are not fully human, are incompetent, and are burdens on society' (sm-Rahman et al. 2021). As in Gove et al. (2016), these authors worried that such stereotypes will put people off seeking help early; and, like Bailey et al. (2021), they worried that the more positive potential for those living with dementia will not be encouraged. In this regard, it is of note that the Alzheimer's Society in England and Wales has produced a dementia-friendly media toolkit to encourage the portrayal of dementia in the media, arts and popular culture to be more positive (Alzheimer's Society 2018).

Moving beyond newspapers and journals, to look at how living with dementia is culturally represented more broadly (for example, in social media, films and television), between 1989 and 2018, Low and Purwaningrum (2020) confirmed the picture already seen. Although there was reasonable evidence of positive depictions of life with dementia, the overall impression was still negative. They concluded by saying that how dementia is depicted and framed in popular culture is likely to influence stigma so that 'we need to be mindful about the social impact of the words, images and messages that we use'; and they ended by quoting from the dementia activist, Kate Swaffer: 'I repeat: "Please don't call us sufferers,"' (Low and Purwaningrum 2020).

In a really interesting book, *Popularizing Dementia: Public Expressions and Representations of Forgetfulness*, Swinnen and Schweda (2015) reflected many of the themes picked out above. They made the point that we need 'a better understanding of dementia as a *cultural* phenomenon' and they went on to say: 'Understanding the multiple ways by which dementia, while biologically influenced, is at the same time culturally constructed contributes to the fight against stigma and can improve the wellbeing of people with dementia and their caregivers' (p. 11). This cultural approach allows a much broader view of dementia and a richness which comes from the input of scholars from gerontology, literature, philosophy and ethics, fashion design, media studies, anthropology and gender theory, as well as healthcare.

The importance of metaphor and the stories we tell about dementia was brought out specifically by Zeilig (2013). She explained that metaphors are a linguistic process by which a relationship is established between one thing and another. 'They also influence the way in which we perceive our worlds and therefore the way we explain and live in them' (Zeilig 2013: 259), which is why they are so important. As an example, Zeilig (2013: 261) quoted the UK Prime Minister, David Cameron, in 2012 announcing an increase in funding for dementia when he talked about 'the quiet crisis, one that steals at lives and tears at the heart of families'. Zeilig aptly commented that this made dementia sound like a primeval monster. In her nuanced account Zeilig (2013) ended by pointing out how stories can tend to distance us from the people we are talking about; they become other, they are 'them' rather than us. We need to question the negative societal stories and stereotypes that encourage stigmatization. As people living with dementia increasingly tell their own stories, this acts as a challenge to the 'mainstream biopics' that associate dementia with 'decline and fall' (p. 266).

Tackling stigma

The problem, therefore, has been identified many times, but how might stigma be addressed? Harper et al. (2019), having identified widespread stigma in association with dementia, went on to suggest that person-centred care, promoting anti-stigma campaigns and policies to improve the lives of people living with dementia and their families would all be of value. But, again to quote Kate Swaffer, to try to do these things without involving people with dementia themselves seems likely to be self-defeating. She wrote:

> I have explored stigma in the literature, looking at it in a new way by questioning whether the researchers exacerbate stigma, even though their intent is to promote positive change. Considering the lack of inclusion of people with dementia in the cohorts being studied, it is still very much 'about people with dementia, without them', which cannot give a true picture of the issues for this group, also serving to reinforce the stigma
>
> (Swaffer 2014: 710).

At the start of this chapter, I said we would put the use of language to one side. It is relevant again now because people with dementia have themselves commented on how they wish to be described. For instance, they have said:

> People with dementia urge you to be thoughtful about your choice of words when talking about what it is like to live with dementia. Any evocative words should be chosen with intent and careful consideration of the message that will actually be received – and the impact it may have on people with dementia themselves
>
> (DEEP 2014: 3 of 3).

The demand for inclusion is being taken increasingly seriously, even if it is not perfect. In a study that elicited responses from 1,172 people living with dementia and 702 caregivers, four themes emerged, all of which showed how developing supportive communities might decrease stigma; they were: 'raising awareness, improving access to support services, providing social events and activities, and supporting people to engage in the community' (Quinn et al. 2021).

Meanwhile, Kim et al. (2021a) suggested that 'The four most promising approaches to reduce stigma are: specialised education on the stigmatised condition; social contact with people living with the condition; targeted public health awareness and messaging; and changes to public policy' (p. 2153). In their study, they looked at both teaching about dementia and at contact with people living with dementia or with their carers, as well as mixtures of both approaches. They found that it was possible to improve knowledge quite quickly, but decreasing stigma came more gradually (Kim et al. 2021a). The study was enough to demonstrate that such programmes (mixtures of teaching about dementia and contact with people with dementia and their carers) could be helpful in reducing stigma.

Hagan and Campbell (2021) looked at 13 people with recent diagnoses of dementia who were involved in empowerment groups and thus became engaged with public consultations about policy and with educational programmes. This sort of engagement provided a sense of purpose, but also allowed people to challenge stereotypical views. Importantly, group identity allowed participants to share a narrative that was positive, as opposed to the frequently stigmatizing narratives that otherwise seem so common: 'The very nature of engagement was sufficiently powerful to overcome the influence of stigmatising media messages. As long as these encounters continue, the opportunity exists for public stigma to be challenged and reconfigured' (Hagan and Campbell 2021: 2374).

Beyond such academic studies, or perhaps we should say before them, are the increasing number of works by people who live with dementia. Keith Oliver, one of the editors of the current series of books and someone living with a diagnosis of Alzheimer's disease, has been a staunch advocate for people with dementia. He has been described as 'tenacious' and 'kind', which he is, and some years ago he gave me the book *Welcome to Our World*, written by members of the Forget-Me-Nots, a group of people living with various types of dementia who had worked together at a creative writing course (Jennings 2014). The perspectives of people with dementia are invaluable in shaping our understanding and in informing our judgements and opinions, including about ethics and morals. In the last few months, I have received a copy of *The Practical Handbook of Living with Dementia* (Parker et al. 2022). Keith has written eloquently in this book too (Oliver 2022). But there is also a chapter by Gail Gregory, who has a diagnosis of young-onset dementia. She describes how she has been helped by writing poetry. In complete contradiction to the stereotyping of stigmatization she asserts that 'You can live your life with dementia' (Gregory 2022: 21).

Conclusion

Stigma can be challenged and there are programmes which help in its reduction. We have seen improvements, certainly in terms of awareness. But there is still a way to go and thinking needs to be varied and practical if we are to make more progress, which will also require political commitment (Bamford et al. 2014).

This seems an appropriate point once again to ask overtly 'So what?'. Stigma is everyone's business precisely because it is a matter of such ethical concern. Practitioners need to beware of stigmatizing language and attitudes in their dealings with the public and with people who live with dementia. Politicians, policymakers, journalists and those who influence our cultural and societal organizations and norms need to eradicate anything that undermines the standing of people who live with dementia or makes them seem 'other'. Family and non-family carers must be advocates and should not inadvertently position people who live with dementia as inadequate. And people who live with dementia must be supported to enable them to live their lives to the full and to flourish so as to dispel the myths and prejudices that surround dementia.

There is much more to say about stigma, but one question raises an interesting ethical point. The question is: what is morally wrong with stigma? If it means that most of the population does not have to face existential anxiety, if unpleasant sights and disturbing behaviour are either hidden or regarded with humour, if public spending can be minimized, is this not a reasonable way to maximize the population's happiness and welfare? This may be right. But it is only right from a certain consequentialist perspective. A deontologist may well see it as a duty to look after people living with dementia properly and to maintain their personhood. The principlist can stress justice, benevolence and non-maleficence, let alone respect for the autonomous wishes of the person living with dementia, as the principles that face down stigma. The virtue ethicist must be compassionate, true and just (that is, non-stigmatizing) to the person living with dementia. Those who use other approaches to make evaluative judgments will be attuned to the requirement for understanding and the importance of building and maintaining caring relationships with those who live with dementia. This brief digression shows that, at least in relation to stigma, one reason for rejecting consequentialist thinking (as opposed to other ethical theories and approaches) is that it allows a morally repugnant attitude to be laudable.

8 From autonomy to relational autonomy

Introduction

We have already come across autonomy as one of the four principles of clinical ethics (see Chapter 3). The word derives from the Greek: *autos* meaning 'self', and *nomos* meaning 'rule'. Self-rule is something most of us are keen on and expect, at least in liberal democracies. Gillon (1986: 60) helpfully summarized 'autonomy' as 'the capacity to think, decide, and act on the basis of such thought and decision freely and independently and without … let or hindrance'. Gillon makes several important introductory points. First, we are not concerned simply with autonomy as such, but with the principle of respect for autonomy. Secondly, that we should distinguish between freedom or *simply* doing what you want to do and doing what you want *in accordance with human rationality*, which distinguishes us from lions roaming free in the savanna. Thirdly, as suggested by his definition above, Gillon points out that we can distinguish autonomy of thought, of will and of action (p. 61).

In this chapter, I shall explore a little further the notion of autonomy and why we should respect it. I shall highlight its problems and a relational solution.

Importance of respect for autonomy

The principle of respect for autonomy is deeply ingrained in liberal democratic societies. It is implicit, for instance, in laws relevant to consent in medical practice. (See Chapter 11 for further discussion of consent, where we shall also confront the problem of what to do if the person lacks the requisite capacity or competence to make a particular decision.) There have been a number of famous cases where judges have stressed that, if the person has capacity (in other words, is competent), then the autonomous wishes of that person must be respected, even if death should follow. A number of cases have referred back to the case of *Malette v. Shulman* et al. which was heard in the Ontario Court of Appeal in Canada on 30 March 1990. The case was to do with a Jehovah's Witness who was given blood against her expressed wishes. Appeal Justice Sydney Robins set out his thinking in the judgment with explicit reference to the notion of autonomy:

> At issue here is the freedom of the patient as an individual to exercise her right to refuse treatment and accept the consequences of her own decision.

> Competent adults … are generally at liberty to refuse medical treatment even at the risk of death. The right to determine what shall be done with one's body is a fundamental right in our society. The concepts inherent in this right are the bedrock upon which the principles of self-determination and individual autonomy are based.
>
> (*Malette v. Shulman* et al. 72 O.R. (2d) 417; at §432.)

The importance and standing of the principle of respect for autonomy undoubtedly stems, amongst many other things, from the serious consideration it was given by Kant and Mill in the second half of the eighteenth and the first half of the nineteenth centuries.

For Kant, the principle of autonomy was fundamental for morals because rational agents, making moral decisions, should be guided by categorical imperatives; in other words, by imperatives which every rational agent would choose autonomously and not for the sake of some other outside influence. Kant said that 'the dignity of humanity consists just in its capacity to legislate universal laws, though with the condition of humanity's being at the same time itself subject to this very same legislation' (Kant 1785: 44). He also wrote: '… autonomy is the ground of the dignity of human nature and of every rational nature' (p. 41). For Kant, therefore, people are autonomous if their choices and actions are not governed by outside factors but only by the imperatives chosen by rational agents.

Mill's account was much easier to understand and more practical. He simply stated: 'That the only purpose for which power can be rightfully exercised over any member of a civilized community, against his will, is to prevent harm to others' (Mill 1859: 135). Self-rule (autonomy) was basic to Mill's conception of liberty. As he said: 'The only freedom which deserves the name, is that of pursuing our own good in our own way, so long as we do not attempt to deprive others of theirs, or impede their efforts to obtain it' (p. 138). But therein lies the rub!

Problems with autonomy

One problem with respecting autonomy is that it becomes difficult to define where pursuing my good in my way illicitly impedes your ability to pursue the things you regard as goods. Tangential issues here are to do with intergenerational transfers and rationing on the basis of age. To what extent should one generation be morally obliged to support another? Should we accept that resources for older people will be less than those set aside for younger people (or the other way around)? Respect for the autonomy of the older generation, say, might seem to be less than respect for the autonomy of the younger generation. Although issues of rationing healthcare and making decisions between different age cohorts are relevant to dementia (see Hughes 2012), they are mainly relevant to broader debates about age and ageism. (These debates are stimulating but complex and I would refer the interested reader to two books edited by Lesser (1999 and 2012a) which cover the relevant territory in illuminating detail.)

Instead, I turn to a more quotidian example of the daughter caring for her mother who is living with dementia. We could take the example of a son, but statistically, daughters more frequently find themselves, more or less willingly, as carers; spouses are more common than daughters, but for my purposes here the spousal relationship changes the dynamics of the argument. (For more about carers see Oyebode and Parveen 2021.) The mother has autonomous wishes – things she wants – but so too does her daughter. Often these may coincide: they both wish to see each other, they both wish to go to the shops or out for a coffee. But sometimes they may not. Perhaps the mother needs increasing care which the daughter can neither supply herself, because of her commitments to her work and to her children, nor afford to purchase. The mother's autonomous wishes can only be met by her daughter providing her with the necessary care. Her daughter's autonomous wishes include helping her mother, but more salient are her wishes to have time for her children and to keep her job. Hopefully, an acceptable solution will emerge which allows both sets of autonomous wishes to be met to some degree. But in terms of principles, there is no way to decide between conflicting autonomous wishes without bringing some further principles into play. We might ask, for instance, what is fair in these circumstances to all concerned (that is, we bring in the principle of justice)? At any rate, Mill's simple statement about liberty is not quite as simple as it seems, because where someone can legitimately complain about my autonomous wishes and actions is open for debate.

There is a further difficulty with autonomy, which is that none of us is fully autonomous. Here we need to be careful and remember the distinction between autonomy of thought, will and action (Gillon 1986: 61). To explore this fully would be complicated. To what extent is my thought autonomous? I seem to think things for myself, but I have to admit my thinking has been moulded by my education, by my social environment, including my family and so on. This also applies to my will or intentions. I can make an autonomous decision to sit down and type. But that I am the sort of person who has such intentions and that this is what I will this morning are not altogether matters over which I have complete self-control: the circumstances under which I will to type also have to be propitious and I do not always have complete self-governance of circumstances.

Certainly, my actions are only fully autonomous in very circumscribed areas. I can only actually type this morning if all sorts of other things are in place: someone has made me a keyboard and is supplying me with electricity and so on. Indeed, once I think what goes into making a computer, the depth of my lack of autonomy is immense. We need to keep in mind Gillon's warning that the issue is respect for autonomy. But when I think of the precious metals in my computer and the people who had to mine those metals, it is uncomfortable to ponder to what extent they did or did not have autonomy of action in deciding to undertake that work. I might feel as if I have autonomy of action in typing this morning and that this should be respected, but that autonomy is dependent on others whose own autonomy of action may well be limited.

Relational autonomy to the rescue

I have identified two problems in connection with respect to autonomy: the problem of drawing limits to one person's autonomy over against another's and the problem that we are rarely fully autonomous in what we do. A solution is to stop thinking of the notion of 'autonomy' and to start thinking in terms of 'relational autonomy'.

Relational autonomy is an idea developed by feminist writers which emphasizes how decisions are typically made in the context of social relationships (Mackenzie and Stoljar 2000; Ellis et al. 2011). Relational autonomy helps to establish that 'a person's sense of self and self-expression should be seen as being firmly grounded in their social and family networks' (Nuffield Council on Bioethics 2009: p. 117, §7.14). The Nuffield Council's report on dementia (which we shall discuss further in Chapter 16) went on to say that when autonomy is understood in relational terms, 'then in order to support a person's autonomous wishes and values it will be necessary to support the whole family and social structure' (p. 117, §7.14).

Just changing the words may not seem like a big deal for the mother being cared for by her daughter, but it reframes the problem. Instead of seeing a clash of autonomous wishes, we can see from the start that the wishes of the mother and daughter are enmeshed. We cannot think about one without the other. It never made sense to try to do so. If we are to be helpful, we always have to see and understand the bigger picture. Similarly, it is ridiculous that I should think of myself as a fully autonomous being and not see myself in a nexus of relationships. People should respect my autonomy, sure, but my autonomous choices have consequences, so it is not as if that respect should be free of all consideration for those who surround me and on whom I depend.

The Nuffield Council's report went further in making links between the richer accounts of relational autonomy and the notions of dependency and self:

A key implication of these accounts is that the dependency of people as a result of their disease does not mean that their autonomy cannot be promoted, nor that promoting autonomy simply involves respecting the wishes and values they had before the onset of dementia. On the contrary, it means that people who have become dependent on others through the development of dementia may need support from those who care for them to help them retain their autonomy, and with it their sense of self.

(pp. 27–28; §234)

I shall leave the self for Chapter 13, but there are some quick comments to make about dependency. In his brilliant book, *Dependence and Autonomy in Old Age*, Agich (2003) made the point that autonomy and dependence can be thought of as two sides of the same coin. My current autonomous actions are dependent on those people who have allowed me to type on my computer. The mother's autonomous wish to get out for a coffee is fulfilled through her dependence on her daughter. Agich put it beautifully in saying that autonomy should be understood as involving:

> ... the way individuals live their daily lives; it is found in the nooks and cran-
> nies of everyday existence; it is found in the way that individuals interact and
> not exclusively in the idealized paradigm of choice ... that dominates ethical
> analysis
>
> (Agich 2003: 165).

This is fully in accord with the notion of relational autonomy. As Agich went on to say, to understand the concept thoroughly we must see people as being '... in essential interrelationship with others and the world' (p. 174).

Conclusion

Autonomy is not an easy concept. Some years ago, Collopy (1988) pointed out that it has various meanings and contains a range of polarities with attendant risks attached to each of them should one particular interpretation dominate. The polarities were between making decisions and being able to execute them, acting on one's own or giving authority to others to make decisions, making competent or incapacitated judgements, being authentic or inauthentic, making immediate or long-range decisions, and between negative and positive conceptions of autonomy (which reflect negative and positive liberties: Isaiah Berlin's freedom *from* and freedom *to* (Berlin 1967: 148)). Autonomy might simply be 'the *liberty* to make one's own decisions' or it might entail that the decisions one makes should reflect 'self-expression' (Craigie 2015). Different understandings and definitions are not without consequence when it comes to the law (Dunn and Foster 2010); and tensions in terms of how broadly and in what way autonomy is conceived underlie arguments about what is or is not relevant when it comes to interpreting the United Nations *Convention on the Rights of Persons with Disabilities* (CRPD) (Craigie 2015), to which we shall return.

Relational autonomy is good for the person living with dementia inasmuch as it forces others (from practitioners to policymakers) to look at the person in a rounded manner in order to understand them fully. It is good for family and other carers in that it does not rule them out; on the contrary, their relationships with the person are seen as vital.

A concluding worry about relational autonomy is that it might be used as an excuse to override someone's autonomous wishes. The wishes of the relatives, having been taken into consideration, might overwhelm any inclination to place the wishes of the person living with dementia centre stage. I think this is a concern. But the reality is that persons are situated in relational contexts. Under all sorts of regimes bad decisions are possible. For instance, someone using the four principles framework (see Chapter 3) might make egregious judgements about what weight to give to each of the principles. Relational autonomy, however, is always the relational autonomy of someone particular. And it seems difficult to deny that we shall do better by that person if their relationships are fully understood.

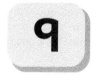

From paternalism to solicitude

Introduction

The increasing recognition given to the importance of respect for autonomy since the 1980s reflects a strong swing away from the dominant attitude, at least in the medical profession, of paternalism. Crudely, this attitude was that the doctor knew best. It used to be the case that people would rarely question what a doctor said. Similarly, I remember as a junior doctor it being made clear to me that I should not address my consultant (he was a surgeon) unless invited to do so. My mother was once given a stern reprimand by our GP because she had raised a question about treatment. The GP was later struck off the medical register for sexual impropriety with a patient. Paternalism was and is not all bad, but it was and is a close bedfellow of power. The doctors' paternalism stemmed from their power, and power can be dangerous.

To the extent that there continues to be a power differential between doctors and those for whom they care, there remains the possibility of paternalistic attitudes. In the case of people living with a diagnosis of dementia, power differentials and the possibility of such attitudes are very real. In particular, just to highlight what is to follow, it seems important to note what was (and is) good about paternalism to see how this might be used in a more beneficial manner. This will lead me to the notion of 'parentalism'; but we need to go further than this, to solicitude, to understand what is actually good about any tendency to paternalism. Eventually, this will bring us to human rights.

From paternalism to parentalism

Medical paternalism has been defined '... as interference by the physician with the patient's freedom of action, justified on the grounds of the patient's best interests' (Weiss 1985). Weiss (1985) characterized what he referred to as 'modern paternalism'. His description of this started well: it recommended that the crucial first step was for the physician to understand the values of the patient. In this he was strongly anticipating VBP (see Chapter 5). But later he suggested that, as opposed to the autonomy-based model, 'modern' paternalism might be better because, first, patients tend to seek 'immediate gratification' (p. 186) and not see the long-term benefits of treatment. He used the example of a young man refusing chemotherapy for testicular cancer and wrote (with emphasis added): 'This situation justifies and even requires the physician's encouraging, or if necessary, *coercing* the patient to complete the therapy' (Weiss 1985: 186). Today, coercing patients into treatment sounds more like the offence of battery than anything else! Modern paternalism is allegedly beneficial, secondly, because patients are not very good at 'decision-analysis' and, thirdly, because 'the physician is likely to be more objective about the patient than the patient will be about himself' (p. 186).

On this basis, 'modern' paternalism seems as bad as what went before. It is worth noting that the description of this approach necessitates a good deal of talk of 'patients' because this hints at the subservience of those who fall under the doctor's care. Weiss (1985) ends by suggesting that the patient-autonomy model emphasizes process and the right to self-determination, whereas 'modern' paternalism looks at outcome and the patient's best interests. The autonomy model 'considers patient values as decisive' (p. 186), whereas the 'modern' paternalist weighs up values amongst many other things. What this ignores is the possibility, embraced by VBP, that the 'many other things' – for instance the scientific matters the 'patient' will not understand! – will also be evaluative in one way or another and should be discussed with the person whom they concern.

We need to move quickly beyond 'modern' paternalism! But is there still not something to be said for the inclination to avoid people making unnecessary mistakes at times of stress, when there are professionals who may be able to cajole (not coerce!) them in a better direction – one which they may themselves choose under other circumstances and may be pleased to have chosen later, whatever their initial inclinations? In a thoughtful piece, Rosenbaum (2015) reflected that facts and knowledge are not the issues at times of crisis. She recalled an accident that had left her with an awkwardly fractured clavicle and although she knew something about surgical procedures, 'being asked by an expert how I wanted my clavicle realigned seemed like being asked by an auto mechanic how I'd like my clutch repaired' (Rosenbaum 2015: 590). Sometimes, what you need is someone to take responsibility and to make a decision because, however well-informed and cognitively competent you might be, emotionally and practically you need help.

Perhaps it is the manner in which help is given that is crucial and that might depend upon the way it is framed. Agich (2003) commended the idea of 'parentalism'. We develop as human persons through our relationships with our parents, relationships which are deeply psychological and social. He continued: 'Parentalism signals the essential interconnectedness of all human persons and is rooted in the basic response to the needy other that such relationships engender' (Agich 2003: 48).

From parentalism to care, concern and solicitude

It is quite easy to be dismissive of paternalism; and yet there is something about it that is of great importance. We might regard the care that a parent has for a child as the epitome of *real* care: authentic care that is intrinsic to the nature of the relationship. Inasmuch as the doctor *really* cares, the inclination to do the best for people is praiseworthy. It is only bad if a healthcare professional starts to ignore the person's actual wishes, preferences and values. This is true, but we are dealing here with something very subtle in the nature of relationships. What we should be after, in my view, is captured by the word 'solicitude'.

At least, it is worth looking at this word and, in particular, at its use in the work of the philosopher Martin Heidegger (see Box 9.1)

Box 9.1 Martin Heidegger (1889–1976)

Heidegger was a German philosopher who wrote in the fields of existentialism, phenomenology and hermeneutics.

Existentialism is not easy to define but suggests a focus on actual existence as the way to characterize human life. Ontology, the study of Being itself, was therefore key to much of his thinking and was the subject of his most famous work *Sein und Zeit*, in English *Being and Time*, first published in 1927.

Phenomenology is also difficult to pin down because it has been differently conceived by most philosophers. But it is something to do with how we understand and frame the experience of consciousness, and for Heidegger this involved, again, consideration of the underlying Being of human existence.

We have already come across hermeneutics in Chapter 4 (see Table 4.1). Put simply, for Heidegger, understanding the human existent is a matter of interpretation, of seeing through to the nature of the Being of human beings.

Heidegger joined the Nazi Party on 1 May 1933, just days after he had been elected the rector of the University of Freiburg (Hitler had become Chancellor of Germany on 30 January 1933), and he remained a member of the Nazi Party until the end of the Second World War. His writings are notoriously hard to understand because of the technical ways in which he uses language.

According to Heidegger, the human existent – referred to as *Dasein* (which literally means 'Being-There') – is always best thought of as 'Being-in-the-World', because this is the basic reality of human existence. More precisely, our type of Being is always 'Being-with' and, in part, this entails being in dialogue with others. Nevertheless, being-in-the-world also entails that we are aware of our finitude: we are 'Being-towards-death'. Now a very basic feature of Heidegger's philosophy is that, once we have perceived what our existence amounts to, our basic affect will be one of anxiety. To cut to the chase, a solution to the state in which we find ourselves in-the-world, is to seek authenticity, which implies that we are genuinely ourselves. And one way we can achieve this is through our relationships with the world and particularly with others in-the-world.

It is here that we come across Heidegger's technical concepts of 'care', 'concern' and 'solicitude'. According to Heidegger, 'Dasein's Being reveals itself as *care*' (Heidegger 1962: 227). Care (*Sorge*) is the general human response to finding ourselves in the world. It is fundamental that we care about our situation. Just to be in the world is to care on this view. Concern (*Besorgen*) is a more developed notion about our relations with the physical things of the world, the things which are 'ready-to-hand'. But solicitude (*Fürsorge*) is our response to other human beings who exist with us. Our Being-with engages with their Being-with, which is where solicitude is encountered.

A little later, Heidegger put it this way: 'But those entities towards which Dasein as Being-with comports itself do not have the kind of Being which belongs to equipment ready-to-hand; they are themselves Dasein. These entities are not objects of concern, but rather of *solicitude*' (p. 157). In other words, human beings are not simply other objects in the world, they are beings with whom we engage because it is part of what we are that we should do so at this fundamental level. 'In short, we are not disengaged beings-in-the-world but are characterized by our worldly engagements' (Hughes 2011b: 217).

There is much more to be said about Heidegger in relation to dementia (see Hughes 2011b: 45–53; 215–220; 233–235). All I wish to insist on here is that the good in paternalism or parentalism should be solicitude, which in turn reflects the inescapable nature of our human relationships. Power is out of the window. It is to do with the essential equality of human beings face-to-face.

Let me give one quick example. I was once visiting an elderly female resident with a diagnosis of dementia in a care home. I was taken to her room by a care assistant who immediately started to talk to the resident who had severe dementia and could not easily respond. The care assistant made her comfortable and started to brush her hair. This was done with the utmost care and concern. It seemed a genuine example of solicitude. The care assistant's response was an immediate expression of her encounter with the resident as a human being. Perhaps another word for 'solicitude' would be 'love'.

Solicitude and human rights

There is a bit of a jump from Heidegger's solicitude to human rights, except that if human rights are not ultimately based on our relationships with one another then what could they possibly be based on? The jump I wish to make is specifically to Article 12.2 to the CRPD (see Box 9.2).

> **Box 9.2 UN Convention on the Rights of Persons with Disabilities**
>
> **Article 12**
> **Equal recognition before the law**
>
> 1 States Parties reaffirm that persons with disabilities have the right to recognition everywhere as persons before the law.
> 2 States Parties shall recognize that persons with disabilities enjoy legal capacity on an equal basis with others in all aspects of life.
> 3 States Parties shall take appropriate measures to provide access by persons with disabilities to the support they may require in exercising their legal capacity.
>
> From: United Nations General Assembly (2006)

It is important to understand that, according to this Convention, dementia is regarded as a disability, so its edicts are applicable. The exact wording of Article 12.2 – '...legal capacity on an equal basis with others in all aspects of life...' – reflects the intuition and determination that any form of paternalism is out of place. People living with dementia are on an equal footing with everyone else. Article 12 has been said to establish a 'philosophical foundation on which to ground the positive duty of the state to maximise autonomy for people with significant intellectual, cognitive and psychosocial disabilities' (Bach and Kerzner 2010: 72).

Without getting bogged down in a discussion of the CRPD (see Donnelly 2014 and Flynn 2018 for informed comment), my aim here is simply to note that fundamental human rights can be regarded *as fundamental* in the sense that they reflect something radical about how we should engage with each other in the world. We do so on the basis of our shared and equal standing as persons.

Conclusion

If there is something good about paternalism it is buried in the interstices of the concept at the level of human relationships, at what Heidegger termed *Fürsorge*, which is translated as 'solicitude'. It is solicitude, or love, that the parent naturally feels for the child. Another way to think of this is to use the distinction made by the Austrian and Jewish philosopher Martin Buber (1878–1965) between 'I-It' and 'I-Thou' relationships (Buber 1937), the importance of which was not lost on Tom Kitwood (2019: 9–11). 'I-It' relationships are distant and detached; 'I-Thou' relationships are warm, engaged and so forth. Whether we are living with dementia or caring for someone who does, our relationships should be authentic and on a genuinely equal basis as human beings-in-the-world. It should also be no surprise that this philosophical and ethical imperative is now explicit in a global legal convention.

10 Dignity and quality of life

Introduction

Talk of autonomy in Chapter 8 and the CRPD in Chapter 9 makes it almost inevitable that in this chapter we should start by talking about dignity. As Donnelly (2014) wrote: 'The principles underpinning the CRPD include respect for the inherent dignity and individual autonomy – including the freedom to make one's own choices – of persons with disabilities' (p. 274). Koppelman (2002) also highlighted a strong connection between human dignity and autonomy: 'When a patient has a voice in decisions regarding her care, when she has the opportunity to express *her* beliefs and values, when she has the opportunity to express *who she is* through choice and action ...., she has dignity and self-respect' (p. 66).

A further link can be made between dignity and quality of life. A loss of dignity is hardly likely to enhance someone's quality of life. Johnston et al. (2016) showed that an approach they had developed, called 'Dignity Therapy', had the potential to enhance dignity and quality of life as well as person-centred care. In brief, this therapy, which is akin to life story and reminiscence therapy, allows someone the opportunity to record and tell others of the meaningful 'events, thoughts, accomplishments and experiences that have been influential in the person's life ...' (Johnston et al. 2016: 110). Previously, Manthorpe et al. (2010) had demonstrated that practitioners have different views of dignity, which will have an impact on debates around quality of life for those living with dementia. But they started with a strong statement about the link between dignity and quality of life, stating dignity is 'an integral component of quality of life' (Manthorpe et al. 2010: 236).

Dignity

The point Manthorpe et al. (2010) made about different accounts of dignity is very important. The term derives from the Latin meaning 'worthy' and suggests that the person is worthy of honour or respect. But the word is perhaps overused, so that respecting someone's dignity can mean almost anything. Macklin (2003) regarded it as a useless concept: she felt it was used as a mere slogan and often meant no more than respect for the person's autonomy. Many people and institutions working in the area of dementia would wish to claim they maintain the dignity of the people they look after, just as they also claim they always provide person-centred care. But what is real dignity? (We shall ask the same question of person-centred care in Chapter 13.) What dignity refers to is, at a conceptual level, hard to pin down.

Woodruff (2016) set out an ontology of dignity. Dignity can be seen as designating either natural or non-natural metaphysical properties. Or perhaps dignity is conferred on someone by others, so it is not a property out there in the world to be discovered at all. This can be referred to as 'dignity of merit' (Woodruff 2016: 228). The idea of a 'universal, permanent, and invariable' metaphysical idea of dignity is summed up by the German notion of *Menschenwürde* ('human worth') (p. 227). Woodruff goes on to suggest:

> The non-naturalistic conception of dignity is attractive to many: insofar as dignity is grounded on being a member of a kind but is not identical to any particular set of natural properties of a particular member of that kind, we have a basis for asserting the equal moral standing of all members of that kind, including those who are treated in undignified ways and those whose natural capacities are diminished
>
> (p. 228).

Woodruff accepted that philosophers have not been able to settle on a correct understanding of 'dignity'. But he commended a 'two-tier model' of *basic* dignity, possessed equally by all, and *refined* dignity 'requiring individual effort and social support to exercise one's species-specific capacities' (p. 230). He then proceeded to develop a concept of dignity as being the capacity to create meaningful lives. On this conception, 'human dignity … is identified first of all with being a member of a kind possessing the capacities to seek and create meaning (basic dignity), and secondly with the development and exercise [of] those meaning-making capacities (refined dignity)' (p. 233). In connection with dementia, Woodruff (p. 236) pointed out that dignity, which involves creating meaning, can be preserved even whilst helping with basic functions; one simply needs – quoting Lustbader (1999: 22) – 'a conversation, rather than a feeding'.

Sulmasy (2013) pointed to three ways in which the word 'dignity' tends to be used. First, there is *intrinsic* dignity; that is, the worthiness and significance which attach to us simply because we are human beings and not because of any other attributes we might have. Secondly, there is *attributed* dignity, where individuals or communities choose to attribute some value or worth to someone. Thirdly, there is *inflorescent* dignity. He explains:

> 'Inflorescent' is not a commonly used word, but it is the adjectival form of the noun 'inflorescence', which means the process of flowering or blossoming. … That is to say, 'dignity' is used in an inflorescent way to refer to individuals who are flourishing as human beings …
>
> (p. 938).

These three ways in which 'dignity' tends to be used are not mutually exclusive. Inflorescent dignity, however, can be regarded as a virtue. It refers to the person whose disposition is to do well humanly (that is, to flourish as a human being) in a manner that is dignified. Despite their detractors, people like Mother Teresa of Calcutta (1910–1997) or Nelson Mandela (1918–2013) are likely candidates for this sort of description. They were also both attributed dignity by being given the Nobel Peace Prize; and, in any case, *qua* human beings, they had intrinsic dignity.

This sort of conceptual analysis is all very well. It is important, because it helps to ward off the rather simplistic tendency to equate dementia ('brain failure') with a loss of dignity (Robertson 1983). Murphy (1984) responded to that particular suggestion by saying that 'Loss of dignity derives from the way we care' (p. 61) and that more than ever in old age people needed their personal identities to be preserved. The suggestion is that we can ignore or undermine a person's dignity, but we can also preserve it in complete accordance with the approach of Woodruff (2016), where meaningfulness is created, and in accordance with the demands of intrinsic dignity as set out by Sulmasy (2013). Nevertheless, it would be good to have some practical direction.

Fortunately, Chochinov (2007) provides some clinical guidance. He first recognized that the more healthcare professionals affirm the value of those they look after, the more the person's sense of dignity is maintained. He then set out the A, B, C and D of dignity-conserving care, as summarized in Box 10.1.

Box 10.1 Summary of Chochinov's (2007) A, B, C and D of dignity-conserving care

Attitude – this is the background predisposition, which we learn, to react in certain ways.
Behaviour – the suggestion is that for healthcare workers this must always be based on 'kindness and respect'.
Compassion – this is based on a profound feeling for the suffering of the person, with the wish that we might be able to relieve it.
Dialogue – allows the professional to recognize the non-physical repercussions of physical illness and the individual's personhood.

Chochinov's article also gives questions, actions, dispositions and tactics to help implement dignity-conserving care. Having the correct attitude might include checking that one's assumptions are correct. Right behaviour would be always to explain any actions to be taken and to facilitate communication in ways that are acceptable to the person. Compassion can be shown by listening to the person's story and by small acts of kindness. Dialogue encourages partnership and allows meaningful relationships to be established through approaches that acknowledge and show an interest in the person.

Attention to the person is the crucial aspect of this sort of care. Maintaining dignity in such ways reflects the ethical approaches described in

Chapter 4. Good care and relationships are central to feminist ethics. Communication is at the heart of discourse ethics. Meaning-making is part and parcel of hermeneutic ethics and narrative ethics involves understanding the person's story. Dignity is, therefore, a core aspect of moral acts towards people living with dementia. As Downs and Bowers (2008) wrote, 'In planning care and support, doctors need to pay as much attention to the essential human worth of a person with dementia and their retained capacity for relationships, pleasure, communication, and coping as they do to deficits and dysfunction' (p. 225).

Quality of life

Whilst discussing dignity, Koppelman (2002) suggested that we need a view of the person's 'whole self'. The same can be said of quality of life. Largely, however, this is not recognized in the research industry that has grown up around the notion of quality of life. It is true there has been some sophisticated thinking about quality-of-life research. But the reality is that the need for whole sight (see Chapter 1 in Hughes et al. 2006) in thinking about people who live with a diagnosis of dementia has not percolated through. Black and Rabins (2017) provided a very useful overview of the conceptual and practical issues around quality of life in dementia. I shall not repeat here the details they set out about the many different quality of life measures. I do not doubt that these measures are useful for particular purposes. The ethical issue I shall pursue is the thought that these measures never capture – and never can capture – exactly what a person's quality of life might be.

For a start, quality of life can be thought of as a political matter. Phillips (2018) has suggested that we should focus more on the meaning of 'life' when we talk of quality of life. This shifts 'the conversation of [quality of life] from one of measurement and administration to one of political order' (Phillips 2018: 9). Later she commends thinking about, not just the facts of our lives, but about the texture. She is suggesting, conceptually, that 'the idea of life as biopolitical is useful to help us explore health care as a series of political and cultural practices' (p. 14). Hence, we may wish to stand back and ask why we are measuring quality of life in the first place: it was never going to be straightforward (Bond 1999). It may be to demonstrate that a particular drug or psychosocial intervention works. But then, exactly what we measure becomes crucial, depending on the intervention; and we should always wish to ask whom it benefits if particular scores improve.

This broader view of quality of life is also visible in the discussion – albeit of older people in general, not older people specifically living with dementia – by Kruse (2016) of the (physical and mental) strengths which older people can bring to the table, which can become 'a social and cultural gain when older people's need or motivation to shape the public space, to worry about and care for other … people is respected …' (Kruse 2016: 402). He continued: 'It is the exchange of received and given care which is so important for the preservation of the quality of life and well-being ...' (p. 402). Again, this stresses that the environment contributes to quality of life.

It also raises the issue of well-being. Briefly, although the two concepts are very similar, I would suggest that well-being contributes to quality of life, rather than the other way round. Kitwood's Dementia Care Mapping was a way to measure well-being and ill-being and, generally, the quality of care, especially in care homes. These ideas are clearly set out and discussed in Baldwin and Capstick (2007: 89–107). Well-being can be understood in three ways: *hedonism* is the pursuit of pleasure and avoidance of pain (as in Utilitarianism, see Chapter 3 above); *desire theories* suggest that the satisfaction of desires or preferences is key to well-being; and *objective list theories* point to the idea that a list can be constructed of items that would bring about well-being. Of course, there is much more to be said about well-being. Griffin (1986) gave it exhaustive philosophical treatment; and Hughes (2014a) discussed maintaining well-being near to the end of life.

I have identified three problems with measuring quality of life (Hughes 2003). First, there is the problem of domains. Do we confine ourselves to questions about health and psychological well-being? Or should we use one of the other instruments with multiple domains and numerous items within each domain? Which domains should we leave out? Secondly, there is the subjective-objective problem. Do we consider the person's subjective account or an objective account of someone's quality of life from an informant? The answer is we need both, but how much of one and how much of the other? Finally, there is the problem of then and now. Should we try to judge quality of life by how things are now, or do we look back at what the person might have said and wanted in the past? The point is that quality of life, as a concept, can never be pinned down.

My intention in this part of the chapter was to pursue the thought that measurement of quality of life never quite captures exactly what a person's quality of life is. Whitehouse (2000) put it perfectly when he suggested that although the notion can be studied scientifically, it goes beyond science. For it brings us back to the initial thought that what is required is whole sight. And it is whole sight of the person living with dementia with all that this entails. We need to see the person in as full a view as possible. We need (potentially) to understand biology, psychology, social and spiritual situations, as well as family, cultural and political backgrounds, which bring in geography, language, aesthetic sense and narrative, amongst other things. The need for whole sight is a guard against glib assertions about someone's quality of life, which may undermine both the person's dignity and human rights.

Conclusion

So, what do these ruminations mean? Policymakers should recognize that quality-of-life studies tell us about statistical realities, but not about individuals and they do not capture everything that might be of value to the person. Professionals, despite any pressures to the contrary, must always see the individual – a person of inherent worth whose individual values and preferences should be of paramount concern. Moreover, there is guidance that could be used to train people to recognize dignity-enhancing care (Chochinov 2007). Family carers must be supported in their efforts to maintain the person's quality of life and to preserve the person's dignity. People who live with dementia should assert wherever and whenever they can – through advance care planning, for instance (see Chapter 12, Figure 12.1) – their own views and values. What is important to them? For what gives them quality of life will also connect to what provides the dignity which is theirs just because they are human beings.

To sum up, it is possible to think of two polarities captured by two German words. In connection with the idea of a metaphysical understanding of dignity we came across the word *Menschenwürde*, signifying human worth and suggesting inherent dignity. Quality of life measurements are conceptually problematic, although for specific purposes they can be used unproblematically. 'Quality of life' can also be used in everyday language, but judgements that a person lacks quality of life should always be made hesitantly for fear that the Nazi idea of *Lebensunwertes Leben*, 'life unworthy of life', might insinuate itself into our thinking. For someone else's poor quality of life may not be poor from their point of view and, in any case, is in some sense my responsibility.

11 Consent and capacity

Introduction

It could be said, on good grounds, that capacity is the main issue to mark out the unique character of ethical difficulties in the care of people living with dementia. Unless people already have mental incapacity from some other cause, with dementia they move, more or less gradually, from a position of full capacity to one of loss of mental capacities, albeit the extent of such losses will be different for different people and will often be debatable at particular times (hence there are plenty of court cases to determine a person's capacity). All of this is important because capacity affects our ability to consent, which affects our ability to make decisions for ourselves. It is important to note in this discussion that decision-making capacity is an issue for everyone. It often crops up with respect to treatment decisions. In addition, however, it is relevant to decisions about where people live, what they eat, what they wear, whether they shower or go out to watch a show. People living with dementia may be aware and understandably nervous that decision-making is becoming difficult and/or that others are trying to take decisions away from them.

This chapter deals with consent and capacity. It is perhaps useful to deal with terminology here. In the USA, 'competence' is a legal term and 'capacity' is 'a more pragmatic concept, referring broadly to the ability to consent' (Fellows 1998). In the UK, capacity is the legal term. I shall have more to say about this later. Capacity is sometimes referred to as 'mental' capacity, as in the *Mental Capacity Act 2005* (MCA) which applies only to England and Wales, but it would be better if it were referred to as 'decision-making' capacity, for that is what it is; and this would also avoid confusion between it and (again in England and Wales) the *Mental Health Act 1983* (MHA) and subsequent mental health acts.

At the end of the chapter, I turn my attention to the notion of 'legal capacity' which is something else again. Legal capacity appears in the CRPD. It reminds us that decision-making is a matter of human rights and takes us back to the importance of dignity and quality of life broadly conceived.

Consent

A useful definition of consent to treatment was set out in the UK by the Department of Health and Welsh Office (1999):

... the voluntary and continuing permission of the patient to receive a particular treatment, based on an adequate knowledge of the purpose, nature, likely

effects and risks ... including the likelihood of its success and any alternatives to it. Permission given under any unfair or undue pressure is not 'consent'
(§15.13).

This helps to emphasize the main components of valid consent: it should be informed; the person should have the capacity to make the particular decision; it should be uncoerced; and it should be continuing throughout the procedure or treatment. However, as with capacity, it is important to see that consent is relevant to almost everything that can be done to or for us. If I do not consent to someone placing a hand on my arm, I can claim that they have assaulted me. Each of the terms involved in the definition of consent can then be interrogated to investigate what they mean and where ambiguities lie (Hughes 2000). We can also form an algorithm, as in Figure 11.1 (adapted from Hughes 2000), to ensure that we follow all the steps to gain valid consent. To simplify matters, Figure 11.1 focuses on consent to treatment, but the same algorithm would apply to decisions about whether I wished to wear my anorak or my overcoat when I go out for a walk.

Figure 11.1 also shows the things to consider if it were felt the person did not have the requisite capacity to make the particular decision. We shall return to these in Chapter 12 when we consider best interests. But let us consider consent in more detail.

First, there is the idea of being informed. An immediate question is the extent to which a person needs to be informed in order to give valid consent. In the UK we have a series of legal cases which show a broadening of the accepted criteria for what does or does not amount to full disclosure of information by a doctor (see Box 11.1).

Box 11.1 Legal standards for adequate information for valid consent for medical treatment

Sidaway v. Board of Governors of the Bethlem Royal Hospital and the Maudsley Hospital [1985] UKHL 1
This ruling established that the legal standard for adequate information is the same as for negligence (referring back to the famous case of *Bolam v. Friern Hospital Management Committee* [1957] 1 WLR 582) where what counted was a practice accepted as proper by a 'responsible body of medical opinion'.

Pearce v. United Bristol Healthcare NHS Trust [1999] 48 BMLR 118
The ruling here was that doctors should disclose, prior to treatment, 'a significant risk which would affect the judgement of a reasonable patient'.

Chester v. Afshar [2004] 4 All ER 587
This case established that a doctor has a legal duty to warn someone, in general terms, of any serious risks that might be involved in a procedure, even if relatively rare.

Montgomery v. Lanarkshire Health Authority [2015] UKSC 11
This case further defined what would amount to a 'material' risk concerning which a doctor ought to inform someone before a procedure. At paragraph 87 the judgment reads:

The test of materiality is whether, in the circumstances of the particular case, a reasonable person in the patient's position would be likely to attach significance to the risk, or the doctor is or should reasonably be aware that the particular patient would be likely to attach significance to it.

Figure 11.1 A simple consent to treatment algorithm

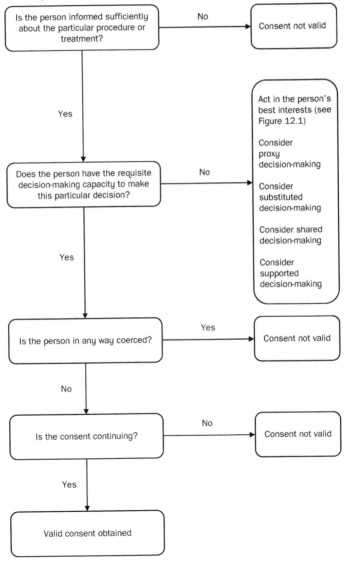

What we see in Box 11.1 is in keeping with Lord Tennyson's poetic idea of a land,

Where Freedom slowly broadens down

From precedent to precedent
[From: *You Ask Me, Why, Tho' Ill at Ease* by Alfred, Lord Tennyson].

Sidaway definitely suggests a profession-based standard: doctors know what patients need to know! *Pearce* and *Chester* change the emphasis to the standards of the reasonable patient, who will wish to know of significant and serious risks. *Montgomery*, which it should be noted is a decision that has been heavily criticized from within the legal profession (Montgomery and Montgomery 2016), reasserts that information should be disclosed if it would be significant to a particular person's decision about treatment. But it goes even further. Four elements can be picked out as encapsulating its model of consent: first, there is the ruling about what counts as a material risk (see Box 11.1); secondly, *Montgomery* advocates that benefits as well as risks should be disclosed; thirdly, the risks and benefits of alternative treatments should also be considered; and, finally, disclosure of information should specifically involve dialogue. We have argued elsewhere that this whole process is in keeping with the principles of values-based practice, as described in Chapter 5 (Hughes et al. 2018).

Montgomery has been hailed as the final nail in the coffin of paternalism in favour of autonomy (notions discussed in Chapters 8 and 9 above). Not everyone agrees with this simple analysis. Dunn et al. (2019) have argued that the ruling suggests doctors must consider a number of factors, including the value of autonomy, but also broader 'subjective, experiential dimensions of well-being' (p. 122). In other words, the process has to be one of real dialogue, not a simple tick box exercise to meet the criteria for autonomy.

I shall come back to capacity shortly, but need briefly to consider the other elements of valid consent. Non-coercion may seem simple enough, but it can be overt or covert and a decision might sometimes be required about where the line is to be drawn between inappropriate coercion and legitimate cajoling. Finally, consent must be continuing. It is relevant to note here the evidence that people living with mild to moderate cognitive impairment 'are able to respond consistently [albeit the study only looked at this over the course of one week] to questions about preferences, choices, and their own involvement in decisions about daily living, and to provide accurate and reliable responses to questions about demographics' (Feinberg and Whitlatch 2001). As we shall see in Chapter 12, people's preferences for life-sustaining treatments tend to remain the same over longer periods too (for example, see Carmel and Mutran 1999).

We certainly should not presume that people living with dementia cannot themselves give informed consent. There is a bigger issue to be tackled from an ethical perspective. Is informed consent the best option for people living with dementia? Some years ago, Whitehouse (1996) wrote hopefully about the importance of more intimate communication in order to get away from the formality of informed consent, instead laying emphasis on assent and trust.

It turns out the notion of consent is by no means straightforward. Alderson and Goodey (1998) provided a very thoughtful account of theories of consent. So, for instance, on the one hand, there is a rather legalistic and positivistic model whereby doctors provide patients with the information (as it were, a thing) and then ensure they have got it, in other words remembered it. If so, they can give valid consent. Or, on the other hand, a social constructionist view of consent suggests 'a process – perceived, experienced, and shaped through interactions between individuals and their social contexts' (Alderson and Goodey 1998: 1315).

Others have also identified the need for a less legalistic formulation of consent. This would be in keeping with Dunn et al.'s (2019) aspirations: to find a way to encourage clinicians to engage at the most human level with the people they care for through sensitive and meaningful dialogue. *Montgomery*, of course, concerned the giving of information to someone with full capacity. But the lessons of the case can be applied to people who lack capacity. There is still the need for careful dialogue. If the person concerned really cannot make the decision, then the dialogue must be with others with significant knowledge of the person, who will usually, but not always, be family members. Issues around giving information, non-coercion and continuing consent remain. But, as so often, it is *how* the task is done that is crucial. Murphy (1988) suggested there was a missing dimension to a legalistic understanding of consent: '… we must make explicit the importance of the style of behaviour and emotional tone in our dealings with patients' (pp. 66–67).

Polden (1989) wrote of 'constructive consent' for people who lacked capacity, by which she implied a thorough and careful form of substituted judgement (see Figure 11.1), which we shall come to in the next chapter. Pursuing the same theme (rather beautifully), Gedge (2004) appealed to the notion of 'collective moral imagination'. She wrote:

> Through imaginative constructions of dialogues, sometimes embedded in plausible narratives, the preferences of intimate others may be 'updated', rendered responsive to current circumstances and wishes of family members, and criticized by relevant ethical norms
>
> (p. 448).

She recognized the obvious worries about proxy decision-makers sometimes being less than trustworthy or heavily burdened by emotional baggage. But she felt that these worries could be ameliorated by hearing a number of intimate voices perhaps conveying contrasting narratives, including the narrative of the person who lacks the particular capacity. She emphasized that in all such discussions, 'Autonomy is only one morally relevant feature' (p. 449). Once again, one sees here the relevance and importance of discourse, narrative, feminist and hermeneutic ethics, as discussed in Chapter 4.

Coverdale et al. (2006), whilst not ignoring autonomy, also brought into the mix the importance of the correct virtues (of which Gedge (2004) was obviously aware too). They pushed the idea of 'geriatric assent' which entailed a four-step process:

i   identifying the person's 'long-standing values and preferences';

ii   with these in mind, considering the person's 'biopsychosocial safety and independence';

iii 'protecting remaining autonomy'; and

iv   'cultivating the professional virtues of steadiness, self-effacement, and self-sacrifice' (Coverdale et al. 2006: 151).

Steadiness is a matter of self-control. It involves, not 'detached concern', but 'stoic self-mastery in the face of the patient's experience of illness, disability and possible death' (p. 155). Self-effacement 'means supporting a patient's personal values' (p. 155). Self-sacrifice is the opposite of self-interest and may often involve tolerating physical risks to people rather than restrictive practices to keep them safe.

In these approaches to decision-making, much effort is put into seeking to understand the person's previous wishes, feelings, beliefs, values and preferences. This will all be relevant to the discussion of best interests in Chapter 12. But for now, there is one further thing to point out about decision-making, which is its distributed nature. Consent is thought of as a means to respect and support autonomy. But as we have already discussed in Chapter 8, we are rarely autonomous in our actions. I suggested it was better to think in terms of relational autonomy. Well, this is relevant to consent as well. In keeping with some of the approaches mentioned above, people living with dementia may need help to consent. This is not to undermine their autonomy, rather it supports it. We shall later discuss supported decision-making. A person's ability to consent may itself need to be supported and may well be distributed over time and between different actors. In an important paper, Rapley (2007) put it this way:

> Knowledge is distributed over encounters with patients and can be distributed over encounters with a patient's significant others. ... decision-making practices are simultaneously retrospective, current and prospective in orientation. ... decision making emerges in and through a web of interdependency in encounters with people

(pp. 437–438).

Capacity

A good place to start in thinking about capacity is Fellows (1998), who made a number of important and useful points. She pointed to the danger of setting the standard for someone to have capacity too high (in order to show beneficence and protect them) and to the alternative danger of allowing almost anything to indicate the person has capacity (to support their autonomous wishes as much as possible). The physician must guard against two errors: we neither wish to allow incompetent people to make harmful decisions, nor to prevent competent people from saying what they want. Here is a very humane sentiment:

> One should err on the side of autonomy when the judgment of capacity is equivocal, respecting the possibility that values and decision-making skills that served these patients for their entire adult lives may persist at some level, even if no longer expressed coherently
>
> (p. 923).

She also commended the idea of a sliding scale, where greater capacity is required for riskier decisions and less for more mundane (less risky) investigations or treatments (a view endorsed by the courts, at least in the UK). She recognized both the importance of families in decision-making, as well as the possibility that there will be areas of concern which have never been discussed within families, such as a person's end-of-life wishes. She stressed the importance of the values a person had previously held when competent, but also the importance of trying to understand the person's current subjective experience. Once again, key to all of this is good communication. If properly undertaken, '… making treatment decisions could become … therapeutic …' (p. 926).

In their discussion of residence capacity (the capacity to decide where to live), Strang et al. (1998) also emphasized how the physician must navigate between Scylla and Charybdis: too concerned to protect, or too concerned to allow the person liberty. In these difficult situations, the multidisciplinary team, with its different viewpoints, can be very useful (Brindle and Holmes 2005). In connection with these two papers, it is worth emphasizing how important judgements about residence capacity can be. The capacity to choose where to live and what care to receive are two capacities that frequently come before the Courts. We shall come back to this in Chapter 20. It should be obvious, however, that decisions about care and place of residence are critically important to people living with dementia and to their families. There are often very real concerns about people and yet, if capable, they should be free to choose for themselves.

I have not yet set out criteria for capacity partly because it seems important to note that 'no concrete formulaic equation can be employed to reliably determine the existence or nonexistence of decision-making capacity' (Zuckerman 1987: 68). The complexity of capacity assessment is shown by a study of capacity to consent to a clinical trial for Alzheimer's disease in which 70 per cent of the caregivers (who were considered to be 'normal') were shown not to have full capacity (Pucci et al. 2001). Decision-making capacity turns out to be a normative affair: there are values at stake in its assessment (Charland 2001). It also involves emotions, because emotions are not irrelevant to the reasons we give for doing things and because consenting to something is a matter of practicality and not solely rationality (Charland 1998).

There is still the difference between 'competence' and 'capacity' to be sorted out. Elsewhere, in discussing the etymology of these words, we concluded that:

> … capacity is the ability to take in or hold information and competence is the ability to use the information to enable the person to have sufficient abilities in the rivalries and demands of life. The etymology also suggests that having a capacity relates to the individual, whereas to be competent is to be able to

do things with others. Competence requires capacity; but capacity without competence is otiose

(Hughes and Heginbotham 2013: 754).

We went on to say that it was possible to think in terms of cognitive, evaluative and volitional aspects of capacity, where the latter two reflect the broader notion of competence. In a more legalistic manner, however, at least in England and Wales, capacity is defined as shown in Box 11.2.

Box 11.2 Definition of capacity in the *Mental Capacity Act 2005* (MCA), for which see HMSO (2005)

'... a person lacks capacity in relation to a matter if at the material time he is unable to make a decision for himself in relation to the matter because of an impairment of, or a disturbance in the functioning of, the mind or brain' (MCA Section 2(1)).

And a person is 'unable to make a decision' if he is unable:

'(a) to understand the information relevant to the decision,
(b) to retain that information,
(c) to use or weigh that information as part of the process of making the decision, or
(d) to communicate his decision (whether by talking, using sign language or any other means)' (MCA Section 3(1)).

It should be added that capacity is always case- and time-specific. We must assess this particular person's capacity with respect to this particular decision (for example a financial one rather than one about treatment) at this particular time, conscious too that capacity can fluctuate and should be tested when the person is in an optimal state.

It is worth pointing out that, in the USA, the criteria are slightly different, there being no specific requirement that the person must retain the information although, in order to understand information, facts would have to be remembered; and, instead of 'use or weigh' the USA criteria talk of 'appreciate and reason', where 'appreciate' means that people must be able to put the information into their own contexts (Grisso and Appelbaum 1998).

The breadth of the interpretation of the words used in these criteria is not without significance. Thus, Kim et al. (2021b) were able to develop from real legal cases a typology of the rationales used in connection with the MCA, which led them to suggest that 'understanding' might usefully be defined narrowly, whereas 'use or weigh' allows room for greater interpretation. There is room, perhaps, for dysfunctions in emotions (Welie 2001) and values (Greener et al. 2012) that also cause a lack of capacity. Greener et al. (2012) suggested we might need to define capacity more tightly, but then allow much broader interpretations of what might be in the person's best interests. (Much more is said about capacity and its assessment in King and Series (2014); in Spencer and Hotopf (2019); and in Emmett and Hughes (2021).) We know that knowledge of the MCA in England and Wales and its legal framework is poor (Shepherd et al. 2018). We also know that the implementation of the MCA has been poor, despite the good intentions embedded in the Act (Emmett et al. 2013; House of Lords 2014; Poole et al. 2014; Penn et al. 2021).

The reasons for the poor implementation were probably many. A good deal of training went on when the Act came into force, but this seemed to lead to people regarding the Act as a tick box exercise. In addition, to implement the Act in the manner that was hoped for would have entailed more resources. In stretched services it is easier to tick some boxes than spend time really engaging with people. However, this is not an acceptable excuse if you are trying to maintain the person's standing as someone of dignity and to honour their real wishes whenever possible.

In a sense, the Act's good intentions were summarized in section 1 of the MCA, where the principles underlying the whole of the Act were set out:

- The assumption should be that the person has capacity.
- All practicable steps should be taken to enable the person to have capacity to make the required decision.
- Anyone can make an unwise decision – this does not mean the person lacks capacity.
- Where there is a lack of capacity, the person's best interests must be pursued.
- Whatever is done, it should be with as little restriction as possible to the person's rights and freedom.

What we see here is an attempt by the lawmakers to respect the person's autonomy and to encourage person-centred care. Those from other jurisdictions (remember the MCA only covers England and Wales) can be forgiven for doubting that this is relevant to them. However, the point is that capacity or competence legislation anywhere, because of the complexity of the notions involved, because it is inevitably much more evaluative than might at first be thought, and because of the intricacies of real-life decision-making, requires to be put into effect with a good deal of rectitude.

Legal capacity

Before concluding, it seems necessary to say something about legal capacity, which is different from mental (decision-making) capacity. Article 12.2 of the CRPD (see Box 9.2) refers to legal capacity: 'States Parties shall recognize that persons with disabilities enjoy legal capacity on an equal basis with others in all aspects of life' (United Nations General Assembly 2006). This is further discussed in General Comment No. 1 on the CRPD (United Nations General Assembly 2014).

Having reiterated the basic general principle of equality before the law, in paragraph 12 the General Comment states that 'Legal capacity includes the capacity to be both a holder of rights and an actor under the law'. Being a holder of rights means that a person has the full protection of those rights by the legal system. Being an actor under the law means that the person is recognized as an agent 'with the power to engage in transactions and create, modify or end legal relationships' (General Comment §12).

It is this second idea, concerning being an actor or agent, that starts to look problematic when we consider people living with the most advanced stages of dementia. In what sense does such a person have 'the power to engage in transactions and create, modify or end legal relationships'? How this power will be effected in severe dementia needs to be determined. Perhaps by some form of advance care planning, but would this be specific enough and clearly applicable? This takes us into the discussion which will follow in the next chapter on best interests.

Moving on, paragraph 13 of the General Comment establishes that 'Legal capacity and mental capacity are distinct concepts'. It repeats that legal capacity involves a person's legal standing (having certain rights and duties) and legal agency (being able to exercise those rights and duties). 'It is', it says, 'the key to accessing meaningful participation in society' (General Comment §13); whereas, mental capacity refers simply to decision-making skills.

Again, 'legal standing' is not problematic. But is it true to say that people with severe dementia have agency to act on their rights and to have those actions recognized by the law? It would seem easier to accept if it stated that all people *potentially* have agency or to say they have situated agency or some such. At least, it would seem sensible to acknowledge that the agency of a person living with severe dementia is circumscribed in a number of ways.

Paragraph 14 of the General Comment asserts that 'Legal capacity is an inherent right accorded to all people, including persons with disabilities'; people have legal capacity '... simply by virtue of being human'. Is this slightly sloppy thinking? As we saw (in Chapter 10), it makes sense to say that dignity issues 'simply by virtue of being human'. This is true even of a very young child. But would it be true to say of a very young child that it had legal agency (it certainly has legal standing – perhaps because it has inherent dignity)? It would be a very precocious toddler who was able to negotiate a mortgage!

In paragraph 14 of the General Comment, we clearly see the philosophical position that underpinned the thinking in this part of the CRPD. Decision-making capacity is firmly portrayed as socially and politically constructed. Be that as it may, the real problem, according to the General Comment, is that 'mental and legal capacity have been conflated' (General Comment §15) and this has been used as a means to deny persons certain rights.

One of the good things about the MCA is that it uses a functional approach to assess decision-making or mental capacity. In other words, it neither simply bases the decision about capacity on something like age (a status approach), nor on whether the decision seems like a good one (an outcomes approach), but rather on evidence of appropriate mental functioning (being able to retain, weigh up and so on; see Box 11.2), which is known as a functional approach. But this approach is condemned,

> ... for two key reasons: (a) it is discriminatorily applied to people with disabilities; and (b) it presumes to be able to accurately assess the inner-workings of the human mind and, when the person does not pass the assessment, it then denies him or her a core human right ...
>
> (General Comment §15).

As far as the second point goes, is it not possible, after all, to say accurate things about the inner workings of the human mind? You could test me to see how many numbers I can hold in my mind (this is the digit span test). Not many is the answer; and you could probably be quite accurate about this, even if I am better at it in the morning than the afternoon. My wife, a physicist, would certainly be much better at it than me. This is to say something about the inner workings of our minds (or is it our brains?). Certainly, my mental mathematics is not as good as my wife's. This is one of the reasons that my wife is better at financial decision-making than I am. I do not feel that my legal standing is thereby undermined, nor my inherent dignity. And as far as my legal agency is concerned, it simply means I need more support when making financial decisions.

Indeed, the CRPD recommends a model of supported decision-making. This is its direction of travel, which I shall pursue further in the next chapter. The point about the functional approach being 'discriminatorily applied to people with disabilities' does carry some weight. Despite the deficits in my understanding of financial matters, if today I went to arrange a new mortgage, no one (I presume) would test my mental capacity to do so. But if I had a diagnosis of dementia, then it is highly likely they would. It could be argued that they would need to test me in order to save me making a terrible mistake. Alternatively, they could simply support me (and my legal agency) in the most appropriate ways possible. Although I might be affronted, should I be allowed to go ahead with a plan that would devastate our finances? My answer is: this depends on whether I have the requisite mental (decision-making) capacity, which requires that I be tested. Testing, of course, should not be carried out in a cavalier fashion. It requires situational support (Welie 2001). The CRPD would not like my answer, but its own answer to such dilemmas seems hopelessly unclear.

Conclusion

Consent procedures and assessments of capacity can be very straightforward. They are carried out every day, thousands of times. Every bit of social support to the person living with dementia potentially involves consideration of capacity and consent. So, too, do medical interventions. The point I have been pushing in this chapter is that the quotidian nature of these assessments should not make us blind to their complexity and importance. This mostly stems from their evaluative and emotional components. These, in turn, reflect the profound connection between consent and capacity and the nature of our standing as human beings. Sabat (2005) nicely illustrated how a person's meaning-making abilities and self-hood, both relevant to capacity and consent, cannot be assessed by standard tests, but require dialogue and real engagement. This is important because it turns out that lay judgements about a person's competence influence their reactions to the person's behaviour, with discrimination (and thereby stigmatization) in cases where competence is doubted (Werner 2006).

Much of the discussion in this chapter has been legal in nature. However, it is what underlies the relevant decisions that is of ethical interest. The law directs us but does not ensure that decisions are right. To go back to residence capacity, it may well be that the professionals involved – the doctor, nurse, social worker, occupational therapist and so on – are very worried about safety if the person were to return home. The family may be split in their feelings, with some worried about safety, but others feeling that the person's independence should not be taken away. At the centre of this dilemma, however, is the person with dementia. The crucial question is whether the person is able to make the decision. This is why the assessment of the person's capacity is vital. It determines whether or not the person can consent to the arrangements that are being proposed. But the assessment can be undertaken either rightly or wrongly. People with dementia and their advocates (whether professional or family) need to ensure that assessments are undertaken in the right way and with the right approach. The MCA, or the equivalent legislation in other jurisdictions, provides a template for decision-making. The CRPD reminds us that the decisions we make and the way we make those decisions must reflect the need to respect the person's dignity.

Gaining consent and the assessment of capacity impinge in important ways on human rights. To be done well (especially in dementia) the assessor requires not only technical clinical skills but also nuanced communication skills that allow genuine dialogue and a variety of virtues to ensure that the person or self is not undermined. Sabat put it perfectly: 'The means by which we evaluate, and arrive at our conclusions about, the afflicted person's competency may well ultimately be a test of our own competency as thoughtful, judicious, humane human beings' (Sabat 2001: 334).

12 Best interests

Introduction

In Figure 11.1 we saw that, if someone lacks capacity to make a particular decision, we should act in that person's best interests. There were then several types of decision-making to consider. In this chapter I shall expand on these considerations.

Definitions turn out, as so often, to be important. Best interests can be spoken of in a variety of ways. It usually indicates that a surrogate decision-maker should be found. At its simplest, this means a proxy, who will often be a family member. But the question is, should proxies say what *they* think? Or should they be making a substituted judgement? That is, should they be putting themselves in the shoes of the person who lacks capacity in order to decide what *that person* would have wanted under these particular circumstances?

My view is that an amalgam of the above options is required. I am taking it for granted that it is right to act in the person's best interests if there is a lack of capacity. My understanding of best interests is summarized by the checklist in the MCA, which I shall come to having considered the issues around surrogate decision-making, which also takes us a little way into the Dworkin–Dresser debate. I shall then discuss shared decision-making, before returning to the CRPD in order to consider supported decision-making. I am commending the MCA best interests checklist beyond its jurisdiction of England and Wales because I think its characterization of best interests makes philosophical sense, albeit with some tiny tweaks.

Surrogate decisions: proxy or substituted?

It is natural enough, when a decision is required and the person is not there to make it, to turn to someone who knows the person to seek their advice ('Will Julian want milk with his Americano?'). Surrogate decision-making is natural and essential. But what role should it play, how far should it extend and how should it be done? The literature contains a number of suggestions.

Famously, Brock (2009) suggested an ethical framework with the intention of promoting well-being and self-determination. The first step is to respect a person's autonomy and see what they would choose. This remains relevant where people have a diagnosis of dementia, because most will still be able to express or indicate their views or inclinations. Where the person lacks the particular decision-making capacity, Brock suggested three principles should be put into effect, although he allowed that more than one principle might be relevant at one time (Brock 2009: 265). The first is the advance directives principle. Any relevant advance directives by the person should be abided by. The second is the substitute judgement principle. So, in the absence of self-determination and of a relevant advance directive, surrogates should use what they know of the person to decide what this individual would have wanted in this particular situation. The third is the best interests principle, 'which looks to what most reasonable persons would want in the circumstances' (p. 265). Elsewhere, Buchanan and Brock (1989) stated the best interests principle in terms of looking at the net benefit of every option facing the person, which should be weighted in line with the various interests that the option would encourage or block, and from which any disbenefits, similarly weighted, should be subtracted.

The whole framework sounds intuitively appealing, even if the best interests principle according to Buchanan and Brock's (1989) formulation seems somewhat limited. Fullbrook (2007) stated: 'those who act on behalf of another must do so from a logical objective attitude, examining all the aspects of the person and establishing the one logical course of action that is best for that person' (p. 683). The focus on the individual is commendable, but seeking the single authentic answer to questions about someone's best interests is problematic (Holm 2001), both conceptually and practically.

Inevitably, discussion of advance care plans, where the person now lacks capacity to make a particular decision, goes back to the Dworkin–Dresser debate. Dworkin (1993) placed great emphasis on precedent autonomy. This followed a distinction he made between experiential and critical interests. Experiential interests are those which depend on us finding some experiences pleasurable or exciting, like listening to music or playing football. It does not matter – as far as my whole life is concerned – if I prefer rugby to football. One is simply an experience I prefer. But people also have critical interests: 'interests that it does make their life genuinely better to satisfy, interests they would be mistaken, and genuinely worse off, if they did not recognize' (Dworkin 1993: 201). Relationships would be an example of critical interests. If I get these wrong – if my marriage breaks up and my children no longer talk to me – my whole life is poorer. The person living with advanced dementia, says Dworkin, even if unaware of them, still has critical interests and we should honour them if they are known, because they shape the person's life as a whole. This is to respect someone's precedent autonomy. Thus, for instance, precedent autonomy could be used to underpin the authority and force of an advance statement to the effect that someone would be willing to participate in research (Buller 2015a – this is further discussed in Chapter 14).

Dresser (1995) took an alternative line, arguing both that (a) it may be critical interests are not as important as Dworkin makes out and (b) more weight needs to be given to the person's experiential interests here and now. If someone living with dementia currently enjoys playing with toys, then so be it. The person's experiences are happy. Why should a worry about previously expressed critical interests usurp or upset the person's happiness here and now?

In a stunning paper, Jaworska (1999) waded into the dispute – sometimes couched in terms of whether we should respect the person's *then*-self or *now*-self – largely on the side of Dresser, but with a new spin, namely that we should respect the person living with dementia as a person who can still value things. In the context of dementia, she suggested that we focus on the person as a valuer. She continued: 'An Alzheimer's patient may be too disoriented to form a life plan or to choose specific treatment preferences, but so long as he still holds values, he is, in the most basic sense, capable of self-governance, and this fact about him commands utmost respect' (Jaworska 1999: 134).

I am going to say little more about the Dworkin–Dresser debate, which is based on the premise that there is a discontinuity of the self, i.e. that the *now*-self is so radically different from the pre-dementia *then*-self that we can say they are different selves and, therefore, that the advance statements of the previous self do not apply to the current self (Buchanan 1988; Hope 1995). Dworkin says that they do, because of precedent autonomy. Dresser says, ignore precedent autonomy, look at the person now. Jaworska asks: what does the person value? Much ink has been spilt over this debate. For instance, Gillett (2019) argued, *inter alia*, that Dworkin's concept of respect for autonomy is limited and that we should consider the person's 'sense of liberty' as important to current decisions.

My reason for not pursuing this debate further now is because in Chapter 13 I shall argue that the presumption of discontinuity can be discredited. Persad (2019), for example, suggested that 'historical embodiment' will sometimes have sufficient force to override concerns about the person's inability to consent now. Roughly, the fact of my body is enough to establish that I am the same self that wrote the advance statement. Further, in a very thoughtful paper, whilst discussing the Dworkin–Dresser debate, Nelson (1995) suggested:

> A conception of the self which takes seriously not only its extension through time but also its relationships to others will entail that at least some proxies – for instance, those intimately related to the patient – may have a *constructive* as well as a hermeneutic task.
>
> (p. 145)

His point is that critical interests might evolve and that a proxy might properly induce in the person 'some form of moral redefinition' depending on the exact circumstances. This requires that the proxy is very close to the person concerned and knows them with a degree of intimacy. He asked who the author of the narrative self might be and replied that, 'At least in part, the narratives that give our life its fundamental structure are joint productions' (p. 146). I think he is absolutely right to point towards the realistic 'complexity of human selfhood' (p. 148) – of which more in Chapter 13.

Before going any further, it is important that we are using the same terminology. Of great importance to assessing best interests is whether or not there has been any advance care planning. Figure 12.1 sets out what we mean by an advance care plan (at least in the context of the MCA – but the terminology can be translated into that of other jurisdictions).

Figure 12.1 Advance care planning

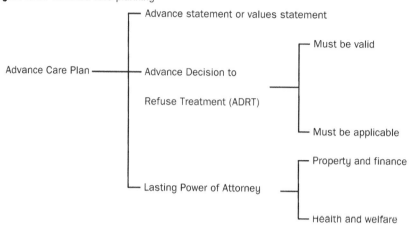

More legal details about advance care planning under the MCA can be found in Hughes et al. (2021: pp. 51–53); and background to advance decisions and advance care planning is also available in Sinoff and Blaja-Lisnic (2014). It should be noted that descriptions such as 'advance decisions' and 'living wills' do not feature in Figure 12.1. They could refer to either advance (or values) statements, which are not legally binding (but should be taken into consideration in best interest decisions (see Figure 12.2)), or (more commonly) to Advance Decisions to Refuse Treatment (ADRTs), which are legally binding as long as they are valid and applicable to the particular circumstances obtaining at the time.

A number of commentators have suggested that the specificity of ADRTs makes them (a) unlikely to be useful and (b) dangerous because, given their legal status, they leave no room for manoeuvre. Shaw (2012) felt the emphasis given to precedent autonomy in the use of instruments such as ADRTs could effectively sentence 'some people who want to live to death' (p. 267). Wolff (2012) argued '… that given our typical lack of insight into how changes in our health condition will affect us in other ways, we should be very cautious indeed in promoting the use of advance directives in end-of-life decisions …' (p. 505). There was caution, too, in the report on dementia by the Nuffield Council on Bioethics (2009): its concern was that '… in many cases an advance refusal of treatment may not operate in the way that the person in fact envisaged' (p. 86, §5.41). Appointing an attorney allows more flexibility. In any case, it seems reasonable to suggest that advance care planning should be broadly based to include lists of things that people value. As Widdershoven and Berghmans (2001) suggested, the important thing is to keep in view 'the interpretative and intersubjective aspects of decision-making' (p. 185).

The main question in this section is, given that some form of surrogate decision-making is sometimes required, should this be proxy or substitute decision-making? Both can be problematic. To reiterate: a proxy decision is where someone other than the person concerned simply makes the decision; a substituted judgement is where the person making the decision is required to try to judge, on the basis of anything written down or said, what the person concerned would have wanted in the current situation. Of course, a proxy could make a substituted judgement, but normally it is presumed that the proxy will more simply make the judgement based on what they themselves feel is best.

One thing to note immediately is that proxy judgements are burdensome (Sugarman et al. 2001). Surrogates find it difficult to know what decision to make (Fetherstonhaugh et al. 2017). Jox et al. (2012) showed that relatives, asked to make proxy decisions about hypothetical cases, tended to decide intuitively on the basis of their own preferences and with reference to the person's age, state of wellbeing and suffering. Professionals, on the other hand, relied on medical and legal authorities and emphasized patient autonomy. In a systematic review of surrogate decision-making, Shalowitz et al. (2006) found surrogates correctly predicted the treatment preferences of those for whom they were proxies with an accuracy of 68 per cent. This result was not improved even if the surrogate and the person concerned had discussed preferences previously! Similarly, Bravo et al. (2018) found agreement between proxies and older adults ranging from 43 per cent (for life-threatening pneumonia) to 70 per cent (for permanent tube-feeding), although it was higher for cardiopulmonary resuscitation (CPR). From their methods, it is not completely clear whether the surrogates were acting as 'mere' proxies or were making substitute decisions.

In any case, substituted judgements have their difficulties too. Torke et al. (2008) claim there are three lines of research that show the weakness of substituted judgements. The first is that preferences regarding life-sustaining treatments change over time, so you cannot rely on what someone said some while ago. However, they cite four works to support this claim: in Weissman et al. (1999) about 73 per cent of people with AIDS with a mean age of 36 years (range 23–60) showed stable preferences for cardiac resuscitation; in Emanuel et al. (1994) stability rates amongst a mixed population of patients was between 71 and 77 per cent; in Carmel and Mutran (1999) the overall stability rate, in an Israeli cohort 70 years of age or over, was 70 per cent; and in Danis et al. (1994) most patients (85 per cent) had not changed their treatment options two years after having made them. Contrary to Torke et al.'s (2008) claim, therefore, it sounds as if you can be about 75 per cent confident that an advance statement about treatment preferences will not have changed, which augurs well for substituted judgements.

Their second line of research suggested that the concordance between patients and their doctors or surrogates was not good (Torke et al. 2008). As recorded above, Shalowitz et al. (2006) found concordance to be 68 per cent. So, on average, you have a 68 per cent chance of deciding in the same way as your relative. One has to say that such odds are not too bad and keep in mind that the studies in the systematic review did not reflect reality, because the 'patient' was always able to give a view. Whereas, in the real situation, the point would be that they would be incapable of expressing their autonomous wishes about treatment. The question is, in that reality, where a frail life hangs in the balance, would concordance then be higher? But casting doubt on the usefulness of substituted judgements on the grounds that family and physicians might well not predict what the person would have wanted is not new (Seckler et al. 1991).

Moreover, there are reasons for arguing that, strictly speaking (logically perhaps), substituted judgements are fictional. Broström et al. (2007) pointed out that we simply do not know 'under what hypothetical conditions the patient is supposed to make his or her decisions' (p. 277). How competent would the person be for instance? Hope et al. (2009) also found the hypothetical questions suggested by substituted judgements to be puzzling; indeed, the required hypothetical question would require a magical answer:

> ... what decision would the person make now, if he or she were "magically" able to regain capacity long enough to make a decision, but that apart from regaining capacity, he or she would remain in exactly the same situation as he or she is in currently?
>
> (p. 735).

Torke et al.'s (2008) third line of research questioned whether patients really wanted 'their prior wishes to be the sole basis for decisions made on their behalf'. The research suggested that people want their families or physicians to have an input into the decisions rather than simply base a decision, perhaps about end-of-life treatment, on something they had possibly written some while ago. One of the recommendations of Torke et al. (2008) was that we should pursue 'a narrative approach to surrogate decisions', which seems to me very sensible.

Hence, although the situation is not hopeless, there are problems with both pure proxy decisions as well as with substituted judgements. But the idea of a narrative approach seems helpful, and it is important to keep in mind the extent to which decision-making for others will be 'interpretative and intersubjective' (Widdershoven and Berghmans 2001: 185).

The MCA best interests checklist

The framers of the MCA felt that no definition of 'best interests' could be given because every case has unique features and the concept should not be pinned down in a legalistic fashion. However, they did provide a checklist, which I would commend, with a few tweaks, to anyone in any jurisdiction. It is set out in Figure 12.2 (see also Emmett and Hughes (2019) for a full discussion of the checklist).

The modifications (shown in italics in Figure 12.2) are intended to bring some accord with the CRPD, to which we shall return shortly. I am not claiming that the slight modifications now render the MCA checklist perfect from the perspective of the CRPD, merely that they make it better. It was never suggested that every step of the checklist should be slavishly followed – it will depend on the case – but these are the things to consider. Very importantly, of course, the person for whom the decision is being made must be centre stage: *that* person's wishes, feelings, values, will and preferences must be paramount.

Figure 12.2 The MCA's (tweaked) best interests checklist (Source: HMSO 2005: §4)

[Alterations derived from the *Convention on the Rights of Persons with Disabilities* are shown in italics; amended from Figure 3.1 Emmett and Hughes (2019: 52–53).]

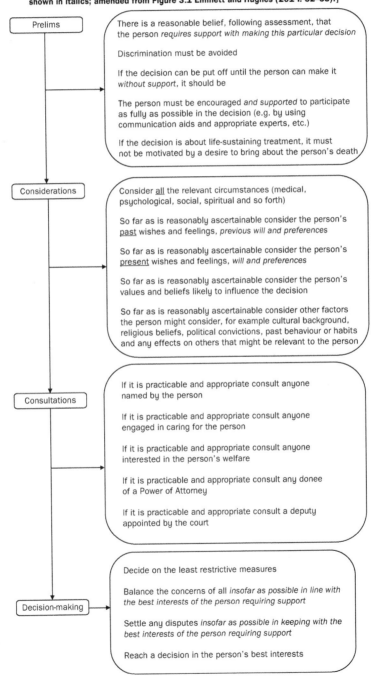

| Prelims | There is a reasonable belief, following assessment, that the person *requires support with making this particular decision* |

Discrimination must be avoided

If the decision can be put off until the person can make it *without support*, it should be

The person must be encouraged *and supported* to participate as fully as possible in the decision (e.g. by using communication aids and appropriate experts, etc.)

If the decision is about life-sustaining treatment, it must not be motivated by a desire to bring about the person's death

Considerations — Consider all the relevant circumstances (medical, psychological, social, spiritual and so forth)

So far as is reasonably ascertainable consider the person's past wishes and feelings, *previous will and preferences*

So far as is reasonably ascertainable consider the person's present wishes and feelings, *will and preferences*

So far as is reasonably ascertainable consider the person's values and beliefs likely to influence the decision

So far as is reasonably ascertainable consider other factors the person might consider, for example cultural background, religious beliefs, political convictions, past behaviour or habits and any effects on others that might be relevant to the person

Consultations — If it is practicable and appropriate consult anyone named by the person

If it is practicable and appropriate consult anyone engaged in caring for the person

If it is practicable and appropriate consult anyone interested in the person's welfare

If it is practicable and appropriate consult any donee of a Power of Attorney

If it is practicable and appropriate consult a deputy appointed by the court

Decision-making — Decide on the least restrictive measures

Balance the concerns of all *insofar as possible in line with the best interests of the person requiring support*

Settle any disputes *insofar as possible in keeping with the best interests of the person requiring support*

Reach a decision in the person's best interests

I have four comments to make about the checklist in Figure 12.2. First, readers might like to consider whether, or the extent to which, the checklist is redolent of the description of VBP set out in Chapter 5 (see Table 5.1). Of course, Figure 12.2 and Table 5.1 are quite different in many ways, partly because VBP indicates a process, whereas the MCA simply provides a checklist. Nevertheless, the emphasis on values, on hearing everyone's views, yet on keeping the person concerned centre stage, whilst trying to reach a consensus, all of these features are shared and, of course, good communication will be essential in judging best interests, as it is in VBP.

Secondly, it is worth noting that there is a rather strange provision, that end-of-life decisions 'must not be motivated by a desire to bring about [the person's] death' (MCA, Section 4(5)). This reflected concerns during the drafting of the Bill that the MCA might herald assisted suicide by the back door. These worries were unfounded. It is interesting to ponder that sometimes we might say with full compassion that death might be the best thing for someone. The question is whether it is ever licit for someone else to aim at a person's death, a point to which I shall return in Chapter 31.

The third consideration is whether the MCA commends pure proxy or substituted decision-making. Mostly, the MCA seems to encourage substituted decision-making. But the MCA's *Code of Practice* (Department for Constitutional Affairs 2007) suggests at paragraph 5.53 that, when consulting others, enquiries should be made about 'what the people consulted think is in the person's best interests in this matter, and if they can give information on the person's wishes and feelings, beliefs and values'. The second part points to a substituted judgement, but the first suggests a pure proxy opinion.

Finally, the reason I am inclined to commend the best interests checklist, with its tweaks, is because it seems to me rational to think that if you truly wish to support someone in the hope that the best possible decision will be made, you had better find out as much about that person as you possibly can. This involves talking to them, about their present and previous wishes, feeling, values, beliefs, preferences and what they willed then and now; it involves talking to others; and it involves considering anything else that might seem relevant. The MCA checklist encourages all of these things. It should do, too, because what is at stake is the standing of the person *as a person*! We shall come on to the notion of personhood in the next chapter.

Shared decision-making

By now, especially in the UK after the *Montgomery* judgment (see Chapter 11), shared decision-making would seem to be the norm. We have moved some way from the sort of blatant paternalism discussed in Chapter 9. And yet, the inclination to avoid throwing the baby out with the bathwater when discussing paternalism persists (Rosenbaum 2015). What is being hankered after is something captured, perhaps, by Agich's idea of 'parentalism' (Agich 2003: 48) discussed in Chapter 9. It connects with the ideas we have already come across in connection with best interests decision-making: the benefits of a narrative approach and the idea that decision-making for others will be 'interpretative and intersubjective' (Widdershoven and Berghmans 2001: 185).

Shared decision-making picks up the idea of intersubjectivity, which should lead to a nuanced understanding of the person's narrative and this in turn should facilitate certain decisions. The extent to which interpretation is required may be more difficult to judge, but where someone is living with more advanced dementia it may become crucial. A question that arises, then, is to what extent is the decision shared if the person helping to make the decision has to interpret too many things, some of them quite subtle?

Shared decision-making has been defined as: 'an approach where clinicians and patients share the best available evidence when faced with the task of making decisions, and where patients are supported to consider options, to achieve informed preferences' (Elwyn et al. 2010). In a useful article, Elwyn et al. (2012) set out the steps required for shared decision-making, but they emphasized too its underlying ethical rationale, which includes both self-determination and relational autonomy, which we discussed in Chapter 8. Unsurprisingly, good communication turns out to be central to the success of shared decision-making. These authors also highlight three steps to shared decision-making:

> *Choice talk* refers to the step of making sure that patients know that reasonable options are available. *Option talk* refers to providing more detailed information about options and *decision talk* refers to supporting the work of considering preferences and deciding what is best.
>
> (Elwyn et al. 2012: 1363)

This is helpful. But when we turn to people living with dementia, in particular those with more advanced symptoms and signs, where talk and the abilities to retain and understand may well be impaired, shared decision-making looks more complex. This should not make us lose sight of the value of the model, which seeks to encourage 'effective clinician–patient dialogue' (p. 1363) in the hope that this will bring about a sharing of minds. The possibility of meaning-making (Widdershoven and Berghmans 2006) and that people living with even marked symptoms of dementia retain semiotic capabilities (Sabat and Harré 1994) must not be forgotten. The human interaction and discourse that is possible in the context of marked dementia is, after all, one of the privileges and joys of working in the field of dementia care.

Still, I have heard it said that 'shared decisions' still sounds as if the decisions are not wholly the decisions of the person who is living with illness or disease; they remain partly the professional's. One response to this is to reply that it simply reflects the reality of the world in which people have relational autonomy and are not fully self-determining. Another response might be to appeal to the need people who are ill or are living with a disease feel to be held and supported by a relationship with an appropriate professional (Rosenbaum 2015). This is, after all, where Agich's idea of parentalism gets a purchase. But maybe we should go further and think of full-blown supportive decision-making.

Supported decision-making and back to the CRPD

This is certainly the direction of travel of the CRPD. As recognized by McGettrick and Williamson (2015), 'the CRPD requires a totally supported decision-making legal regime which poses significant challenges in terms of operationalising this for people with very severe dementia and those with profound learning disabilities' (p. 11). Section 12(4) of the CRPD talks of respecting 'the rights, will and preferences of disabled persons'. The worry is that the MCA (and similar legislation in other countries) is incompatible with the CRPD specifically because it does not – in its substituted (best interests) decision-making – refer to rights, will and preferences (Bartlett 2012). The concern is that, having judged you lack capacity, someone else can make a decision for you in your best interests, but this may not be in accordance with your will and preference (Alghrani et al. 2016). An example might be where we (the multidisciplinary team and your family) decide that it is best for you to go into a care home, but your will and preference would be to go back to your own home.

However, there is an argument that it shows a narrow and incorrect understanding of what best interests entails, at least in the MCA, where its checklist stipulates that in judging best interests we must consider the person's past and present wishes and feelings, his or her beliefs and values and any other factors likely to be considered by the person. This sounds very much like respecting the person's will and preferences, which could also be easily emphasized as in Figure 12.2. I think we see the same point in Donnelly's (2016) call for 'a stronger legislative endorsement of will and preferences', as well as greater supportive mechanisms, but not at the expense of all substituted decision-making (p. 318).

In a typically stimulating paper, Donnelly (2016) made a different point, which is against using the social model of disability in an unthinking way. The CRPD strongly endorses the social model of disease, which in many lights is to be applauded. But Donnelly sagely pointed out the obvious when she said, 'the model fails to take account of the realities of embodiment—ie people exist as bodies and experience disability both socially and corporeally' (p. 320). Nevertheless, the CRPD is setting benchmarks for a rights-based approach to the whole area of capacity and incapacity and has stressed the importance of support structures to enable the person's rights to be realized (Donnelly 2014: 275).

Scholten and Gather (2018) made the point that there are problems in realizing the ideal of supported decision-making in the comatose patient or in people with severe dementia or psychosis. They argued that supported decision-making 'does not make competence assessment and substitute decision-making superfluous' (p. 231). But they went on to say, sensibly and very importantly, that 'reasonable accommodation requires health professionals to exhaust the available resources of [supported decision-making] before they take recourse to substitute decision-making' (p. 231). They advocated a combined competence and supported decision-making model, where decision support incorporates three aims: 'It must be provided (1) to enhance a person's [decision-making capacity], (2) to improve advance care planning and (3) to improve substitute decision-making' (p. 230).

By the bye, Scholten and Gather (2018) also provided some interesting statistics: on the one hand, 'the accuracy by which substitute decision-makers predict the treatment preferences of patients is low, namely around 68%'; but, on the other hand, '83% of patients whose treatment preferences were overridden when incompetent approved of the received treatment in retrospect' (p. 232). So, it is not completely clear that substitute decision-making is as bad as some studies make it out to be.

Conclusion

So where are we? On the one hand, the direction of travel of the CRPD towards supported decision-making and a more rights-based approach seems in many ways exemplary (Cahill 2018). On the other hand, how this is put into effect when decisions are required in the more advanced stages of dementia is a puzzle. If we have recourse to advance care planning, this will be helpful – but advance care planning cannot be regarded as determinative *sans phrase*.

We must remember that best interests decisions can be about medical treatment, but also about social issues, such as where to live or what to wear. The discussion above about shared and supportive decision-making and how best to achieve this is relevant to whoever is making the decision. This might be a medical doctor, but could equally be a social worker, a spouse or child of someone living with dementia. In any event, the focus on best interests in this chapter should emphasize how useful it can be for people living with dementia to communicate – and to be supported in communicating – their past and present wishes and feelings, beliefs and values, will and preferences in whatever manner suits them.

For we need close acquaintance with the narrative of the person's life. We need the interpretative skills of a hermeneutic approach and the communicative skills required for authentic dialogue. All of this depends on genuine relationships and care and engagement with the biological (embodied), psychological, social and spiritual realities of the person. Underlying the legal approach to incapacity and best interests, therefore, there are not only ethical approaches (as described in Chapter 4), but also philosophical issues to do with our standing as persons with rights. It is to personhood and citizenship that we turn next.

13 Personhood and citizenship

Introduction

Given the involvement of ethicists and philosophers (not to mention sociologists and psychologists) it should be no real surprise to hear that the literature around personhood is contentious. Should we be talking about persons or selves? Should we be aiming at person-centred or relationship-centred care? What do we mean by personal identity? Is it better to be seen as a person or a citizen? If as persons (or citizens) we have rights, what are the correlative duties? And whose duties are they?

Personally, I like to think of myself in different terms under different circumstances. Sometimes I am a citizen; sometimes a person with a self. The main thing is that we treat people living with dementia and each other well. But the semantic questions are not trivial. They could literally be a matter of life or death. If X is not a person, not a self and has no rights as a citizen or anything else, there seem no good moral, psychological or social reasons for X's life to be defended very strongly. Except of course, X can still be a sentient being, just like a cockroach. Arguably, however, the extermination of cockroaches can on occasions seem required!

We need to understand what these words mean (personhood, selfhood and the like), as well as the consequences of using them in certain ways. We shall move from such terms to consider person-centred care, different views of the person living with dementia and then the SEA view (which will be explained), before ending with thoughts about citizenship and rights. My hope is that we shall end up with a humane account of what it is to be a person like you and me.

Persons and selves

'Personhood', according to the SOED, is 'the quality or condition of being a person'; and 'person' is defined variously as 'the individual human being' and as 'the actual self or being of an individual'. This latter definition seems to make 'person' and 'self' synonymous and they are often used synonymously. The SOED also gives a philosophical definition of 'person': 'A self-conscious or rational (esp. embodied) being'. The self seems to be what it is that makes people individual; according to the SOED, 'self' means 'a person's or thing's individuality or essence'. The self also seems to refer to the inner being: 'true or intrinsic identity; personal identity, ego'.

In a thoughtful paper, Millett (2011) noted that the possession of personhood is frequently regarded as what is needed to be 'morally considerable'. But his concern is that criteria for personhood tend to emphasize the sort of rationality of which the SOED speaks and which is easily perceived to be absent in dementia. He asked that we put aside personhood. 'One effect would be that we could focus on the idea that there is a being with an inner life confronting us, a being with value simply because he or she has a 'life-world' – a constructed meaningful world revealed to him or her through their senses' (p. 515). Rather than loved ones thinking about persons (or selves) living with dementia as 'an ontological unity in decay' (p. 520), they might do better to conceive of an inner life-world (*Lebenswelt*) continually being created. It is a nice idea but is open to the charge that inevitably this *Lebenswelt* is itself prone to be compromised by dementia.

Tieu and Matthews (forthcoming) have set out a critique of the current notion of 'person' which they then argue undermines the moral goals of person-centred care. Instead, they suggest that 'selfhood' is a better concept. Their understanding of selfhood is that it is formed in the context of relationships with carers and care environments. Such a concept needs to withstand the worries about the decline of the self, which is a real prospect if the self depends on some form of recognition or self-reflective awareness. Such worries exist for personhood as well as for selfhood.

However, it need not be that we accept the premise that personhood or selfhood will inevitably decline and disappear in dementia. In a very convincing paper, Holton (2016) pointed out that equating memory too closely with personhood, and thereby with inevitable decline in dementia, is too quick a step. For memory is more than one thing. Whilst '… the kind of confabulation that occurs in dementia can seem very alien', empirical work on different types of memory suggest it is not, because '… a creative process akin to it is something we all do all the time' (p. 260). Holton (2016) went on to suggest that the construction of memories is not something that inevitably comes from within. We can all contribute to the genesis of memories. He ended by saying that, 'even if we focus just on memory, the social will inevitably intrude. Keeping a personality going in dementia … is a job for us all' (p. 260).

If personhood and selfhood are moral ideas, they can also be considered as having a metaphysical status. This is seen particularly in debates about personal identity. What is it to be the same person over time (Lesser 2006)? Two different ways of thinking about personal identity have been considered: quantitative and qualitative. The quantitative (numerical) view – long debated by philosophers – seeks to establish how we can say that someone is the same person now and then, whereas the qualitative view is more to do with the qualities that make this the same person – that determine *who* a person is, not just that the person is the *same* one (McMillan 2006). The philosopher Paul Ricoeur (1913–2005) talked in terms of *idem*, or sameness, that is numerical identity, and *ipse*, implying the self, that is qualitative identity, with *ipseity* implying selfhood (Radden and Fordyce 2006). It is then possible to debate the extent to which one type of identity should take precedence and whether (and how) the two interact. Is it that some of my qualities as a person are what demonstrate that I am the same person? So if I lose those qualities, do I cease to be the same person? These issues are discussed in much more depth in Hughes et al. (2006). Part of their importance is because the notion of personhood underpins Kitwood's conception of person-centred care.

Person-centred (and other types of centred) care

I need not give an exhaustive account of person-centred care in this book given its place in a series stimulated by the work of Tom Kitwood (2019). Luckily, one of the editors of the series, Dawn Brooker, has answered the question 'What is person-centred care in dementia?' (Brooker 2004) and this has been followed by a successful book, now in its second edition (Brooker and Latham 2016). A convenient summary of person-centred care is provided by the acronym VIPS, which stands for:

- Valuing all human lives
- Individualized approach, recognizing uniqueness
- Perspective of the person needing support
- Social environment that supports psychological needs (adapted from Brooker 2004: 216; and Brooker and Latham 2016: 12).

The VIPS framework is essentially ethical. Brooker (2004) commented that Kitwood had used the notion of person-centred care in order to emphasize its Rogerian roots in client-centred care, where communication and authentic relationships were central. Again, this is redolent of the ethical approaches we discussed in Chapter 4.

On a slight tangent, given that we have invoked both person-centred and client-centred care, it is interesting to look more closely, albeit very briefly, at a variety of types of centredness. Nolan et al. (2001: 757) suggested that the next logical step beyond person-centred care was relationship-centred care, the benefit being that it recognizes 'caregiving can only be fully understood within the context of a relationship'. Well, but does person-centred care negate 'the context of a relationship'? And what about patient-centred care (as opposed to person-centred) and family-centred care, which also have a significant literature?

Box 13.1 Ten themes derived from five different types of centred care (person-, patient-, relationship-, client- and family-centred care)
[Adapted from Table 2 in Hughes et al. 2008. For fuller explication of the themes, please see original article.]

Respect for individuality and values
Meaning
Therapeutic alliance

Social context and relationships
Inclusive model of health and well-being
Expert lay knowledge
Shared responsibility
Communication
Autonomy
Professional as a person

Some years ago, we looked at the care literature around all of the five types of centredness just mentioned (Hughes et al. 2008). We established two things. First, that different types of centredness could be summarized by ten themes (see Box 13.1); and, secondly, that each of the types of centredness showed all of the themes. There are differences between the types of centredness, for they are used in different contexts. But it is erroneous to argue that one type of centred care is better than another on the grounds that it encompasses a missing theme. We concluded that the unifying themes of these different approaches suggest 'a movement in health and social care' away from a narrow view to one 'which involves increasing the social, psychological, cultural and ethical sensitivities of our human encounters' (p. 461).

Kitwood saw very clearly how persons were undermined by what he described as 'malignant social psychology'. In discussing the dialectical interplay of neurological and psychosocial factors, he said: 'The social psychology is malignant because of its effects upon the person who is neurologically impaired; that is all' (Kitwood 1990: 186). Reflecting (perhaps unconsciously) the distinction found in the work of Karl Jaspers (1883–1969) between the sort of explanation (*Erklären*) provided by science, and that provided by understanding (*Verstehen*), which relies on empathy (Jaspers 1923: 27), Kitwood demanded 'inter-subjective understanding' and not the 'form of explanation' generally provided by 'medical science alone' (Kitwood 1990: 194). (For further details on the explanation–understanding distinction in Jaspers, see Hoerl (2013).)

Davis (2004: 375) quoted Kitwood saying that there is an obligation 'to treat each other with deep respect' (Kitwood, 1997a, p. 8) because of the unconditional regard that is due to each person. This, with Kitwood's real commitment to the importance of relationships, led to his now famous formulation that personhood 'is a standing or status that is bestowed upon one human being, by others, in the context of relationship and social being' (Kitwood,1997a: 8). We shall return to this formulation shortly. Person-centred care is premised on this foundational understanding of personhood. If the psychosocial environment is right, the person with dementia will do well; there may even be some *re-menting*, whereby cognitive function improves.

There is much here to make person-centred care an ethical imperative. A deontologist (see Chapter 3) might well stamp a foot and assert that of course there is a moral obligation to maintain the person by affording dignity and whatever is required. But qualms have been expressed. Davis (2004), for instance, suggested that the corollary of the insistence on the possibility of an ideal psychosocial environment maintaining personhood is that carers might feel a sense of guilt which then compounds any sense of anticipatory grief. They might feel themselves 'directly involved in the dissolution of personhood' (p. 376). Hence, there is a genuine worry about suggesting that personhood can be maintained. Many would tend to agree with Davis's concluding sentiment: 'There must be a greater honesty in determining the violence that dementia does to the substance of the person and absolve [sic] those closest relations of the guilt of overseeing this decline' (p. 378).

Nevertheless, it could be argued that this is all to do with presentation. If family carers, as a whole, were to be told that any decline in the person's state would be a poor reflection on them, not only would this be untrue, it would also be unkind and ignorant, for it lacks charity and practical wisdom. If, alternatively, carers understand the approaches commended by the VIPS framework, not as a means to eliminate the possibility of decline, but to ameliorate it and to improve the person's quality of life by improving quality of care, then it seems much more acceptable; the person-centred care approach thus has an aim which we can accept as a moral duty. We know that much care falls short of the ideal of person-centred care, but we also know that such care can be achieved and there would seem to be no ethical reason not to work towards the ideals established by Kitwood (Brooker 2019).

Narrower and broader prospects

In any case, I would wish to push back against the idea (in Davis 2004) that there is inevitable decline in the 'substance of the person', or that we see the 'dissolution of personhood' in dementia (Hughes 2001). The idea that personhood diminishes in dementia has firm philosophical roots. For example, there is John Locke's (1632–1704) characterization of a person: '… a thinking intelligent being, that has reason and reflection, and can consider itself as itself, the same thinking thing, in different times and places; which it does only by that consciousness which is inseparable from thinking, and … essential to it' (Locke 1964: 211). Locke went on to say that in consciousness 'alone consists personal identity, i.e. the sameness of a rational being' (p. 212). In a similar vein, a more contemporary account was given by Derek Parfit (1942–2017), who argued that personality is not what matters, rather it is psychological connectedness and/or psychological continuity (Parfit 1984: 216–217). This is also reminiscent of David Hume (1711–1776) and his bundle theory, namely that we are just bundles of particular experiences: 'Had we no memory, we never should have any notion of causation, nor consequently of that chain of causes and effects, which constitute our self or person' (Hume 1962: 311).

It should be obvious that these philosophical ideas pose a threat to the personhood of people living with dementia. Reviewing the stories that we tell about ageing and about Alzheimer's disease, Herskovits (1995) was able to show how complex the concept of 'self' is, but also how 'loss of self' was implicit in constructs of Alzheimer's. Allegedly, if you cannot remember certain things, then you cannot be the same person and if you can remember nothing, then you cannot be a person at all. Brock (1988), for example, argued that 'the severely demented have been cut off from the self-conscious psychological continuity with their past and future that is the basis for the sense of personal identity through time and which is a necessary condition of personhood' (p. 88). The loss of psychological continuity and connectedness, as we saw in Chapter 12, is a threat to the standing of advance directives. Buchanan (1988) discussed this problem and in doing so noticed that the person with profound dementia 'is a being with morally considerable interests' because they have the capacity for pleasure and pain, but is nonetheless not a person (p. 299). Not everyone, however, fears that the personal identity problem undermines advance directives, because there may be other normative (utilitarian or rights-based) reasons to honour them, even in the face of the worry about disrupted psychological continuity (Furberg 2012).

In Chapter 12, I said I would argue that the presumption of discontinuity can be discredited, so we do not have to be sucked into the Dworkin–Dresser debate. We do not have to presume the discontinuity between the *then*-self and the *now*-self and this is because we neither have to accept that the self radically changes into a different self nor that it may even disappear. Why not? Well, in large part because of the definition of personhood supplied by Kitwood. Remember, that definition stressed the context of relationship and social being. Locke, Hume and Parfit were wrong inasmuch as they only considered psychological phenomena, especially consciousness and memory – and keep in mind that 'memory' signifies a whole lot of things (Holton 2016) – as the defining features of personhood. Kitwood's suggestion was that I am the person I am partly because of my interrelationships with others. This should remind us of Heidegger's notion of the human existent as essentially *being-with* (see Chapter 9). In any event, if personhood 'is a standing or status that is bestowed … in the context of relationship and social being' (Kitwood, 1997a: 8), then it is not necessarily lost if 'memory' (whatever that is) fades.

The literature certainly reflects this belief, that it is possible to maintain personhood despite poor cognitive function (Stein-Parbury et al. 2012; Johnston and Narayanasamy 2016). For instance, Lindemann (2009) talks (in a profound and touching paper) about 'holding the person in her identity' (p. 417). In a review of the literature, looking at the impact of dementia on the self and identity, Caddell and Clare (2010) concluded that, 'Overall, the vast majority of evidence points to the persistence of self, at least to some degree, throughout the course of dementia' (p. 125). It is easy to imagine, however, how the methodology of such studies is problematic, with different models and concepts of the self being used. The same researchers investigated the views of a group of people living with a diagnosis of mild Alzheimer's or vascular dementia. They showed that people are aware of tension over the issue of continuity and change in their lives, but the study highlighted 'the potential role for others and for the environment to play a part in maintaining the identity of a person with dementia' (Caddell and Clare 2011: 396). Cowley (2018) extended rather nicely Lindemann's notion of 'holding the person' to speak of friendship and of how this can both be a criterion of identity and 'partly *constitutive* of identity' (p. 260). Friends and family members can sustain the identity of the person living with dementia even as that person declines.

Before pressing on with this broader view of the person, it is useful to remind ourselves how pervasive the narrower view is, at least in the philosophical literature. Tooley (2009), for instance, writing about personhood acknowledged that 'a number of considerations strongly support the idea that the concept of a person is crucial for the formulation of many basic moral principles' (p. 129), which seems reasonable, although I tend to think there is something more metaphysical going on to support the importance of personhood conceptually. Tooley then stated:

> For while there is widespread agreement that certain combinations of psychological properties … suffice to make something a person, there is considerable disagreement among philosophers both concerning which of those properties are the morally significant ones, and concerning which properties constitute a minimum basis for personhood.
>
> (pp. 132–133)

Tooley went on to list 17 properties which make something a person. He discussed the difficulties associated with such a list. But the real point is that the list is made up of 'psychological properties'. It is a highly rationalist list. It does include, at the end, the abilities to interact socially and to communicate. But by this he intends the cognitive ability to communicate and to be social, not the possibility and metaphysical implications of social interaction and communication.

This cognitive bias has not gone unnoticed. Stephen Post, a pioneer in the field of ethics and dementia, first used the term 'hypercognitive' in the first edition of his book *The Moral Challenge of Alzheimer Disease* (Post 1995). In the second edition he wrote: 'Too great an emphasis placed on rationality and memory, arguably the cardinal values of modern technological societies, wrongly suggests an exclusion of people with dementia from the sphere of human dignity and respect' (Post 2000: 4). Reflecting on his earlier work and commenting on writers such as Brock (1988), mentioned above, Post (2006) says: 'The philosophers of hypercognitive personhood seem to state that if we do not wear the personae dictated by their intellectualist leanings, we count less or not at all under the protective principles of non-maleficence and beneficence' (p. 231).

What has to be seen is that there is much more to the person, and to the person's self, than is implied by hypercognitivism. Social constructionism – implicit in Kitwood's (1997a) formulation, where the status of personhood is 'bestowed' – highlights the extent to which the narrow view of a self or person is not simply mistaken, but is also egregious.

For me, reading two papers by Steve Sabat and Rom Harré (1992, 1994) was intellectually determinative. They are predicated on a social constructionist account, according to which:

... selfhood is publicly manifested in various discursive practices such as telling autobiographical stories, taking on the responsibility for one's actions, expressing doubt, declaring an interest in care, decrying the lack of fairness in a situation, and so on

(Sabat and Harré 1992: 445).

Their research supported the suggestion that selfhood can be undermined or supported by the discursive practices of those around the person living with dementia. Furthermore, they showed that, even when people are significantly impaired according to cognitive tests, they can still convey meaning and understanding (Sabat and Harré 1994).

Sabat (2001) set out three concepts of 'self'. Self 1 is the self designated by the use of personal pronouns ('I', 'me', 'my' and so on) or by gestures (pp. 276–277). Clearly, Self 1 can survive – as Sabat's verbatim recordings of his conversations over extended periods of time with people living with dementia show – late into the course of dementia. Self 2 is the unique set of mental and physical attributes that distinguish us from others (pp. 290–294). Even if some of these might change and disappear over time, some will remain, possibly to the end of the person's life. Selves 3 are 'the variety of different social personae and patterned and coordinated forms of behaviour, the display of any of which depends upon the social context within which one finds oneself at any one moment' (p. 294). Thus, yesterday I was the submissive patient at my dental check-up in the morning, a dutiful husband and academic during the day and host at a drinks party in the evening. I behaved in certain (different) ways in response to those around me. People living with dementia are no different. If they are confronted by others who undermine them, they behave in one way (perhaps with anger or a sense of defeat); if they are supported and treated with respect, they behave in another way (perhaps with vitality and felicity).

The importance of Selves 3, therefore, is that it develops Kitwood's idea of 'malignant social psychology'. Sabat (2001) spoke of 'malignant positioning' whereby caregivers' questionable assumptions colour attitudes and undermine the person's self-esteem (pp. 124–125). Indeed, this is also the effect of formal cognitive testing, which Sabat (2001) characterized as presenting 'an extremely influential and mainly 'defectological' picture – a laundry list of things he or she cannot do' (p. 93), along with 'often unwarranted inferences' about the person's incapacities (p. 94). Elsewhere, Sabat et al. (2011) have aimed the same critique at those who are inclined to refer to people with a diagnosis as 'demented' saying that once we use such language '... we not only diminish their sense of self-worth and sense of selfhood, but we also fail to see the very same persons as being able to act meaningfully in the world' (p. 289).

The social constructionist model of dementia gives us broader prospects than, say, a disease model, where everything is explained by and reduced to neuropathology; or a cognitive neuropsychological model, where cognitive dysfunction is explained in terms of computer analogies (Hughes 2011b: 119–152). There are, however, philosophical doubts about the social constructionist model (Thornton 2006; 2007: 139–164). The doubts involve the constructionist claim that meanings arise from (are caused by) social practices (discourse), rather than seeing that discourse, in order to be meaningful, requires that the normativity of language (the fact that certain things must mean certain things in order that meanings can be understood and language can work) is constitutive of our understanding of meaning (and other psychological phenomena) (Hughes 2011b: 168–180). If it is to be meaningful, we cannot just make up language. Nevertheless, the social constructionism, inherent in Kitwood and much plainer in Sabat and Harré, moves us to the uplands where we gain a much broader perspective on personhood and selfhood.

The SEA view

What we have been seeking is an account of personhood which is robust enough to be both 'morally considerable' (Millett 2011) and metaphysically broad. For some time, I have suggested that the Situated Embodied Agent (SEA) view gives us these characteristics (Hughes 2001, 2011b: 29–54). The SEA view of personhood in dementia does not supply a definition of what it is to be a person, but a characterization that provides necessary and sufficient conditions for the ascription of personhood. Even if the specific use in connection with dementia were novel, the terms are not new, but have been gleaned from philosophers who have written about issues relevant to personhood for some while.

Here are some examples. Taylor (1995) wrote of our embodiment: 'Our understanding is itself embodied. ... My sense of myself, of the footing I am on with others, is in large part also embodied' (pp. 170–171). Earlier, he had given a sense of our situated (and embodied) agency when he encouraged: '... an understanding of the agent as engaged, as embedded in a culture, a form of life, a 'world' of involvements, ultimately to understand the agent as embodied' (Taylor 1995: 61–62). Slors (1998), too, suggested that 'My body can play the part that is usually ascribed to the immaterial ego; it can provide a deeper psycho-biographical unity ...' (p. 68). In 1999, MacIntyre emphasized the point about embodiment by saying: '... it is true of us that we do not merely have, but are our bodies' (MacIntyre 2009: 6). And our embodied situatedness was captured by Merleau-Ponty in 1945 when he famously wrote in the Preface to his *Phenomenology of Perception*: 'The world is not what I think, but what I live through' (Merleau-Ponty 2002: xviii).

So, we are situated as persons in a variety of fields: physical, psychological, social, spiritual, aesthetic, familial, geographical, cultural, moral and legal. The point is that we cannot be circumscribed. There is always a further way in which I can reveal my self as a person in the world. We are also bodies, which locate us but also explain the way we do things. Finally, we are agents, acting in and on the world, and we can be agents in a variety of ways, sometimes acting intentionally and sometimes not. But we are not just agents or just embodied; we are situated agents, situated bodies and embodied agents all at once. My embeddedness in the world with others is a source of morality. My being-in-the-world as a situated embodied agent is a metaphysical ground.

The SEA view is reflected in the literature. O'Connor et al. (2007) looked at the notion of personhood in dementia and considered how to organize research to broaden the vision. On the basis of the literature, they came up with 'three interrelated and intersecting domains of inquiry: the subjective experience of the person with dementia, the immediate interactional environment and the broader socio-cultural context' (p. 121). The broader socio-cultural context itself could be split into: questions about race and ethnicity; socioeconomic status, gender and sexual identity; organizational culture; and the importance of societal discourses in shaping the experience of dementia. All of this attests to the situated nature of the person living with dementia.

Harrison (1993) had previously cited Alasdair MacIntyre's *After Virtue*, where he wrote about selfhood as, 'a concept of a self whose unity resides in the unity of a narrative which links birth to life to death as narrative beginning to middle to end' (MacIntyre 1985: 205). Later MacIntyre indicated that narrative history provides us with 'the characterization of human actions' (p. 208); and he pointed out that 'The narrative of any one life is part of an interlocking set of narratives' (p. 218). Harrison commented: 'The narrative view reinforces the notion that personhood is more than just the cognitive abilities or characteristics typically associated with personhood' (p. 434). So, again, we see the importance of being situated in narratives, which make our lives intelligible.

Heersmink (2022) discussed 'the distributed nature of memory and narrative identity' and was sympathetic to the SEA view of the person with dementia, although he wished to push further to recognize the importance of 'evocative objects' in the environment, which might also help to secure personhood. I think the point is a good one, although not one that causes significant problems for the SEA view, for we can be situated in the world of objects as much as anything else, and the SEA view can be combined with an externalist notion of mind, that the mind is not just in the head (Hughes 2011: 107–111). We can also go back to MacIntyre, who noted that a setting – including (he might say) one containing evocative objects –

> … has a history, a history within which the histories of individual agents not only are, but have to be, situated, just because without the setting and its changes through time the history of the individual agent and his changes through time will be unintelligible
>
> (MacIntyre 1985: 206–207).

Turning to the notion of embodiment, Phinney and Chesla (2003) wanted to explore how dementia is 'experienced as a phenomenon of the lived body' and how 'symptoms are experienced by the person with dementia' (p. 285). They conducted in-depth conversational interviews over the course of two to six months with five women and four men with a diagnosis of Alzheimer's disease. They described, rather poignantly, how 'The everyday grace of engaged activity is lost' (p. 296). Influenced by Heidegger and Merleau-Ponty, they talked about how 'a ready-to-hand practice is the act of a skilled body in smooth flow' (p. 296) and went on to say that their findings show 'that we as human beings exist in and through our skilled bodies that are involved in the world as both explicit and implicit understanding' (p. 297). Rather than simply thinking, dualistically, of there being a deteriorating mind and a separate body, they commended the idea of 'Incorporating an understanding of how the self is essentially embodied' (p. 298) in order to understand the experience better. It is the whole person – the embodied self – that counts.

The call to take more seriously our embodiment has clearly been heard in the writings of Pia Kontos, strikingly in her early paper reflecting on her ethnography in an Orthodox Jewish long-term care facility (Kontos 2004). It is a rich and profound account which draws (again) on Merleau-Ponty, suggesting (for instance) that selfhood is disclosed in the 'rhythmic flow and fluent form' of the gestures of residents in the home, as well as in their verbal exchanges, which exemplify Merleau-Ponty's 'assertion that communication dwells in corporeality or, more specifically, in the body's capability of gesture' (p. 841). She wrote: 'During interactions, words assume a gestural significance to the extent that their conceptual meaning is formed by inference from the gestural meaning' (p. 840). The phrase 'gestural significance' is striking and brings to mind Sabat and Harré's (1994) idea of the semiotic subject, where meaning is possible despite decline in formal cognitive testing scores. In Kontos (2004) we clearly see how meaning is embodied.

The paper also introduced to the world of dementia studies the work of Pierre Bourdieu (1930–2002) and his notion of *habitus*. *Habitus* refers to the dispositions we acquire in response to the social world around us. It is how we perceive and react to the world, but it is embodied and pre-reflexive. Kontos (2004) suggested 'selfhood resides in the dispositions and generative schemes of *habitus*' (p. 842). She continued: 'Thus embodied selfhood owes its coherence not only to the foundational unity of the body, but also to the embodiment of culture-specific conditions of primary socialisation', as shown by 'the residents' mastery of their social world' (p. 842).

Kontos (2005) pushed the notion of 'embodied selfhood' and showed how this moves beyond Kitwood's simpler idea of personhood being 'essentially social' (Kitwood and Bredin 1992: 275). A purely social account of personhood misses out a vital component, '... the existential expressiveness of the body in its relation to the world, and our sociocultural ways of being-in-the-world' (Kontos 2005: 567). Kontos concluded: 'Personhood persists as an embodied dimension of human existence and, as such, must be embraced in dementia care' (p. 567).

Kontos is not alone in being critical of Kitwood's formulation of personhood, nor in having doubts about the usefulness of the concept of person (see Tieu and Matthews forthcoming, mentioned above). Higgs and Gilleard (2016) have argued as follows:

> Kitwood's approach fails to distinguish between maintaining the moral standing of persons and preserving their capabilities of performing personhood. The failure to recognise this distinction places the burden of responsibility upon other persons for sustaining the personhood of individuals with dementia,

not just in sustaining moral concern for them (their moral status as persons), but in preserving their capabilities for personhood (the metaphysical components of personhood). The failure to achieve the former is too easily treated as a failure to realise the latter.

(p. 779)

An implication here is that the inevitability of decline in terms of the person's capabilities is not being squarely faced. Instead, Kitwood is saying (in effect) that we have to remember the person's standing as a moral being and, when the person inevitably declines, it is as if this might not have happened had we been better at buttressing the moral standing of the person. The metaphysical decline is, after all, what could be taken to sanction a change in our moral concern. As a second point, Higgs and Gilleard (2016) suggested that invoking notions of personhood (moral or metaphysical) is confusing and it would be better to focus on the recognition of 'a common humanity and the taking of due care' (p. 779).

One positive thing to emerge from this discussion is the importance of not simply blaming the carers. In addition, I would argue that the emphasis on persons is no bad thing. On the ground, it is not rocket science. First, see that this is a person like you and like me (recognize a common humanity); secondly, treat them as you would wish to be treated in this situation (take due care). The problem is not at this basic day-to-day level. Nor, I think, is it at the level of philosophy. It is no bad thing that we see the complexity of personhood or self-hood. Indeed, I think it is more complex than Higgs and Gilleard (2016) have suggested, because the metaphysical stance is not merely a matter of preserving capabilities. The metaphysical stance is the suggestion that even when capabilities have deteriorated, the person still exists as someone situated in a history, a narrative, a family, a culture, and so on – that these things are in some way constitutive of personhood – and moreover might still exhibit 'gestural significance'; but even if no significance can be identified, the person would still exist intersubjectively and meaningfully in the context of engagement between persons (Aquilina and Hughes 2006: 154–158).

But the problem Higgs and Gilleard (2016) have correctly identified is not at the level of philosophical understanding, which has to be constantly worked out, it is rather at the level of societal organization. It is to do with adequate training, education, payment, support, leisure, advancement and so on. If we cannot get carers (professional or non-professional) to act as if this is a person like you and me and to see that the person should be treated accordingly, it is an economic and political issue rather than one to do with the philosophical framework that underpins the ordinary use of the word 'person'.

Finally, there is the notion of agency. In a study of agency in people with dementia, Boyle (2014) found that even people living with advanced dementia 'sometimes expressed their perceptions, feelings and desires in habituated, embodied or emotional forms. ... even when their capabilities for language, deliberation and social (inter)action are extremely limited, people with dementia may still demonstrate imaginative agency' (p. 1140). In our own discussion of agency in severe dementia, we made the point that acts are carried out in the embedding context of the world, so that agency is situated and has to be understood in this way (Aquilina and Hughes 2006: 154–158). The 'gestural significance' is understood (or not) in a context, which includes the history of the relationships involved.

Of course, it is often presumed that people living with dementia will not be able to act as agents. However, as Zeilig et al. (2019) stated: 'The capacity to act and to effect change in the external world is a fundamental part of personhood'. In the context of work in a co-creative arts group for people with dementia, Zeilig and her colleagues argued that agency (and well-being) should be thought of as relational. The interdependency brought about by co-creative practices allowed agency to ebb and flow (Zeilig et al. 2019).

Baldwin (2010) indicated a number of ways in which narrative agency can be maintained and enhanced. He defined it as 'having the ability and opportunity to author one's own story' (p. 247). Art and the co-construction of stories are examples of some of the practical ways to help narrative agency. He commented: 'A focus on small stories can be seen as an antidote to the fragmentation of narrative and a means of establishing small restitution narratives' (p. 248).

In this section I have outlined the SEA view of the person with dementia and suggested some of the benefits of this perspective. I have shown how the notions of being situated, being embodied and being agentive are reflected in the literature. And, of course, these three facets of personhood always interact. Much of the literature on embodiment, for instance, is also about agency; and agency is embodied and situated: '… the notion of agency itself involves a sense both of the embeddedness and the embodiment of human persons' (Hughes 2001: 89).

Zeilig et al. (2019) noted that 'The systemic assumption that people with dementia can no longer 'do' or 'act' necessarily results in their citizenship being challenged' (p. 17). The potential for agency in people living with dementia to be enhanced or undermined, therefore, now leads us to consider citizenship and rights.

Citizenship and rights

In Chapter 2, we looked at how politics relates to ethics and said that politics is ethics writ large. Well, just as we are situated in our narratives, our families and communities, so too we are situated in the *polis*, which originally meant the Greek city state, but can be taken to mean the body politic. As persons, therefore, we are situated in political society: we are citizens; and, as citizens, we have rights, which relate to those we also have as human beings.

Bartlett and O'Connor (2007) argued that we need a broader lens in connection with dementia to include both the notions of personhood and citizenship. Their view was that personhood was too limiting, being apolitical and concerned with psychosocial issues. Citizenship, meanwhile, also seemed to offer too narrow a view because it seemed to depend on the ability to exercise rights and responsibilities, which might be problematic in dementia.

My immediate response is to ask why the notion of personhood has to be apolitical. By my lights it is utterly political, because we are situated in particular societies and political systems. My political beliefs are part of who I am. Bartlett and O'Connor (2007) also stated that the lens of personhood does not promote the idea of agency, but we have already seen the extent to which this is not true. However, they also state (which I think is a good point) that '… a shift to citizenship would ensure people with dementia were seen and treated as people with power …' (p. 112), this being particularly relevant to the research agenda.

Although I hold that personhood as a notion is enough, because of its uncircumscribable breadth (at least from the perspective of the SEA view), I think there are reasons to encourage the idea of citizenship. It does bring into focus larger social and political concerns, which might otherwise be ignored. Apart from anything else, it alerts us to issues around human rights, which we shall come to. But it also helps to emphasize the standing of the person as a member of society.

This can be seen purely in terms of political citizenship, where the focus is on membership and participation in a particular *polis*. An obvious example of this is voting, where there is the danger that either the person living with dementia, for instance in a care home, might be disenfranchised, or that people who lack the requisite capacity might be allowed to vote or might have their voting preferences manipulated (Redley et al. 2010). Thinking about testing for the capacity to vote is very challenging and would be regarded as deeply undemocratic. But participation and representation in democratic institutions is problematic and needs further consideration and recognition of its decidedly normative nature: '… there should be not only awareness, but also discussion on these democratic challenges for, and with, citizens with dementia' (Sonnicksen 2016: 339).

Beyond purely political citizenship, however, there is also a notion of social citizenship, which has been deeply developed by Bartlett and O'Connor (2010). For them, in connection with dementia, social citizenship is: '… a relationship, practice or status, in which a person with dementia is entitled to experience freedom from discrimination, and to have opportunities to grow and participate in life to the fullest extent possible' (p. 37). The relational nature of social citizenship chimes with earlier concepts of relational autonomy (Chapter 8) and relational agency (Zeilig et al. 2019). So, too, social citizenship can also be conceived as inherently relational (Kontos et al. 2017).

There is no doubt that talk of citizenship helps to shift our ways of thinking about people living with dementia (Gilmour and Brannelly 2010). Part of the aim of Bartlett and O'Connor (2010) was 'to reposition people as active citizens, as opposed to only welfare recipients, and to show the contribution people with dementia can make and do make to everyday life' (p. 123). Bartlett (2016) noted how the literature on citizenship and dementia has expanded and she made connections between it and dementia friendly communities. There is certainly evidence of people living with dementia being able to engage with their local communities, through artistic practice (Dupuis et al. 2016), through dance (Kontos and Grigorovich 2018), through gardening (Noone and Jenkins 2018) and through the hairdresser (Ward et al. 2016)! On this basis, it would be reasonable to argue that citizenship helps us to realize just how much more broadly personhood must be conceived. Bartlett (2021) looked at how access to the outside world is achieved in real-life by people living with dementia. There are practical challenges, such as learning how to use technology, moral challenges around autonomy and freedom, as well as neurological challenges. 'Therefore, our primary responsibility should be to engage with those living with dementia to recognise these challenges and find solutions, so that inclusive (social) citizenship can be mediated in even more pluralistic ways in the years ahead' (Bartlett 2021: 13). Once again, there is an ethical ring to these words: citizenship is also a moral requirement.

Thinking in terms of human rights is a way to sharpen the focus that the citizenship lens provides. Despite the rhetoric about citizenship and human rights, 'the reality of practice is that practitioners often do not think in terms of rights' (Kelly and Innes 2013: 67). There are a number of specific human rights that are relevant to dementia, set out in the UK's *Human Rights Act 1998* (Home Office 1998), which incorporates the *European Convention on Human Rights* (Council of Europe 1950): the right to life (Article 2); the right not to be tortured and to be free from inhuman or degrading treatment (Article 3); the right to liberty and security (Article 5); the right to respect for private and family life (Article 8); and the prohibition of discrimination (Article 14) (for further details see Hughes et al. 2021a: 47; and Donnelly 2014: 274).

It is important to realize that part of the point of claiming a right is that rights have correlative duties, so that once a right is established, there is a duty for someone to make certain that the conditions required to realize the right should be in place. Rights must be (in principle at least) enforceable. So dementia rights, like disability rights, suggest moral and political duties. Sometimes these duties will apply at the local level – to neighbours and friends who should make sure that the person living with dementia next door to them is kept safe – and sometimes they will apply at a political level, where lawmakers can legislate against discrimination and in favour of equality.

In 2015, the Mental Health Foundation produced a report, *Dementia, Rights, and the Social Model of Disability*, (McGettrick and Williamson 2015) which described the social model of disability and the influence this has had on national and international law. As the report stated: 'In the social model, people with dementia are centre stage, with their voices elevated, and are recognised as equal citizens with rights. They are the agents of change and their agency is valued and recognised' (p. 1). The CRPD, which we have already discussed at several points, is an example of where the social model of disability has had an impact. The social model of disability can be regarded as the response of the disability rights movement to what should be described as the disease model (but is unfortunately usually called the medical model, not that a reference is ever given for such a model!). The point of the disability rights movement is that it embodies what people living with disabilities wish to be: 'empowered citizens with rights and the ability to live a life of their own choosing' (McGettrick and Williamson 2015: 14).

It is worth noting that there are intellectual tensions within the disability rights movement (Shakespeare 2014), but the direction of travel is towards greater recognition of the inherent rights and dignity of people with disabilities as equal citizens of the world. Recognizing that people living with dementia can also be regarded as disabled is a way to encourage their standing as citizens with equal rights (Cahill 2018). Shakespeare et al. (2019) stated: 'The banner under which other disability communities have united is opposition to inappropriate medicalisation' (p. 1078). They went on to recognize that people living with dementia are activists too and that a relational and social model sits easily in the context of dementia. Even if there are some tricky issues in bringing together dementia and the disability rights movement, the marriage of the two has a purpose. Shakespeare et al. (2019) later said (rather movingly):

> If we are beginning to understand the voice that people with dementia retain, and the possibilities for a more expanded understanding of personhood, then we open the doors to a more powerful articulation of the rights of people with dementia and thus their ability to retain their humanity to the end of their lives.
> (p. 1084)

Efforts are being made to create and maintain citizenship for people with dementia around the world (Nedlund and Larsson 2016; Keogh et al. 2021; Steele et al. 2021). This can be challenging: to what extent are people living in care homes with dementia 'incarcerated' and how prevalent is 'torture' and 'violence' within the homes? There is no doubt that incarceration and violence occur, but should all care homes be closed? What then? And how much activism can there be in the context of a deteriorating neurological condition? I think there are answers to these questions: people with dementia can do well in different types of environment and care staff can be motivated, under the right circumstances, to provide person-centred care which honours the rights of the citizen residents; and, of course, you can be an activist for as long as possible. In some ways, the length of time is not the concern, which is more properly that you should be able to flourish, to participate and exercise your rights as a citizen whenever you want.

Conclusion

A rights-based, social citizenship model of dementia takes us in the direction of respect and enablement, of agency and dignity. The assertion of rights for people living with dementia seems crucial. However, the realities of dementia must be kept in mind too; as must the conceptual limitations of claims about rights (to which I shall return). Still, when the arguments about models have ended, we find ourselves *being-with* a person – a bearer of the rights that we wish to confer, but definitely a citizen – in the world. Here is someone for whom the African notion of *ubuntu* is apposite: 'an authentic individual human being …

part of a larger and more significant relational, communal, societal, environmental and spiritual world' (Mugumbate and Chereni 2020). It is seeing people thus that is the basis of our morality.

Having reviewed in Part 2 a range of concepts relevant to ethics and dementia, I shall now move on to discuss research and ethics in relation to dementia.

Part 3

Research Ethics and Ethics Research

14 Research ethics

Introduction

Research ethics is a big topic. My aim here is not to set out all the details of the various laws, directives and regulations that concern research on people who lack capacity to consent or are in other ways vulnerable. These can be found in links to some of the references to this chapter and elsewhere (see for example Emanuel et al. 2008a, Comstock 2013 and Friedman et al. 2015: 25–48). Of course, ethical practice – including novel approaches to dementia treatment such as invasive brain surgery (Gilbert et al. 2022) – must take account of all the relevant laws and regulations. This is because there have been famous and terrible examples of research being undertaken unethically – we only have to think of the Nazi experiments during the Second World War (Lifton 1986). The main point is simply that concern for the person as a legal and moral agent is central to research ethics and this is no different for persons living with dementia.

In this chapter, I shall start by highlighting the inequities in research funding for dementia, move on to mention the *Declaration of Helsinki* and then consider specific ethical dilemmas that arise in research to do with dementia. In particular, but briefly, I shall look at research on genetics, biomarkers and medicines and say something about psychosocial research. I shall end with some reflections on the implications of this for the different groups relevant to dementia research.

Research inequities

In the Nuffield Council's (2009) report (see Chapter 16 below), it was stated that more funding was required for dementia research. Despite improvements, funding for dementia still lags behind the funding of other conditions, which seems wrong on the grounds of fairness. On the one hand, in the UK in 2019 dementia cost about £35 billion, which is estimated to be more than the combined costs of cancer and heart disease (Social Care Institute for Excellence 2022). And yet, on the other, in the year 2017/2018, the UK government spent only £82.5 million on dementia research, or 0.3 per cent of the total annual cost of dementia; whereas government funding for cancer research was £269 million in 2015/16, which is 1.6 per cent of the annual cost (£16.4 billion) of cancer (Alzheimer's Research UK 2021).

Perhaps these inequities reflect a type of stigma. We know that the prevalence of dementia, both in the UK and in the USA, is greater in those of lower socioeconomic status (Arapakis et al. 2021). Hence, disadvantaged people are more likely to get dementia, to be stigmatized and to receive the least in terms of government resources for research.

The Nuffield Council (2009) also felt that more research was required on care and support and on the lived experience of dementia. The importance of qualitative research was emphasized. Quantitative research is based on numbers and statistics and asks, for example, whether, or to what extent, one treatment is better than another; or it asks epidemiological questions about the incidence and prevalence of diseases in populations. Qualitative research is more interested in the experience of living with conditions: how are they described and what do they mean to the person? More recently we have seen that innovative qualitative research, especially using a participatory approach (where participants in the research play a role in its design and interpretation), can enhance 'inclusion, empowerment, self-expression, flexibility, and communication' (Phillipson and Hammond 2018). The report suggested that more funding was required on non-Alzheimer's dementia too. It emphasized that we should not underestimate the ability of people living with dementia to make their own decisions about research. The use of advance decisions in research could also be encouraged. Further, the report suggested researchers need to consider the effects of a trial beyond its end.

In line with a greater recognition of citizenship in dementia (see Chapter 13), we have indeed seen the emergence of greater participation on the part of people living with dementia in research. The importance of accessing the perspectives of people with dementia was recognized even 30 years ago (Cotrell and Schulz 1993), as well as more recently (Dowlen et al. 2018). But still, we only infrequently see genuine co-production, as opposed to having a few people living with dementia and their carers on an advisory panel after the research protocol has already been conceived by the professional researchers. Nonetheless, a good example of co-production is Crutch et al. (2018), where the idea and much of the impetus for the research came from people with lived experience of the condition (posterior cortical atrophy, often thought to be a variant of Alzheimer's disease). We have also seen people living with dementia developing their own gold standard for ethical research (DEEP 2020). As Kitwood (1995) said in commenting on the ethics of research in dementia: '... we must attend not only to the content of research, but also to the process' (p. 657).

Declaration of Helsinki

The *Declaration of Helsinki* is the cornerstone of ethical guidance for research on human subjects. It was first adopted in Helsinki by the World Medical Association (WMA) General Assembly in June 1964 (WMA 2013). It has been amended nine times, which includes two notes of clarification, the last time being in Fortaleza, Brazil, in October 2013. We shall start with the declaration and its legal spin-offs.

The *Declaration* is not a law, but its authority is undoubted and it has universal clout. Many laws reflect its precepts. It is clear in its commitments: 'While the primary purpose of medical research is to generate new knowledge, this goal can never take precedence over the rights and interests of individual research subjects' (WMA 2013: §8). It is also clear about research involving vulnerable people. Such research is only justified if the research is in response to their health needs or priorities and if the research cannot be carried out in a non-vulnerable group. Further, the particular vulnerable group should 'stand to benefit from the knowledge, practices or interventions that result from the research' (WMA 2013: §20).

As an example of how the *Declaration* has been adopted into national and international laws, we can see the same provisions appearing in England and Wales in the *Mental Capacity Act 2005* (MCA)(HMSO 2005), in sections 30 to 34, which relate to arrangements for research in those who lack the capacity to consent. For instance, the MCA states that there must be potential benefit without disproportionate burden to those involved and, if there are risks, they must be negligible and not interfere with the person's freedom of action or privacy, or be unduly invasive, or restrictive (MCA section 31). The MCA makes it clear that if the person undergoing research does anything to suggest a wish to be withdrawn from the project the person must be withdrawn without delay (MCA section 33(4)).

Meanwhile, Directive 2001/20/Ec of The European Parliament and of The Council of 4 April 2001 relates to 'the implementation of good clinical practice in the conduct of clinical trials on medicinal products for human use' (European Parliament and European Council 2001). This directive also deals, in Article 5, with clinical trials on incapacitated adults not able to give informed legal consent. Similar themes appear as those in the Helsinki Declaration. For instance, it states that there must be 'grounds for expecting that administering the medicinal product to be tested will produce a benefit to the patient outweighing the risks or produce no risk at all' (Article 5 (i)). The clinical trial must be 'designed to minimise pain, discomfort, fear and any other foreseeable risk' (Article 5 (f)); and its protocol must be endorsed by a properly constituted ethics committee (Article 5 (g)).

Specific ethical dilemmas in dementia research

As well as the general ethical problems in research, such as how to gain fully informed consent, there are issues that are specific to dementia, such as whether it is necessary to have fully informed consent in all research projects involving people living with dementia. Götzelmann et al. (2021) carried out a systematic literature review. From 110 references they gleaned 105 dementia research-specific ethical issues (DRSEIs). These they grouped according to eight accepted principles for ethical research (Emanuel et al. 2008b). Table 14.1 lists the number of DRSEIs falling under each principle (there were sometimes subcategories) and provides one example from each principle.

Table 14.1 Dementia research-specific ethical issues (DRSEIs) [derived from Götzelmann et al. 2021]

Principles for ethical research	Number of DRSEIs (n=105)	Examples of DRSEIs
Respect for participants	11	Risk of dependency of the participant on the researcher
Independent review	3	Risk that research ethics committees might systematically exclude people with dementia
Fair participant selection/recruiting	5	Risk that gatekeepers might hinder participation
Favourable risk–benefit ratio	16	Risk of insurers or employers discriminating against people found to have risk of dementia
Social value	2	Challenges associated with gaining access to Information on predisposition to develop dementia
Scientific validity	20	Risk that non-spousal research couples have higher drop-out rate
Collaborative partnership	5	Risks associated with not taking different perspectives into account
Informed consent	43	Risk of therapeutic misconceptions

Rather than delving further into the examples included in Götzelmann et al. (2021), I shall now focus on specific areas of research. Interested readers may, however, wish to access the full list of DRSEIs in Götzelmann et al. (2021). There are also other review articles of ethical issues in dementia research (for example, Chandra et al. 2021).

Genetic research

In the 1990s there was a host of articles published about genetic testing in dementia. The science of genetics need not detain us; more details can be found in standard texts on dementia (Hye and Velayudhan 2021). There has been no consensus in favour of genetic screening for dementia in non-symptomatic individuals (Post et al. 1997; Blennow and Skoog 1999; Smith 2017). This is because the causative genes are so rare and susceptibility genes provide such limited information for the individual.

Burgess (1994) considered the effects of telling a person their genetic status by comparing people with Alzheimer's disease to those with Huntington's disease. In Huntington's, families generally know they are at risk, which may help to prepare them. Burgess (1994) noted that people with dementia will be more prone to have someone with them when their status is revealed, in order to help (perhaps later) with substituted decisions. However, the substituted decision-maker might, if a family member, also be affected by the news about the risk, so they too would require counselling along with the person living with dementia. Interestingly, Götzelmann et al. (2021) identified a relevant ethical risk as being that 'of not considering that proxies have major self interest in dementia research, e.g., because they have [the] same genetic traits, which could influence their proxy decision, and their manipulative behaviour may be difficult to detect' (p. 8 of 11). Post (1994a) argued we should not be misled into thinking that every genetic defect was a sign that the person could not lead lives that were 'creative and meaningful' (p. 785). He suggested that we need to overcome stigma and 'accept difference in our midst', for such people can teach us about 'equality and commitment' (p. 785).

Cassel (1998) continued the theme, warning that genetic advances should not suggest 'the implication of perfectibility', that we might be able to create 'perfect human beings' (pp. S19–S20). With great wisdom she warned against falling for 'a reductionistic model that lets us forget that we have tremendous responsibility and impact over the quality of our human society by what we do together ...' (p. S20). Redolent of the *Helsinki Declaration*, she said we must remember that 'what is fundamentally human is bigger than biology and, in some ways, more exciting' (p. S20). Kitwood (1997a) also put matters into perspective when he wrote: 'In general, the gene has been accorded a causal power that goes far beyond the evidence; it is, after all, simply a template on the basis of which proteins are assembled. The dynamics of cell function must be explained in other, and far more complex ways' (p. 33).

Whilst ethical discussion has tended to circle around the issue of disclosure, both to people with genetic traits and to their families, the literature I have highlighted above offers something of a corrective, suggesting that fundamentally our lives are not about our genes.

Biomarker research

The science has moved on. 'Biomarkers are naturally occurring markers of the underlying pathological process of a particular disease' (Lilford and Hughes 2018: 422). In dementia biomarkers can be detected, amongst other things, by cerebrospinal fluid (CSF) and neuroimaging. Such techniques have helped to establish that a disease like Alzheimer's exists on a continuum, from a preclinical asymptomatic stage to the full-blown disease. It becomes possible, therefore, to detect non-clinical disease. What are the ethical implications of this?

In a review of the literature, we identified four themes (Hughes et al. 2017). First, there are concerns about stigma (see Chapter 7). Someone who volunteers as a research participant might discover that they carry a significant amount of Alzheimer's pathology. If they have to reveal medical information for insurance or for employment purposes, they may face discrimination, which has led some to suggest we need changes in the laws on privacy and confidentiality.

Secondly, there is a variety of issues that arise in keeping with standard ethical theories. Knowing your risk for dementia on the basis of your biomarker status might be helpful (that is, beneficent), although Bunnik et al. (2018)

concluded that biomarkers in Alzheimer's disease could not have personal utility and would not help with the participant's autonomy because of their uncertain clinical significance.

An important ethical question is to do with the consequences of disclosure of biomarker results. Participants in the REVEAL study were told their risk of Alzheimer's disease on the basis of their ApoE status (Christensen et al. 2011). They were initially found not to have an increased risk of anxiety, depression or distress in comparison with those where a prediction was simply based on age, family history and gender; but when they were followed up after a year they were more sensitive to the limitations of disclosure and worried about the possibility of discrimination, although they still felt that the benefits of being told outweighed the risks.

The third theme to emerge from the review was to do with the psychological burden of knowing one's own risks of future dementia, which has been referred to as 'existential dread'. All this suggests the need on the part of researchers and RECs to ensure there is careful counselling prior to a person consenting to participate in trials which might lead to disclosure.

The final theme was to do with language. Not only are good communication skills required to convey sensitive and complicated news about risks, but also the language used should not itself be stigmatizing. For instance, younger healthy people found to have significant brain amyloid, putting them at risk of Alzheimer's disease, should not have anything said to them which might suggest that they are ill. For one thing, they still might not develop Alzheimer's (even if the risk is high); and for another it would be wrong to say anything that might induce depression, anxiety, stigma or self-stigmatization. These four themes suggest ways in which researchers and RECs need to consider more carefully the implications and potential burdens of biomarker research.

In summing up, we suggested that 'we need to know more about the values that might be at play here (including the public's values), which will touch on attitudes towards medicalization, on what we regard as normal or as pathological and, consequently, on what counts in the good life' (Hughes et al. 2017: 33). We ended by quoting Karlawish (2011): 'The discovery of preclinical [Alzheimer's disease] may be how we prevent the tsunami of dementia, but we must not drown in the challenges created by our own discovery'. It is a good quote, even if we should be suspicious of the metaphor (see Chapter 7) which has science saving us from what is portrayed as a devastating catastrophe.

Alpinar-Sencan et al. (2021) established, indeed, that notions of the good life were relevant to whether or not someone would wish to know their risk status. They felt their data showed that debates about personal utility, over against clinical utility, were less relevant as moral motivating factors in favour of testing than concerns about physical and psychological well-being, responsibilities within families and the desire for self-determination, as well as visions of the good life. Overall, their study, more than some others, revealed scepticism about the value of testing.

Alpinar-Sencan et al. (2021) also touched on worries about suicide and how these differed in different countries. There is certainly evidence that suicide rates go up after a diagnosis of dementia. In a study of over two million people in the USA, compared to the general population, the rate of suicide was about 53 per cent higher in the first year in people with a new diagnosis of dementia (Schmutte et al. 2021). The risk of suicide and euthanasia following an early diagnosis of dementia is something that has been discussed for over a decade (Draper et al. 2010).

Davis (2014) argued in favour of pre-emptive suicide when faced by dementia and suggested that biomarkers might help with the 'predictive challenge'. In other words, the challenge (according to Davis) is to predict when would be an appropriate time to die by suicide (it being felt by Davis (2014) that suicide would be a positive step); one would neither wish to do this too early, when there was still life to enjoy, nor too late, when it may become impossible to pursue one's intentions because of cognitive or physical difficulties. In an editorial, Powell (2014) said that 'The key philosophical question is whether preventive suicide is ever a rational response to learning that one has a certain risk of developing dementia' (p. 512). Davis (2014) thinks it is. In a response to her paper, however, Dresser (2014) thought otherwise.

There is an empirical point, which is that the likelihood of a predictive test authoritatively sanctioning someone to commit suicide is not currently secure enough to make this a rational plan. Still, the accuracy of the predictions is improving and once the person also starts to experience symptoms it may well be that some will see suicide as rational. Dresser (2014) suggested that clinicians have a responsibility to point out the alternatives to suicide. Further, 'If people use preclinical diagnosis as a trigger for suicide, the absence of an adequate societal response to [Alzheimer's disease] will be partly to blame' (p. 550). Her sensible paper concluded: 'Pre-emptive suicide and precedent autonomy may supply a way out for some individuals, but they are inadequate responses to the larger moral challenges that dementia presents' (p. 551).

The point is that one of the ethical consequences of research on biomarkers might be that people will consider euthanasia and suicide as a reasonable response to bad news. Although the results of the REVEAL study argued slightly against this concern (Christensen et al. 2011), research protocols should consider how to mitigate the risks to the mental health of research participants by disclosure of their biomarker status. In many ways, this reflects the earlier ethical debates about genetics.

Pharmacological research

Many people living with dementia will be enrolled in drug trials, which are a subset of clinical trials. A clinical trial is 'a *prospective study comparing the effects and value of intervention(s) against a control in human beings*' (Friedman 2015: 2). In Europe they fall under the Directive referred to above (European Parliament and European Council 2001). A clinical trial need not be of a drug; it could be of a device or procedure. Such trials engage with the principles set out in Table 14.1 (Emanuel et al. 2008b). Again, space does not allow a full discussion of all the ethical issues, but important factors to be considered are:

- randomization (how it is decided that a participant will be in the treatment group or the placebo group, or in the standard treatment group or the novel treatment group)
- the nature of the control group (active treatment or placebo)
- conflicts of interest (which might bias the results)
- informed consent (discussed in Chapter 11)
- recruitment to the trial (fairly and without coercion)
- monitoring of safety and efficacy
- criteria for early termination of the trial
- privacy and confidentiality
- data falsification
- publication bias, suppression and delays (Friedman 2015: 25–48).

Focusing on drug trials, I shall pick out only two ethical issues and mention the worry about a new drug for the treatment of dementia before some further reflections from the literature on consent. First, there is the issue of clinical equipoise (Freedman 1987), which is where there is genuine uncertainty about which treatment in a drug trial, say, is better. If it were known for sure that drug B was better than drug A, then it would be immoral to give people in the trial drug A because it is wrong knowingly to give inferior treatment when better treatment is available. So there must be equipoise. Researchers must be genuinely uncertain as to which treatment is better; and potential participants must be aware that this uncertainty exists. In my experience, some participants in drug trials for the treatment of dementia take part because they have strong beliefs or hopes that the treatment will be effective. The consent process, which involves informing potential participants about the lack of knowledge about the drug, as well as about randomization (so that in a placebo-controlled trial they may be receiving a substance of no anticipated value) does not always seem to temper this enthusiasm. The instinct to keep hope alive and to remain optimistic influences both researchers and participants.

Secondly, it is hard to avoid the issue of money. When drug companies have spent millions of pounds developing a drug, they are keen that it should be shown to work. They will say that this is to benefit people with the particular condition, but the real responsibility of those at the top of the drug company is to their shareholders, who will want to see a profit. Hence there have been worries that trials run by drug companies are more likely to be successful than independent trials, that researchers who are financially sponsored by drug companies do not maintain complete impartiality, and that drug companies will stop trials for financial and not for purely scientific reasons (Chopra 2003). More recently, there have been grave concerns about numerous aspects of research by the pharmaceutical industry in low- and middle-income countries (Mtande et al. 2019).

The newest drug for the treatment of dementia at the time of writing is aducanumab. This is a novel drug, a monoclonal antibody said to remove amyloid from the brain. Unlike the other available anti-dementia drugs, which only provide modest benefits, this looks as if it might tackle the underlying pathology. However, there have already been numerous studies of monoclonal antibodies which have failed. The concern around aducanumab is that it has been licensed in the USA for use in Alzheimer's disease on grounds that seem shaky (Alexander et al. 2021; S. Walsh et al. 2021). The effect is inevitably that the hopes of those who live with the diagnosis are raised. But if the process by which the drug has been licensed is flawed, there will potentially be a considerable loss of confidence, as well as concern that people have been subjected to unnecessary risks at a very high cost. The cost of the drug is about $56,000 (or £41,000 or €43,000) per person each year.

Finally, in this section on drug trials, when looking at the literature on consent, the Dworkin–Dresser debate is again in evidence. Buller (2015a) argued that precedent autonomy should allow someone to consent to research in the future, even if 'greater than minimal risk' (p. 701) is involved, just as it allows people to refuse life-saving treatment. Jongsma and van der Vathorst (2015) took a different view, arguing that we can neither assume that 'research participation is a critical interest' nor that critical interests can overrule experiential interests (p. 708). Similarly, Hallich (2015) argued, like Dresser (2014), that 'experiential interests may … sometimes negate the authority of critical interests' (p. 710). Buller's response, in part, was seemingly to agree that if a person were objecting to research participation, despite what was stipulated in that person's advance directive, it would be wrong to enforce it, but suggested the same would then apply to advance refusals of treatment (Buller 2015b). This is a little disingenuous because whereas a person living with dementia might actively fight against being given an injection as part of a research study, a person is unlikely to show any signs of battling against life-saving treatment being withheld. If, in the latter case, slightly inconceivably, the very ill person with advanced dementia suddenly indicated they wanted to be actively treated, this wish would (at the very least) have to be seriously considered.

Meanwhile, in some nuanced research undertaken by Shepherd et al. (2021), which harkens back to our discussions about best interests in Chapter 12, it was shown that the decisions made by proxies about their loved ones being enrolled in research are subtle. Whilst proxies wanted to do what was 'best' for the person and to keep them safe, they also wanted to make the 'right' decision, which they regarded 'as being authentic to the person's values and life' (Shepherd et al. 2021: online). It is noteworthy, given some of the emerging themes in this book, that Shepherd et al. (2021) stressed relationships, virtues (such as trust), values and (we can add) authenticity as key to proxy decision-making.

Psychosocial research

The Nuffield Council (2009) report commended qualitative research, which is often psychosocial in nature. Overall, the risks of such research are not as great as the risks in, for instance, a drug trial. However, ethical issues still exist. As well as worries about recruitment, consent and so on, there is the concern that relationships will be established that cause dependency. This is an issue for researchers who build up friendships partly to encourage individuals to join the research and then to stay in it. There can be a falsity about this, one which is keenly felt when the study ends and the researchers cease contact with the participants.

A separate ethical issue is that RECs can apply the same strict criteria to some qualitative psychosocial research as they apply to clinical trials. This might seem fair enough at first blush, but it can also impose a considerable burden on researchers and be a block to quite benign research which is likely to be pleasurable and of benefit to participants. It can reasonably be argued that the ethical nature of some psychosocial research depends critically on the virtuous character of the researcher. Of course, fraudulent activity in clinical trials is also avoided by employing virtuous researchers, but the character of the researcher is much more to the fore in qualitative research than it is in quantitative. Social science research can be more about integrity than about regulatory compliance (Israel 2015).

Conclusion: what should be done?

I shall end by considering the ethical nitty-gritty of what all this means for the different stakeholders in the research process.

First, there are the policymakers. We have seen that their role is vital in ensuring that research is conducted ethically: through regulatory bodies they set the standards. This is complex when research is being undertaken in different centres and different countries, especially where the regulatory authorities are not well funded or organized. But there is also the ethical requirement that their regulations should not stifle research or themselves place a burden on potential participants. For example, it can be unrealistic to stipulate that people living with advanced cognitive impairment (or even their proxies) should have to read exceedingly long information leaflets and sign consent forms they may not fully understand. When people with dementia themselves undertake research, it is no surprise that they complain about the bureaucracy involved in gaining ethical approval. (T. Davies et al. 2021).

Then there are the researchers. They must be fully aware of any inclination towards bias, including the bias that people will be better off in their studies. Beyond the regulations, one thought is that the process of research can – and should – be considered a relationship. In Hughes et al. (2009) we set out the A to G of Research as Relationship, which is adapted here:

- **Acquaintance:** is to do with getting to know someone
- **Being with:** signifies that it is not solely a question of 'doing to' people
- **Contiguity:** means physical (or virtual) closeness

- **Dependency:** where researcher and research participant rely on one another
- **Exchange:** which is mutual, with commitment and the promises involved in consent
- **Fruitfulness:** indicating the hope of good outcomes with data provided for a purpose
- **Gift:** where there is reciprocity and where even the relationship is given as a gift.

Above all else, it is well for researchers to recall Kant's dictum: 'Act in such a way that you treat humanity … always at the same time as an end and never simply as a means' (Kant 1993: 36).

For families and other close carers of people living with dementia, the lesson is both that research can be beneficial for the person and should be encouraged; but also, that it can be harmful and depressing if it turns up unexpected and unwanted results or simply does not work. In addition, it can be painful or just inconvenient. Those close to the person living with dementia, therefore, have a real role as advocates. They need to be supportive of the person, allowing them to make decisions for themselves but, if this is not possible, they need to think very hard about what is going to be best for the person and not allow false hopes to permeate their thinking. They must demonstrate the virtue of prudence in deciding what might be enjoyable or in keeping with the person's overall values and preferences.

People living with dementia are already showing that they are able to lead, as well as participate in, dementia research, which can be seen as part of the citizenship movement (T. Davies et al. 2021). Their views on research are so obviously crucial, it now seems amazing that for so long they have been ignored. How the interactions between professional researchers and people with expertise by experience (that is, those living with dementia) are negotiated is something that needs careful consideration. In many instances, the expertise and experience of researchers will be crucial if progress is to be possible.

People living with dementia can find themselves under pressure to participate in research. They might be willing to help for altruistic reasons and they might benefit from research participation, but they must feel comfortable with what is going on and know that they can withdraw from research at any stage for any reason and for none. The argument is sometimes made that there is a duty to participate in research on the grounds that the current generation has benefited from the participation of others who went before, so now it is this generation's turn. This argument has some merit in that altruism is as good a reason to participate in research as any other. I do not think, however, that it should be regarded as universally compelling. We should recall the *Declaration of Helsinki*, that 'new knowledge … can never take precedence over the rights and interests of individual research subjects' (WMA 2013: §8). And, to adapt Cassel (1998: S20): '… what is fundamentally human is bigger than [research] and, in some ways, more exciting'.

15 Ethics research

Introduction

The previous chapter was about the ethical principles that guide research. This chapter is about research on ethical issues in dementia. Over the last 20 to 40 years, research on dementia has burgeoned. In one sense, any writing on ethical issues is itself research; but increasingly there have been empirical studies with the aim of telling us something useful about ethical issues: what do different people think about particular issues? What do people do under certain circumstances? What can we conclude from what they say or do? Much of the research on ethical issues is qualitative. We want to understand why and/or how people do particular things or think in certain ways. Qualitative research may involve ethnographic techniques, for instance, with observations taking place in a care home to see how person-centred care is put into effect. But the research can be quantitative too. As an example, we might undertake a survey to find out how many people approve of the use of robots in a care home for people living with dementia.

It is worth lingering over these initial points just a little because it is a complex area. It is reasonable to question how any research (quantitative or qualitative) that produces facts can then tell us what we ought to do, which is what is required of ethics. This reflects a well-known problem in moral philosophy known as the is-ought problem, which was first brought to prominence by David Hume, whom we came across in Chapter 13. He pointed out that no amount of stating what *is* the case will tell you what *ought* to be the case: you cannot derive an 'ought' from an 'is' (for a slightly old but full discussion of the is-ought question, see Hudson 1969). Say a survey showed that almost all nurses thought that feeding by hand in the advanced stages of dementia was the most ethical way to go about things, would this mean that such feeding was ethical? What if the recorded verbatim comments of a focus group agreed, would that clinch the deal and allow us to say that feeding by hand was always ethical in advanced dementia? It is not clear that the issue is solved by a majority vote! (The issue of feeding will be discussed in more detail in Chapter 28.)

The philosophical issues, including the is-ought problem, were discussed by McMillan and Hope (2008), who argued that we need empirical study *and* ethical analysis, and by Widdershoven and van der Scheer (2008), who similarly argue that we need empirical *and* normative ethics. Indeed, the book edited by all four of these authors, *Empirical Ethics in Psychiatry*, which contains these works, also contains examples of empirical ethics in connection with dementia: how responsibilities for care are organized (Goldsteen 2008), issues for family carers (Baldwin 2008), philosophical issues around advance care planning

(Hughes and Sabat 2008) and legal issues to do with decision-making when the person lacks competence (Welie 2008). Empirical research does not tell us what is right or wrong, but it contributes to the discussion and provides data to inform our normative deliberations.

My aim in this chapter is to consider the breadth and nature of the research on ethical issues in dementia. I shall start by looking at some general overviews of ethical issues in dementia. The works I have chosen to consider reflect (what could be called) a convenience sample. They are simply examples I have to hand. I wish then to highlight the breadth of the issues that can arise and I do so by looking at research we undertook some years ago with family carers. I shall, before some concluding thoughts, highlight a systematic review of ethical issues which seem specific to dementia.

Overviews

I introduced Stephen Post in Chapter 13 as a leader in the field of ethics and dementia (see 'The Ethicists' in Killick 2017). *The Moral Challenge of Alzheimer Disease* (Post 1995) was described in the British Medical Journal as a pioneering book and as a medical classic (Bartley 2009). Post was already established by then as an ethicist interested in dementia. With colleagues Robert Binstock (1935–2011) and Peter Whitehouse, he had co-edited *Dementia and Aging: Ethics, Values and Policy Choices* (Binstock et al. 1992), which contained sections on different perspectives on dementia, treatment decisions, advance directives and euthanasia, caring, justice and public policy. Post (1994b) had covered the topics of care, justice, cost, genetics, diagnosis, independence, research, pre-emptive suicide, autonomy, quality of life and treatment limitations, behaviour control, nutrition and hydration. In the UK, Jones (1997) covered some of the same issues but stuck fairly closely to the framework of the four principles (as in Chapter 3) and included relevant law.

A book which helped to open up a whole area of discourse, *Ethical Foundations of Palliative Care for Alzheimer Disease*, appeared in 2004 (Purtilo and ten Have 2004). The title suggests it is mainly to do with the end of life, but the book is much broader than this and discusses a variety of moral and philosophical issues from decision-making to the management of pain, from research to autonomy, from the moral self to advance directives. Shortly afterwards, in Hughes and Baldwin (2006), we focused on making decisions and the great variety of issues that arise for carers of people living with dementia (see below), but also included discussion of ethical principles and theories, truthfulness, treatment, safety and quality of life.

Gauthier et al. (2013) provided a good overview of ethical issues around the diagnosis of dementia, including in connection with research, as well as where symptoms are minimal or the diagnosis based on biomarkers might be uncertain. The review also touched on end-of-life care and stigma.

Meanwhile, *The Law and Ethics of Dementia* was published in 2014 and provided an authoritative account of several legal and ethical issues in connection with dementia, whilst also including the perspectives of people living with dementia and their carers (Foster et al. 2014). The book discussed the determination of best interests and substituted judgements, along with personhood, precedent autonomy and proxy decision-making, truth-telling, research, genetics, perceptions of dementia, end-of-life issues, resource allocation, sexuality, the use of new technologies and the issue of abuse.

Johnson and Karlawish (2015) reviewed the ethical issues in dementia and picked out: (a) the risks associated with diagnosing preclinical dementia, which might include stigma and discrimination; (b) research and capacity; and (c) living with dementia, which included discussion of treatment and care, as well as civic privileges and rights, where the focus was on driving and voting. More recently we have also written a book on law and ethics aimed mainly at nurses which reflects, more succinctly, the themes and issues in the current volume (Hughes et al. 2021a).

The breadth of ethical issues

Some years ago, we undertook research that involved asking family carers of people living with a diagnosis of dementia what difficulties they faced as carers. We did not ask them to name 'ethical' difficulties, but in more or less every case their difficulties were essentially ethical in that they always raised questions about what was right or wrong, about what the person ought or ought not to do (Baldwin et al. 2004).

In the course of the pilot project for this study we recorded the issues raised by the family carers (Hughes et al. 2002a); and we undertook a non-systematic review of the literature about ethical issues for carers (Hughes et al. 2002b). In the main study we undertook a more systematic interrogation of 14 bibliographic databases (Baldwin et al. 2003). The issues that emerged from this work are recorded in Table 15.1

In Table 15.1 I have attempted to group some of the issues, but only lightly. Quality of life and dignity are not the same thing, but they are related (as in Chapter 10). Similarly, wandering and technology are not coterminous, but the use of technology often crops up in connection with wandering. (I should quickly add that the word 'wandering' reflects usage at the time of the study and many professionals would now avoid its use – see Chapter 19.) It should be noted that the items entered under the right-hand column for Baldwin et al. (2003) represent the broad ethical categories and not the detailed issues that came to light in the literature search.

Also, not obvious in Table 15.1, but more obvious in the actual papers, are the differences between the issues that arise for family carers and issues that arise for professionals. They can be as different as, on the one hand, not wanting to take over tasks because you risk undermining the person's self-esteem and, on the other, research ethics. Not wanting to take over tasks is also a nuanced issue, reflecting the nature of a particular relationship and requiring a nuanced response depending on the relationship (see the case of Mr and Mrs Carter in Chapter 3).

Table 15.1   Ethical issues emerging from family carers and from the literature

Issues derived from Hughes et al. (2002a)	Issues derived from Hughes et al. (2002b)	Issues derived from Baldwin et al. (2003)
Assessment		
	Autonomy	
Avoiding infantilization		
	Best interests	
		Feeding
Communication		
		Research issues
Community resources		Planning
Compulsion and coercion	Need for constraint	
Confidentiality		
Consent		Informed consent
Constant telephone calls		
	Intimate (sexual) care	Sexuality
	Carers' needs	
		Resource issues
	Dignity	Quality of life
Difficult behaviour		Behavioural issues
	Need to share care	
Driving		
Conflicting loyalties		Patients' rights
End of life decisions and euthanasia, right to die and palliative care		
	Duty and religious conviction	
	Previous beliefs	Advance directives
Feelings of guilt		
Giving up care		
Genetics		
Lack of support	Standards of care	
Letting them down		
Misunderstanding		
Need for information		
Professionalism and professional relationships		Professional care and ethics
Providing personal care		

(*continued*)

Table 15.1 (Continued)

Issues derived from Hughes et al. (2002a)	Issues derived from Hughes et al. (2002b)	Issues derived from Baldwin et al. (2003)
Public embarrassment	Possibility of moral growth	
Recognizing vulnerability		
	Surrogate treatment and decision-making generally	
Treatment issues, including withholding, withdrawing, over-sedation and covert medication		
Self-care		
Sleep deprivation		
Taking over tasks	Responsibility for finance	Legal and planning issues
Talking about person as if not there	Loss of personhood	
Taking risks		
	Reciprocity	
Telling the diagnosis		
Treating the person as a person	Vulnerability	
		Research issues
Truth-telling		
Use of respite care	Placement in long-term care	
Wandering		Technology

It cannot be resolved by recourse to the *Helsinki Declaration*, which would help with some questions in research ethics, nor even by looking in a textbook of medical ethics. General ethical principles and theories could be applied, but the solution to the problem in real life would need to be subtle and individual.

The other point to note is that the list of ethical issues which arise is long and broad. Real life throws up more than can be imagined. An example would be the wife caring for her husband who felt the need to use sedating medication to keep her husband calm. Her rationale was that if he were to be agitated at night, as he had been, she would no longer be able to cope with him at home. She knew his wish would be to remain in his own home, so she reasoned that she had to sedate him, but this caused her considerable worry. It was an ethical worry: was she doing the right thing?

Embarrassment in public, feeling guilty, reciprocity (the feeling that 'my mum looked after me, now I must look after my mum') and conflicting loyalties ('I have to look after my mum, but also my husband and children') – these are all issues for family carers which are particular to their unique perspectives. They have to be dealt with in their own contexts and are examples of the breadth of ethical issues that arise in connection with dementia.

Table 15.2   The spectrum of disease-specific ethical issues in dementia care. Adapted from Strech et al. (2013)

Major categories	First-order disease-specific ethical issues	Second-order disease-specific ethical issues
Diagnosis	Complexity of diagnosis	Diagnosis being made prematurely or too late
		Difficulties around MCI definitions
		Need to avoid underestimating the views of relatives
	Point of diagnosis	Ignoring evidence of illness and advance planning
		Acknowledging the burdens of bad news
		Not seeing the views and experiences of relatives
	Need for treatment	Thinking current drugs are better than they are
		Need to balance benefits and risks of treatment
		Ignoring views of relatives
	Understanding the patient	Considering the patient's personhood
		Considering the person's wishes and preferences
		Considering the person's autonomy
Assessment of capacity		Ambiguity around capacity
	Problems	Poor assessment
		Need to consider the setting or substance of decisions
		Problems around what might be authentic
		Underrating the views of relatives
Particulars and disclosure		Respecting autonomy
		Suitability of information
		Participation of relatives
		Reflection on influence of culture
Decision-making and informed consent	Enhancing person's capacity to make decisions	Need to involve the person
		Need to foster decision-making capacity
		Need to build relationships with the person to encourage autonomy
		Need to avoid rushing the person to make a decision
		Need to avoid infantilizing the person
	Sound surrogate decisions	Suitable 'best interest' and 'substituted judgements'
		Proper contact with relatives
		Appropriate use of information from relatives
		Attention to advance planning
		Importance of legal advice or input
	Proper attention to living wills or advance directives	Problems with interpretation
		Problems knowing whether or not to abide by content

(continued)

Table 15.2 (*Continued*)

Major categories	First-order disease-specific ethical issues	Second-order disease-specific ethical issues
Considerations of social context		Concern for relatives
		Concern for professionals
		Risks of harm
		Worries about resource allocation
Professional issues	Ongoing evaluation of risks and benefits	
	Empowering the person	Appropriate settings
		Appropriate motivation
	Carers' attitudes	Towards people living with dementia
		Regarding conflicting interests or values
		Education and encouragement of carers
	Judgements about abuse and neglect	
Specific circumstances involving decision-making		Driving
		Intimate relationships
		Genetic investigations
		Monitoring
		Use of antibiotics
		Use of antipsychotics
		Need for neuroimaging
		Covert medication
		Restraint
		Artificial feeding
		End of life and palliative care
		The risk of suicide

They also tend to raise the ethical approaches I discussed in Chapter 4: in the gendered examples I have just used, feminist and care ethics would loom large with an emphasis on relationships and communication, as well as on the virtues. In short, real people raise a raft of issues that do not always readily engage with the major ethical theories (apart, I think, from virtue ethics).

Dementia-specific ethical issues

Can we be more specific about the ethical issues that arise in connection with dementia rather than in connection with other conditions? Luckily,

Strech et al. (2013) have tackled this question and concluded that there are 56 ethical issues that crop up in clinical dementia care (see Table 15.2). (By the way, Daniel Strech was also involved in Götzelmann et al. (2021) showing a persistent commitment to the usefulness of this sort of systematic qualitative review.)

Table 15.2 again points to the breadth but also to the depth of ethical issues that arise in dementia care. Here is not the place to discuss these issues further. Some have already been mentioned in earlier chapters, such as capacity, decision-making, advance decisions and consent, as well as autonomy, stigma, values, risks and benefits. Many of the remaining issues will be tackled in Part 4 of this book on dilemmas in practice. For specific examples of the issues, it is worthwhile consulting Table DS1 (The spectrum of disease specific ethical issues in dementia care), which is complemented by quotations from the original literature and appears in the online supplement to Strech et al. (2013). For further comment on the issues see Hughes and Strech (2017).

One spin-off from this research has been studies that have looked at the extent to which these disease-specific ethical issues are picked up and considered in national dementia guidelines. Knüppel et al. (2013) found that the proportion of ethical issues identified in national clinical guidelines ranged from 22 per cent to 77 per cent, with a median of 49.5 per cent. In other words, guidelines varied quite considerably in terms of their guidance on ethics. A later review of Danish guidelines reached a similar conclusion, suggesting that practitioners need more guidance on ethical issues (Schou-Juul et al. 2022).

Conclusion

The literature shows that the predominant conversation about ethics has been from the point of view of professionals, both practitioners in health and social care as well as ethicists and other interested academics. The views of family carers are reasonably well represented too. The perspectives of people living with dementia are largely, although not entirely, absent. This will change, at least as far as people in the mild to moderate stages of dementia are concerned. Understanding the views of people living with severe dementia will remain a challenge.

In this chapter I have sought to consider the breadth and nature of the research on ethical issues in connection with dementia. It is of note both that there is change in the issues and that, to some extent, they remain the same.

In Baldwin et al. (2003) we were able to demonstrate: (i) issues which seem to remain central to ethical discussion in connection with dementia, such as decision-making and end-of-life care; (ii) one issue that seemed to appear, disappear and then re-appear, namely genetics; and (iii) one – quality of life – that appeared briefly and then disappeared. Quality of life remains an issue in the dementia literature, but its ethical nature is scarcely as discussed as it once was.

Another interesting thing to emerge from the research was that, by the year 2000, issues were being discussed discretely rather than in connection with other issues. An exception to this was the pairing of research and consent: two issues that continued to be discussed together. But consent was not being discussed so much in conjunction with other issues such as those around treatment. This reflects the professional-focused nature of the literature at the time. I doubt this has changed much, although it should do as research increasingly starts to reflect the views of people living with dementia and their close carers.

The content of the discussion of some issues might also have changed. Notably, in connection with technology, around the year 2000 we were discussing electronic tracking and tagging devices. Now the spectrum of technological possibilities – from robots to smart homes – is much broader (see Chapter 19). Nevertheless, the ethics remains the same. There will inevitably be new things to think about, but the basis of what is right and wrong, what makes some things good and some things bad, has not changed even if our conclusions about moral issues have shifted.

Part **4**

Dilemmas in Practice

16 The Nuffield Council's framework

Introduction

The Nuffield Council's report, *Dementia: Ethical Issues*, has already been mentioned several times in this book (Nuffield Council on Bioethics 2009). At the start of the report, it sets out a framework which informed the way it approached particular ethical issues. Here I shall present an overview of that framework as a prelude to further discussion in this part of the book of dilemmas in practice.

The intention is not to present further details of the report. Readers are encouraged to consult the full work which is freely available online (see Nuffield Council on Bioethics 2009). It is worthwhile doing so because the report is in itself akin to a textbook on ethical issues in dementia and it certainly demonstrates the breadth and depth of dementia-specific ethical issues. The report picked up 43 of the 56 dementia-specific ethical issues identified in Strech et al. (2013), which was more than any other publication they reviewed. The framework I shall discuss will not be to the fore in Part 4, but its influence will be apparent. It sets us off in the right direction.

Having said this, I should declare an interest, which is that I was fortunate enough to be on the working party that produced the report (and I was later on the Council). So, my enthusiasm for the report cannot be called wholly objective, even if the report has been highly regarded (Hughes 2020a; Knüppel et al. 2013).

The framework consists of six components, which I shall discuss in turn, albeit briefly.

Component 1: A case-based approach to ethical decisions

This takes us back to Chapter 5 and the discussion of casuistry. The report commended the approach of Jonsen and Toulmin (1988) and highlighted a three-step process. The first step was to identify and clarify the relevant facts. If a person living with dementia is starting to become agitated, the ethical response will be determined by, for instance, knowing whether or not there is a urinary infection. If we also learned that the person had recently been bereaved, this would suggest other ways in which we might be helpful. There can be a variety of ethical responses, but these will be determined by being clear on the facts.

The second step is to identify, interpret and apply relevant ethical values. We would not wish to restrain the agitated person unless there were some danger to that person or to someone else. In other words, autonomy, beneficence and non-maleficence are all applicable. If there were a urinary infection and antibiotics seemed necessary, but the person was refusing to take them, we might have to consider the use of covert medication (see Chapter 23). What would the person have thought about this? How do the staff feel about using this deception? What are the views of the family? These questions are questions about values: around truth-telling, trust, care, relationships and so on.

The third step involves comparison with other similar (paradigm or sentinel) cases where it has been clear what should be done. In the case of a bereavement, it might be that staff have experience of a family visiting more frequently and bringing photo albums, including pictures of the deceased person. If this helped in the past, it might help now, partly by encouraging talk about the person who has died. But this will depend on temperament and on the severity of dementia, which will differ from case to case. Perhaps in other cases an anxiolytic medication at a low dose for as short a time as possible has helped. Or perhaps a mixture of approaches would be helpful.

Component 2: The nature of dementia

Because dementia results from a brain disorder it is reasonable to regard it as a harm. Of course, as with a disease such as diabetes, there is a mild stage when the quality of someone's life will hardly be affected, but even mild effects are not good. Regarding dementia in this negative way is not the same as regarding the person negatively.

Three things follow: (a) research is important, not solely with a view to curing dementia, but also to improve the quality of the lives of people living with dementia; (b) slowing the rate of decline in dementia, as long as side effects do not outweigh benefits, must be a good thing; and (c) when there are decisions about resource allocation, dementia should be regarded in the same way as other diseases and funded accordingly.

Component 3: Quality of life in dementia

The report took the line 'that quality of life with dementia can, given proper care, be positive overall for most people, even though the onset of dementia will inevitably lead to the loss or diminution of some valued aspects of a person's life' (Nuffield Council on Bioethics 2009: §2.20, p. 24). The report went on to recognize that some people might value 'a certain level of reflective and deliberative awareness' to such an extent as to feel that there could not be any good quality of life in dementia. They may even then feel that life with dementia would not be worth living. But the report rejected this view for three reasons: (a) a person's life is of value even if there is severe cognitive impairment (this has been Stephen Post's line for many years (see Post 2006)); (b) in dementia the person's quality of life depends largely on the input of those caring for the person, so education and support are vital in order to maintain quality of care and thereby quality of life (this was Tom Kitwood's view (Kitwood 1997a)); and (c) we should take a positive approach to quality of life in dementia because this is more likely to enable people to live well, whereas a negative view is likely to encourage poor quality of life (this is connected to Steve Sabat's argument about malignant positioning (see Sabat 2001: 124–125)). As I argued in Chapter 10, if we have whole sight we can guard against glib assertions about a person's quality of life, which can undermine both the person's dignity and human rights.

Component 4: Promoting interests in autonomy and well-being

According to the report, 'negative' and 'rationalistic' accounts of autonomy are 'not only insufficient in the context of dementia but also problematic. They are problematic because they may promote a negative view of dependence ...' (§2.30, p. 27). The working party wished to emphasize three perspectives. First, to enable autonomy we have to give active support in order to encourage the person 'to retain and express their sense of self, rather than simply being protected from harm or interference' (§2.31, p. 27). Secondly, because we are situated in relationships it is important that we also enable and promote autonomy by 'enabling and fostering relationships that are important to the person' (§2.32, p. 27). And, thirdly, we should pay attention not solely to the rationality of decision-making, but to its emotional side too. Hence, if someone is happily engaged in an activity, then we can presume that the person is consenting to that activity even in the absence of a formal consent procedure. For a variety of reasons, therefore, the report encouraged the idea of relational autonomy, which we discussed in Chapter 8.

Moment-to-moment well-being is something that can be ensured by positive interactions. It is the sort of thing picked up by Kitwood's observational tool, Dementia Care Mapping (see Chapter 10 and Kitwood 2019: 52 – 54; as well as the discussion by Bob Wood in Kitwood (2019): pp. 138–140). Even if the person's recall is so poor that a brief conversation will soon be forgotten, such a conversation supports well-being whilst it lasts and continues to have an influence on the person's overall sense of well-being. Cognitive dysfunction, on the other hand, can erode the person's ability to take part in enjoyable activities. So both moment-to-moment well-being and cognitive function need to be balanced in estimations of a person's well-being. Generally, meaningful activities will increase well-being.

Component 5: Solidarity

In a separate report for the Nuffield Council on 'solidarity', Prainsack and Buyx (2011) provided this working definition: 'solidarity signifies shared practices reflecting a collective commitment to carry 'costs' (financial, social, emotional, or otherwise) to assist others' (§5.3, p. 46). They emphasized that solidarity is a set of practices, not simply an internal sentiment, that can be carried out at various levels from the personal to the national and international. Nevertheless, differences can be detected between solidarity at the national level, where welfare arrangements accept that we have obligations towards anonymous others, and solidarity at the personal level, where a free choice is made on the basis of a sense of love and duty with respect to someone who is known. Two members of the Nuffield Council's working party regarded these differences as reflecting sociological and moral conceptualizations of solidarity (ter Meulen and Wright, 2012). It may be, however, that – rather than two concepts – we simply have different manifestations of Prainsack and Buyx's (2011) 'costs' under the one umbrella concept of solidarity.

In the dementia report, it stated:

> When considering the idea of solidarity, those receiving care and support should not be seen simply as people with particular rights or as victims of disease or disability, but rather as citizens with both their own needs and a societal role. People with dementia may need assistance in order to be empowered and given a voice, but they should also be included as citizens with their own views on how solidarity should be practised, and with their own contribution to make.
>
> (Nuffield Council on Bioethics 2009: §2.45, p. 30)

We are, as the report says, 'fellow travellers' with those who live with dementia, with duties to support and care for them. 'Solidarity is relevant also to individual relationships: personal solidarity, in the form of love, loyalty and compassion, is the basis and motivation for giving care to one's partner, parent or friend' (§2.44, p. 30). Solidarity can be regarded as a virtue, both as an inner disposition and as a way of acting by which we flourish as human beings (see Chapter 3). The notion also links to justice and the requirement that there should be a just (fair) allocation of resources. Thus, it is a rich notion and one that is relevant to many aspects of dementia care, indeed it is the basis of care itself.

Component 6: Recognizing personhood

We have already discussed personhood in Chapter 13. It is interesting to note that citizenship has emerged as relevant to solidarity. Our interconnectedness is a feature of solidarity, but (as we have seen) is also deeply embedded in the nature of personhood. The report latches on to the ideas of bodily identity and social connections, but also mentions emotional and spiritual aspects of a person's life. These facets of our lives as persons come together to suggest that the value and values of a person's life must always be respected. We require Heideggerian solicitude (see Chapter 9). It is personhood that gives us our moral and legal standing.

Conclusion

The Nuffield Council's framework can be used to support many decisions in dementia care and it sends us in the direction of recognizing the human rights of persons who are living with the diagnosis. They need to be seen as persons, like you and me, who can express their autonomy, usually in relation to others, even if they are hindered by infirmity. People living with dementia can be encouraged and helped to engage with society if the environment allows them to do so; and to be enabled in this way – through solidarity – is potentially to boost their well-being, their personhood and their citizenship. The components of the framework provide a background against which we can decide the merits and demerits of a variety of arguments around dilemmas that occur in the lives of people who live with dementia and of their carers. It is to such dilemmas we now turn.

In the chapters that follow, which each consider particular dilemmas that arise in dementia care, I shall largely follow the same format. First, I shall present a vignette: a fictional story (albeit one concocted on the basis of real experience, whether my own or reported in the literature) to highlight the ethical dilemma. Secondly, I shall discuss the relevant research literature (convenience samples rather than systematic reviews). Thirdly, I shall reflect on the dilemma or dilemmas using the notion of patterns of practice as described in Chapter 6.

17 Diagnosis

Introduction

The first area I shall discuss centres on ethical issues in connection with the diagnosis of dementia.

Vignette: Freda Smith's reluctance to be diagnosed

Mrs. Smith, a widow who lived on her own, had shown signs of increasing cognitive impairment for some while. Her daughter was very worried about her. The GP visited her at home (she would not attend the surgery and had become annoyed when her daughter tried to make an appointment for her) and tried to persuade her to accept a referral to the local memory clinic. She refused, saying there was nothing wrong with her, that it was just her age, but that she was coping perfectly. The GP did notice some deficits in terms of her recall and orientation but felt it best not to push matters. Six months later, one cold night she locked herself out of her house and her daughter was worried sick. The GP made a referral to the local old age psychiatry team asking for an assessment at home.

When the team (a psychiatrist and nurse) visited and revealed who they were, Freda became extremely annoyed. She denied any problems and gave semi-plausible excuses for the various things that had happened. She told them they were not to discuss her personal business with her daughter, whom she claimed was just 'after her house'. When the psychiatrist gently tried to suggest that there were now some noticeable difficulties with some aspects of her memory, Freda screamed at him to get out of her house and said she was not interested in hearing anything about her memory, which was, as far as she was concerned, good enough. She said it was her right to live as she chose. The doctor and nurse left, but the nurse visited again a week later having promised the daughter to do so. Freda was then more placid, but the moment the nurse started to say anything about memory, or forgetfulness, or difficulties around the home, she started to become irate and agitated. If they spoke about non-threatening issues, she was calm and pleasant and was happy for the nurse to help her with a few tasks, such as throwing away some food items from the fridge which had started to rot.

Ethical issues in connection with diagnosis

Freda is an extreme case in that she decidedly does not wish to have a diagnosis, but she was not exceptional at the turn of the century, when

Marzanski (2000) found that 9 out of 30 participants did not wish to know what was wrong with them or receive any information. These days, many people do wish to know what is wrong with them when they sense there is something amiss. But it is not uncommon to find people who are ambivalent about receiving a diagnosis or who, because they do not recognize any problems, do not quite understand why they are being seen by a doctor or other professional. Perhaps an initial place to start our discussion of Freda and of the ethical issues around diagnostic disclosure is to recognize that it is not totally irrational to wish to avoid a diagnosis. The almost globally accepted professional or official mantra is that early diagnosis is a good thing, but it is not clear this is always the experience of those who actually live with a diagnosis.

We have already discussed stigma (Chapter 7). In Chapter 14, we discussed the use of biomarkers to make earlier diagnoses and the possibility of making a prodromal diagnosis of non-dementia Alzheimer's disease (that is, where there is evidence of Alzheimer's pathology but an absence of illness). We also have to recognize that the absence of curative treatment, and the marginal utility of the current relatively few medications, undermines to some extent the value of a diagnosis. All that can be said is that post-diagnostic support might be valuable. But someone as feisty as Freda might question what this actually entails. She may or may not welcome the suggestion that she could make a Lasting Power of Attorney (LPA) or, if she were lucky, join a group to discuss the diagnosis she does not wish to receive.

To say that the mantra in favour of early diagnosis is the conscious or subconscious result of a cabal of researchers (who seek funding for the next research project), drug companies (who wish to make profits) and governments (intent on keeping the pharmaceutical industry based in their countries), inevitably sounds like mere conspiracy theory. But to raise questions about the drive for early diagnoses is certainly not unethical (Le Couteur et al. 2013). It may be that generally, at a public health level, it is a good thing to diagnose people earlier, but at the individual level the person's wishes and values should be heard without the pressure of the public health message. As so often, it is the nuance of individual cases that is crucial, even if on the whole an earlier diagnosis is better than a later one.

It also throws into light the accepted but controversial diagnosis of mild cognitive impairment (MCI), mentioned in Chapter 1. Lohmeyer et al. (2021) showed a good deal of uncertainty amongst those diagnosed with MCI. The participants were uncertain about the meaning of 'MCI' and about the validity of specific biomarkers. This reflects concerns and uncertainties about the concept of MCI highlighted some years ago: about how the label might affect the person's sense of self (Corner and Bond 2006); about the status of the concept itself (Graham and Ritchie 2006) and its clinical standing (Gaines and Whitehouse 2006). It is a diagnosis, which in practice is loosely defined, but not a disease, and in itself carries no certainty for the individual – not even the certainty of future dementia. It is true that 'MCI' has become accepted parlance, part of normal practice, and that the fifth edition of the American *Diagnostic and Statistical Manual* (DSM-5) has embraced it under the rubric of 'mild neurocognitive disorder', but the conceptual problems with the terminology persist.

Freda, who does not wish to hear the word 'dementia', might be impressed by the thought that we should get rid of it. Hachinski (2008) declared that 'The concept of dementia is obsolete. It combines categorical misclassification with etiologic imprecision' (p. 2172). Meanwhile, Trachtenberg and Trojanowski (2008) argued that 'dementia' was a word to be forgotten. It is unkind and 'can easily rob patients of their humanity in the eyes of others and, more important, in their own eyes'. They continued: 'At its unkindest, it is a word without hope, which is a crucial tool when faced with a devastating illness' (p. 593).

I have also advocated that 'dementia' should be replaced by some other words (Hughes 2011b: 12–19). This is partly because it is simply insulting to tell someone they are out of their minds, which is what the etymology suggests. So 'dementia' encourages stigma. But it is also, as Hachinski (2008) suggested, diagnostically imprecise. Hearing that someone has dementia does not tell you what is going on. They may have movement problems, difficulties with speech, behavioural disinhibition or whatever.

In place of 'dementia' I commended (Hughes 2011b: 16–19) a descriptive syndromal diagnosis: acquired diffuse neurocognitive dysfunction (ADND). I argued this was no more complicated to understand than attention deficit hyperactivity disorder (ADHD) and serves to explain what is going on. The exact type of ADND could then be specified as Lewy body disease, vascular disease and so on. Some were critical of my suggestion, but DSM-5 no longer refers to 'dementia' and instead uses the label 'major neurocognitive disorder' (American Psychiatric Association 2013). The point is that the word 'dementia' can be regarded as otiose. There are ethical reasons to discard it. Indeed, some go further and say that even the more specific label of 'Alzheimer's disease' should also be discarded; in its place we should talk of brain ageing, which occurs in different ways in us all (Whitehouse and George 2008).

Turning to the question of diagnostic disclosure, until the end of the 20th century the tendency was to be paternalistic; this became gradually less so in the 1990s (Rice and Warner 1994; Gilliard and Gwilliam 1996; Clafferty et al. 1998). Many practitioners felt it was not necessary or would be too upsetting to tell people they had dementia. By the end of that decade, in a research environment, carers expressed the view that patients and families can benefit from being told the diagnosis (Smith et al. 1998). The researchers noted that one carer had felt abandoned after diagnosis, emphasizing the need for post-diagnostic support; and they pointed to the ethical issues of autonomy, the right to know and confidentiality.

Even at the start of the decade, Drickamer and Lachs (1992) had posed the question: should patients with Alzheimer's disease be told their diagnosis? On the whole, they thought they should because of the need to maximize autonomy which requires that people are given the best available information (even if it is uncertain) and enabled to make advance decisions. They highlighted the fundamental requirement to be truthful. Nevertheless, they also recognized that the erosion of decision-making capacity in dementia might make things difficult and that there had to be sensitivity to the possibility of the diagnosis causing harm, such as depression. Certainly Husband (2000) found worries that giving the diagnosis seemed likely to cause low self-esteem, self-stigmatization and impaired quality of life, although the possibility of helpful interventions was also noted. The suggestions of Drickamer and Lachs (1992) about the ethics of diagnostic disclosure remain convincing.

The studies in the late 1990s and around the turn of the century almost certainly reflected the new pressure to be open with people because of the licensing of the cholinesterase inhibitor drugs and later of memantine. Valid consent to take the drugs required honest diagnostic disclosure. Pinner (2000) stated in an editorial: 'It is not a question of whether to tell the truth or not; we must be truthful to our patients. When and how are the questions that need to be explored, with the help, of course, of our patients' (p. 515).

At the start of the new century, there was still evidence that in many cases people were not being given the diagnosis, even if rates were improving, often because of concerns about the consequences for the person's mental health (Marzanski 2000; Jha et al. 2001; Pinner and Bouman 2002). A study in Finland seemed to show an improvement: 93 per cent of carers confirmed that a diagnosis had been given openly to the person living with dementia (Laakkonen et al. 2008). Nevertheless, 55 per cent of those with Alzheimer's disease had developed depressive symptoms. Recall that Schmutte et al. (2021) showed a 53 per cent increase, compared to the general adult population in the USA, in the suicide rate in the first year after diagnosis. Contrariwise, more than 10 years previously Purandare et al. (2009) found a relatively low prevalence of suicide in people with dementia in England and Wales and fewer psychiatric symptoms before death when compared to controls.

Many of those writing at this time were able to give ethical arguments to support their commentaries. Marzanski (2000) gave arguments in favour of truth-telling: respect for autonomy, the need for trust in the doctor-patient relationship and acknowledgement of reciprocal obligations, fidelity and promise-keeping. He also gave arguments for limited truth-telling or lying. First, the therapeutic privilege: 'Honesty should not be confused with cruel openness' (p. 112). So, if there is the threat of harm following disclosure, 'benevolent deception' might be justified. Secondly, there may not seem to be an ethical imperative to tell the truth if the person is unlikely to understand the information. Thirdly, some people simply do not wish to know their diagnoses. Marzanski's very sensible conclusion was that we should ask people if they wish to be given information about what might be wrong.

Pinner and Bouman (2002) found that older people generally wanted to be fully informed, but the views of people living with dementia were largely unknown – a point confirmed by Bamford et al.'s (2004) systematic review of the literature. Pinner and Bouman (2002) highlighted the place of the ethical principles of autonomy, beneficence and non-maleficence (see Chapter 3) in deciding whether or not to disclose the diagnosis. They also outlined their practice, which was (as suggested by Marzanski 2000) to ask people if they wished to know a diagnosis. Where the relatives did not wish the person living with dementia to know the diagnosis, they commended a 'patient-led' discussion – involving the family and the person with the diagnosis. They wisely suggested that 'disclosure must not be seen as a one-off event, but as an ongoing, dynamic process and a fundamental part of the care of a patient with dementia' (p. 133).

On the basis of ethnographic research, Hillman (2017) agreed with this point: 'Focusing on a distinct moment of diagnosis disclosure … fails to recognise the negotiated nature of ethical decision-making that occurs over time and in collaboration…, and the ethical interest in broader contextual issues beyond the 'moment' of disclosure' (p. 57).

The Nuffield Council's report encouraged the idea of a 'timely' diagnosis (Nuffield Council 2009: §3.17, p. 43). This was suggested to the working party which produced the report by the Alzheimer's Society (footnote 134 on p. 43). A 'timely diagnosis' can be defined 'as when people with dementia and those around them are ready for and will benefit from it' (Brayne and Kelly 2019: 124). In Brooker et al. (2014) a diagnosis is 'timely' when it can be used by people to '… make sense of what is happening to them, make lifestyle changes and plan for the future' (p. 686). This was in the recommendations of the European Union's ALCOVE project, which also set out four principles 'to maximise benefit and to reduce harm associated with diagnosis at an earlier stage' (Brooker et al. 2014: 682). They were:

1 Diagnosis should be available and accessible to all when changes in cognitive function are first noticed;
2 Fear and stigma need to be decreased in order to increase diagnosis;
3 The person's rights and wishes about diagnosis should be centre stage;
4 Giving and receiving a diagnosis of dementia should be seen as part of an adjustment to living with dementia (pp. 686–687).

It is incontrovertible that when people are seeking help they should be diagnostically assessed. The worry, however, is that – despite the benefits of an early diagnosis – we are witnessing the medicalization of normal ageing. If we look for changes in cognitive function as we age, we shall find them. This does not mean that we require a diagnosis of dementia. When that diagnosis is required is an evaluative judgement which must be largely guided by the person concerned. The worry is that societal pressures will overrule individual judgement. The ethical point is that caution is required rather than blanket policies. Of course, blanket policies can produce benefits at a societal level which are not seen at a personal level.

Just to pick up one remaining thread from the story of Freda Smith: confidentiality. She does not wish her daughter to be involved in discussions about her health. During evidence-gathering for the Nuffield Council's report (see Chapter 16), we heard that some family carers were upset when doctors would not involve them in decisions about the person they cared for because of the need to maintain confidentiality. The report suggested that 'the appropriate attitude of professionals and care workers towards families should be that of partners in care, reflecting the solidarity being shown within the family'

(Nuffield Council on Bioethics 2009: §3.12, p. 41). Of course, if someone living with dementia has the appropriate capacity, then that person's refusal to share information must be respected. But if they lack capacity – for instance if they have no idea of the risks they have been taking or of the multiple times they have been calling their relatives with the same request – and cannot understand why their families might need to be involved, then a decision can be made in the person's best interests and for the sake of their well-being, which may or may not involve sharing confidences, for example about the diagnosis. Elsewhere, we have suggested that, although confidentiality is an important principle, it 'is less important than the respect and trust implicit in the nexus of caring relationships that surround and aim to support the person with dementia' (Hughes and Louw 2002a: 150).

Patterns of practice and Freda Smith

Freda does not want a diagnosis and does not seemingly want help, although she is happy to see a friendly face. Thinking of patterns of practice leads to a focus on coherence. First, there is the need for internal intra-practice coherence. What does the practice of giving a diagnosis entail? Well, it needs to be done in a certain way. Practitioners need to understand the person's own understanding or expectations and 'warning shots' need to be given, rather than the bad news being blurted out. Whitehouse (2004) said: 'The conversation about diagnosis sets the stage for what will hopefully be a healing relationship between patient and clinician' (p. 124). Forcing the issue with Freda, therefore, will never do. Frisoni (2004) made the discerning comment that 'patients with anxiety-related behaviours do not ask for the diagnosis because they do not wish to know – vaguely and indistinctly they know already and their anxiety would increase intolerably if the verdict were made explicit' (p. 125). It is a question of starting where the person is and moving on to discover what the person can tolerate, a point recognized in the ALCOVE principles set out above (Brooker et al. 2014). Freda has made it obvious that she cannot tolerate the implications of an assessment. Post (2004) regarded compassionate disclosure of the diagnosis as 'a moral act of respect for patients', but he also went on to say it is 'an opportunity for human resilience and community, and a necessary practical step toward future planning' (p. 126). Respecting Freda implies keeping clear of the diagnosis: she does not wish to show resilience beyond what she is already showing.

Similar considerations are in play when it comes to intra-personal internal coherence. Many commentators have made something of the analogy with diagnoses of cancer. Some years ago, that diagnosis would have been avoided if possible; but not now. Breaking bad news in cancer care is a reasonable paradigm for dementia care (Maguire 1999). The question to ask is: what would I do in other circumstances? Employing compassionate and sensitive techniques, I would not seek to impose investigations or diagnoses on people. Of course, there might be extreme examples where compulsory care is inevitable. One can imagine this eventually in Freda's case if things do not go well. For now, a casuistic path can be trod (see Chapter 5). Are there in fact differences between cancer and dementia? Some cancers are curable, dementia is not. Cancers can be regarded as extrinsic to the self, whereas dementia threatens something more intrinsic to the self perhaps. So whilst, to be coherent, our practices might be more like cancer, the need to push a diagnosis might well be regarded as less of an imperative in dementia care.

But what about external coherence, where we wish to establish coherence between a person's patterns of practice and the moral norms that define and constitute the good life for human beings? That is, what virtues are required in this pattern of practice? The virtue of practical wisdom is frequently going to be relevant and may be seen in the notion of a 'timely diagnosis', discussed above.

But we need more than this. We also need compassion, honesty, bravery, genuine warmth and hope. The team need to engage with Freda Smith, as the nurse is now doing, in an unthreatening manner, to provide a sense of security, friendship and hope. This may also help her daughter to feel less stressed, which in turn may help their relationship. The aim is to allow Freda to continue to live an independent life for as long as possible. This is to respect her autonomy; but we also need to be cognisant of her dependence. The importance of the relationships established at this point cannot be over-emphasized (not least because the professionals need to confirm the good intentions of Freda's daughter). Being-with now will ease any doing-to in the future. But more than this, making the journey to a diagnosis, and possibly not to a diagnosis, in a low-key, harmonious, supportive and loving manner coheres with the intention of allowing Freda to live as good a life as she can, given the reality of the situation for her.

Conclusion

Getting diagnostic disclosure correct is a complex yet crucial task. Practitioners must attune to the individual dynamics of the person's situation. People have a right to know their diagnoses, but only if they wish to, which most will. How, when and where are the crucial questions, as well as by whom? Much will depend on the quality of the relationships that are or can be established and the trust and hope that such relationships engender (Merl et al. 2022). Giving the diagnosis is not detached from the rest of our practices. So our approach to the person to whom we can give a diagnosis of a particular form of dementia must sit within and square with our general approach to other people who are potentially vulnerable, anxious or threatened.

18 Independence and driving

Introduction

The diagnosis of any serious illness can pose a threat to one's independence. Especially in dementia – where there may be the feeling that your standing as an independent autonomous agent is being undermined, that your opinions and wishes are being ignored, that you are simply being protected and where stigmatization and self-stigmatization are a reality – worries about independence naturally emerge. A potent symbol of the loss of independence comes when a person is told they can no longer drive. I have even heard it sardonically said that the main function of a memory clinic is to stop people from driving; and this is certainly one of the things that people dread when they attend such clinics.

Here are some of the things we heard in the research we did with family carers:

- 'It was one of these great ethical dilemmas, because my husband's whole life was driving'
- 'I knew that would be the beginning of the end. I knew that when my mother lost her driving licence, she'd lose her fight to carry on, which is what happened really. Losing the car was incredibly traumatic because her car summed everything up for her. It was about independence, freedom, being in control. Driving symbolised all that' (Baldwin et al. 2005: 24–25).

If driving is a potent symbol of independence, it is not the only one. In a moving story, which emerged from research on quality of life carried out by Lynne Corner, Bob had always enjoyed running, but now had a diagnosis of dementia. Friends he had run with promised to take him out for a run, but then became hard to contact. His wife said: 'I don't think he ever got over that' (Corner and Hughes 2006: 92). Bob's wife, however, also felt there were unacceptable risks associated with him running, even though he was physically fit: 'Professionals legitimized the carer's feelings and no attempts were made to take on board just how important running was to Bob's self-concept'; all of this had 'a catastrophic effect on how he perceived himself' (p. 93).

This chapter briefly considers ethical issues around how the perception of risk affects independence, particularly in relation to driving.

Vignette: Misael Fischer's driving

Misael came to England when he was three years old with his parents who were fleeing Nazi oppression in Europe. He was a driver all his adult life. His first job was as a lorry driver, but later he became the manager of a successful transport company. When he was 76 years old, he was given a diagnosis of dementia. The following year, whilst visiting his GP, he was seen to reverse into another car in the surgery's car park causing minor damage to both cars. The GP took this as a sign that Misael was no longer able to drive and contacted the Driving and Vehicle Licensing Agency (DVLA). Misael's licence was revoked. He was furious but felt there was nothing he could do. He stopped going out and became increasingly depressed.

Ethics of risk-taking and driving as part of independent living

The Nuffield Council's report contained a recommendation that, instead of talking of 'risk assessments', we should always think in terms of 'risk-benefit assessments' (Nuffield Council on Bioethics 2009: §6.17, p. 101). This would ensure that, for any particular action, resource or service, the benefits would be considered as well as the risks and, moreover, the risks associated with *not* doing or providing whatever it might be would also be factored into relevant decisions. The reason for stressing the benefits as well as the risks was in order to maximize the person's autonomy and well-being. If we think of Bob, the runner (whom I described above), restricting his running – not allowing any risks attached to running – meant that he lost the benefits of open-air exercise and friendship. Similarly, Misael became depressed when he could no longer use his car. It might be surmised that the risks were great enough in one or other of these cases to justify the loss of autonomy and well-being. But even in the case of Misael, we do not yet know how great the risks might have been since he has not been fully assessed.

The Department of Health (2010) produced a report, *'Nothing Ventured, Nothing Gained'*, which also picked on this theme and spoke of 'risk enablement', which it regarded as a more person-centred approach to risk, where practitioners are encouraged to seek the least restrictive alternative to any intervention. All of this is aimed at supporting people with dementia to live at home.

In a very useful review of the literature, Bailey et al. (2013), as well as pointing to the ethical tension between non-maleficence and respect for autonomy, highlighted two narratives. One was the official narrative about risk enablement, whilst the other narrative reflected personal worries amongst professionals and families about risks. They also pointed to the 'growing recognition that risk needs to be considered as a subjective, experiential, dynamic and changing aspect of everyday life that concerns not just the individual but also their wider contexts' (p. 397).

Turning to driving, it remains the case that the extent to which dementia contributes to the overall chances of crashes occurring is uncertain (Fallon and O'Neill 2017). Obviously, safe driving becomes more difficult as cognitive function worsens, although there are no definitive neuropsychological tests that pin down exactly when driving becomes dangerous. In Great Britain, the DVLA (it is the Driver and Vehicle Agency (DVA) in Northern Ireland), in its official guidance, states: 'It is difficult to assess driving ability in people with dementia. DVLA acknowledges that there are varied presentations and rates of progression, and the decision on licensing is usually based on medical reports' (DVLA 2022: 87). Different countries will have different laws. In the USA, different states have different regulations. My interest, however, here and in other chapters, is to do with the underlying ethics rather than the particular laws and regulations, albeit I tend to draw on the laws from the jurisdiction with which I am most familiar. The difficulty for practitioners is to assess when risks become untenable (Wilson and Pinner 2020). The evidence suggests that in early dementia the risks associated with driving are no greater than those for other groups, such as young men (between 16 and 21 years old) and those with low blood alcohol concentrations (below 0.08 per cent) (Dubinsky et al. 2000).

Post (2000) stated:

> Although there is an indisputable duty to prevent people from driving if they clearly threaten community safety, this principle should not be applied prematurely or without individualized risk appraisal demonstrating impairment of driving ability
>
> (p. 47).

Bartlett and O'Connor (2010) pointed out that a free citizen can travel and use the transport system; but they also set the issue in a broader stage:

> From a disability perspective, the problem that needs to be addressed here is not how someone with a cognitive impairment copes with not being able to drive but how society must start to address the transport needs of a growing subsection of society
>
> (p. 100).

Recognizing the potential social impact if driving must cease, some have recommended specific conditions under which people with milder dementia might still drive, even if they should stop when dementia is more severe (Freedman and Freedman 1996; Shua-Haim and Gross 1996). In a sense, this suggests the difficulty with risks generally: we want to encourage the individual, but only up to a certain point, after which we become more draconian.

Patterns of practice and Misael Fischer

Healthcare practitioners of any sort practising in the UK are bound to tell anyone who has dementia of their responsibility to inform the DVLA or DVA of their diagnosis. There are also circumstances under which it is permissible for doctors to break confidentiality and inform the DVLA of the diagnosis (General Medical Council 2017). Some practitioners seem to regard protecting the public as an overriding responsibility, which can be a manifestation of power or a sign of low risk-tolerance.

A coherent practice would be to see confidentiality as an overarching responsibility, which is only negated by serious risks concerning which a judgement is required. This, after all, would be the practice in other areas of clinical work. The judgement about when driving is too risky to be tolerated in turn requires diligent and broad enquiries (Wilson and Pinner 2020).

But rather than having too readily to be judge and jury, my practice, where people were convinced of their driving abilities, was to encourage them to be assessed at a driving assessment centre. In the UK, as in other countries, there are networks of such centres. People seem to find it easier after a proper driving assessment to accept if they are told they cannot drive. At least there has then been a fair test. If the person refuses to be tested, persists in driving, does poorly in a number of key cognitive areas on testing and, crucially, if the family or others are concerned, then there would be a duty to inform people that they need to tell the DVLA about the diagnosis and the worries. If they do not inform the appropriate authority (and remember that there are also implications for the person's insurance), given a certain level of risk, professionals may then have to break confidentiality and inform the authority themselves.

In terms of external coherence, this sort of approach can show propriety, integrity, a sense of justice, honesty, prudence and realism. In the case of Misael Fischer, the seemingly peremptory manner in which the DVLA was informed did not show the sort of coherence required by a pattern of practice seeking to be person-centred. McKillop (2016) describes the real-life experience of losing your driving licence and how frustrating this is for the person living with dementia if proper assessment is lacking.

Conclusion

The responsibilities of all clinicians in the UK are outlined above. These might be slightly different in other countries. What about families? Well, if there is a concern about someone's driving, it makes ethical sense to say that this should be discussed and reported. There are more or less ethical ways to do this; it will depend on the circumstances. It may be possible to discuss the matter with the person concerned who might very reasonably then decide to give up driving. But it may be impossible to discuss it without causing a lot of anger, in which case it may be better for families to raise the issue with healthcare professionals. In any case, it always seems fairer to me to seek a driving assessment, unless the person's inability to drive is obvious. People living with dementia need to listen carefully to advice, but they should be informed that the option of formal testing of their driving is a possibility (presupposing that it is a possibility in the country in which they live).

Risks, including risks associated with driving, are rarely easy to judge with certainty. A degree of humility is required by all concerned. For what is at stake is both the safety of the public and the standing of the person as a citizen with rights, whose relational autonomy and dignity should be protected.

19 Technology

Introduction

On the one hand, assistive technology promises to improve the well-being and decrease the risks that potentially face people living with dementia. On the other, there are fears that technology reduces the quality and extent of human relationships. As was said in a study of healthy couples over the age of 70 years living in Sweden:

> Technical devices, regardless of the form in which they are used, are still only devices and cannot replace human relationships ... There was a fear that the person would be reduced to *a thing*, with relational coldness, detachment and instrumentality ... elders regard human encounters as fundamental in care
>
> (Harrefors et al. 2010: 1530–1531).

In this chapter, I shall look at the ethical principles and discussions around the arguments in favour of and against assistive technology, which is defined as 'any device or system that allows individuals to perform tasks they would otherwise be unable to do or increases the ease and safety with which tasks can be performed' (World Health Organization 2004: 10).

Vignette: Margaret Strathbone's robot

Mrs Strathbone lives in a large home on her own. She has a diagnosis of vascular dementia. Her son lives over 150 miles away. His mother insists on her independence but will accept no external help. A cause of much concern is that she needs to take her medication three times a day. Her GP feels she should be in a care home. Her son, however, buys a robot for her. The robot can tell her when she needs to take her medication. It can also offer her entertainment on its screen and can ask her questions to check she is all right and is not lonely. Mrs Strathbone loves the robot, but her brother feels it is demeaning for her to be holding conversations with a machine and feels that his nephew is trying to avoid his duty to look after his mother.

Ethical issues around assistive technology

A good way to start is to recognize how varied assistive technology now is: it is not simply electronic tagging and tracking, nor just alarms to remind you of this and that, it is whole smart homes, robots and a great variety of technical products which we now take for granted, from smartphones to virtual assistants such as Alexa. Not only has the range of products significantly increased in recent years, but so too has the literature. The aim here is to emphasize the relevant ethical issues.

Evans et al. (2015) undertook a systematic review of assistive technology aimed at dementia. They found such technology was helpful with activities of daily living, monitoring safety and helping with healthcare. Fewer devices were found to help with the social aspects of dementia, such as behavioural issues and recreation. Pappadà et al. (2021) also found that the technology was well-accepted and helpful, although they noted the lack of common methodologies in the research. They made the interesting observation that assistive technology is likely to be particularly useful during a pandemic when human contact is otherwise restricted. Di Lorito, Duff, et al. (2021) showed how an exercise programme could be delivered to good effect by video during the coronavirus disease (COVID-19) pandemic. Certainly, in their scoping review Budak et al. (2021) were confident enough to suggest that the provision of psychosocial interventions by assistive technologies might be a useful way to combat loneliness.

A further systematic review, by Sriram et al. (2019), provided a handy list of the many types and uses of assistive technology. The most commonly used devices were for safety and security. They suggested that people living with dementia and their carers should help to co-design devices. Sriram et al. (2019) specifically considered ethical issues. They recorded that carers weighed up a sense of security against autonomy. Indeed, they found that concerns over safety seemed to negate all other ethical issues. Carers agreed that people living with dementia should be as involved as possible in decisions about the use of assistive technology. But there seemed to be unresolved issues around who had the power to start and end the use of technical devices.

Lynn et al. (2019), in a systematic review that looked specifically at care homes, also detailed the types of intervention using assistive technology. As others have done, they noted 'methodological heterogeneity' in the studies. On the whole they found a broad range of positive outcomes, from complementing the work of staff, to providing a sense of independence and enhancing well-being and social interaction. Assistive technology also provided some challenges, such as false alarms, problems with reliability, staff ignoring alarms when they were too repetitive or being anxious about using technology. Also, the devices did not reduce falls and there were worries about costs. It was clearly vital that devices had to be acceptable to the people living with dementia. The authors raised the important ethical issue of privacy.

Kruse et al. (2020) were largely positive on the basis of their systematic review. They found that the commonest facilitators to the use of assistive technology were that the carers wanted it and it enabled independence. (This fits with the case of Mrs Strathbone of course.) The top two barriers to the use of technology were its cost and the fact that people with dementia did not want it. Medically, in the studies they scrutinized, they found improved cognitive function, increased activities of daily living and improved autonomy, although the validity of any claim to increased autonomy can be called into question. Indeed, the references to autonomy seem odd in that in one study mentioned by Kruse et al. (2020) it is said to have increased autonomy, but the study also says that people living with dementia did not want assistive technology! Other studies simply state that independence has increased, which suggests autonomy has too. In any case, an ethically significant point is that the paper noted a dichotomy between carers, who tend to want assistive technology, and people living with dementia who do not. The question of power – and whose autonomy is improved – is to the fore.

One important message from Sanders and Scott (2020) is that assistive technology does not provide a 'one size fits all' solution. As in other reviews, a relative lack of good quality evidence could be detected. Again, it was seen as important that people living with dementia should be involved in the design of devices. They also highlighted a lack of trust in the devices. However, importantly they were able to distinguish between assistive technologies that were used 'by', 'with' and 'on' the person with dementia. It is easy to see how these distinctions also sketch out three different ethical approaches to the technology. People living with dementia and using technology themselves would seem to cause few problems if this represents genuinely autonomous choices. People working 'with' others, their carers, to find technological solutions is obviously a way to build trust in each other and in the technology. Where technology has to be used 'on' people living with dementia, a raft of problems emerges, presumably as dementia becomes more advanced. All of the issues to do with capacity and consent (Chapter 11) and best interests (Chapter 12) become apparent.

In a study of robotic pets, which can be regarded as social robots whose aim is to interact and communicate with the human being by following behavioural cues, Koh et al. (2021) found positive associations between the use of these robots and the domains of mood and affect, communication and social interaction, companionship, and other indicators of well-being. These reflect ways in which the pets can be regarded as ethically beneficent. On the other hand, there was also evidence of the worrying (maleficent) effects of the robotic animals in that they could be misperceived as live animals, people could become too attached to them, there were some negative reactions and there were concerns about hygiene and cost.

In an important study, Lariviere et al. (2021) looked at how assistive technology was actually used in practice. They showed that, in real-life situations, devices were not always used as designers had perhaps intended. Yet, carers and people living with dementia could devise ways to use the technology to suit their needs. How effective a device might be depended on the relationship between the carer and the person with dementia, how they had understood the instructions about the use of the technology and how they had adapted it to their environment. Value judgements would inevitably affect how people navigated the decisions required to acquire and use assistive technology.

In an exemplary randomized controlled trial, Howard et al. (2021):

> ... found provision of home-based technology, installed following an individual needs assessment within current practice in England, had no significant effect on the time that people with dementia were able to continue to live independently in their own homes. There was no evidence of cost-effectiveness ...
>
> (p. 887).

In itself, this study is a warning – an ethical one and one that has had to be learnt many times – that it should not be presumed that a good idea necessarily works. As John Hunter (1728–1793) wrote to Edward Jenner (1749–1823) in a letter of 1775, 'Why not try the experiment?' (Wells 1974: 144). It is better that we ascertain the facts before we commit to interventions which may, after all, prove costly and of little real effect. Facts will help to shape our values (see Table 5.1). There is a worry that the technology itself is leading the way, whereas the real needs of people living with the diagnosis should come first.

This leads us to consider the ethical issues more specifically. We have already highlighted above the notions of safety and beneficence, non-maleficence, autonomy, privacy and trust. Elsewhere, in connection with electronic tagging, we found concerns about civil liberties, stigma and dignity, especially amongst community psychiatric nurses; most people, however, did not have objections to electronic tagging, especially when this was weighed against alternatives, such as close observation (with a view to restraint) and locked doors (Hughes et al. 2008).

In a sophisticated overview in connection with using assistive technology in the community for people living with dementia, Zwijsen et al. (2011) were able to categorize and summarize the ethical issues, as shown in Table 19.1.

In discussing their research, Zwijsen et al. (2011) make the point that assistive technology is often presented in the community as the way to avoid long-term care, so it may not be a completely free choice (it is an 'adaptive preference'). As discussed above, Howard et al. (2021) would tend to suggest that the choice is not even relevant. In any case, we have to recognize that assistive technology is used in long-term care too. Zwijsen et al. go on to highlight, quoting Agich (2003), the extent to which 'actual autonomy' has to be grounded 'in the concrete social world of everyday life' (Zwijsen et al. 2011: 425). Here, assistive technology acquires layers of complexity (as shown by the ethnography of Lariviere et al. 2021) so that declaring it simply good or bad is misplaced. Rather than stressing an abstract notion of autonomy, it would be better to view people as 'social, dependent and reciprocal' (p. 425). We are embedded as persons in complex biopsychosocial and spiritual realities, which are also economic, political and so on (see Chapter 13).

In another innovative study (involving some of the same team as Zwijsen et al. 2011), Niemeijer et al. (2011) considered how surveillance technology was viewed by care professionals and ethicists. They highlighted 'an inherent duality rooted in the moral conflict between safety and freedom' (p. 307).

Table 19.1   Ethical themes and sub-themes in connection with assistive technology and dementia (adapted from Table 1 in Zwijsen et al. 2011)

Theme	Sub-theme	Description of ethical themes
The personal living environment	Privacy	Many are concerned that privacy would be invaded by the use of assistive technology. Privacy may even be impossible. There is a concern that data captured by devices might be stored and used in ways which contravene a person's right to privacy. However, it is also argued that the need for surveillance outweighs concerns about privacy.
	Autonomy	It is argued both that devices will increase freedom and autonomy, but also that surveillance might lead to interventions that will restrict autonomous choice and freedom. Some people would wish to be able to cope on their own, even if they were to fall, rather than have someone else intervene. Is the device for the person living with dementia or for their carers when it comes, for instance, to people 'wandering' (Hughes and Louw 2002b)? Do tracking devices allow autonomous decisions about where to go, or is the person restricted in their ability to decide?
	Obtrusiveness	Obtrusiveness is said to be 'context specific' and it is a matter of subjective judgement whether or not something is obtrusive. A device is obtrusive if it is either physically or psychologically too noticeable or too prominent in a manner that is undesirable to the person concerned.
The outside world	Stigma	I have discussed stigma in Chapter 7. Elsewhere, we argued that 'Being lost and half dressed in the middle of the night near a dual carriageway is hugely stigmatising, and electronic tagging may avoid this' (Hughes and Louw 2002b: 848). On the other hand, being electronically tagged like a felon is also stigmatizing (recall the possibility of self-stigmatization).
	Human contact	Loss of human contact may be the flip-side to the independence aimed at by assistive technology. 'What is more, health professionals also feel that good care is linked to genuine relationships and social interaction' (Zwijsen et al. 2011: 423). Social isolation and loneliness might follow and some worry that robots designed to combat loneliness will still not replace human contact.
Design and application of the device	Individual approach	People should not be monitored simply because it is possible, but because of a concrete need individually identified. The users of these devices need to be involved in their design.
	Affordability	High technology will not be affordable to those on low incomes.
	Safety	Some older people feel more secure knowing that they are being monitored. But monitoring in itself does not guarantee safety. We know that close carers are often more concerned about safety than the people living with dementia.

In addition, those involved felt the technology should be beneficial and aimed at the needs of individual residents, and that individual rights and privacy should be respected.

In Chapter 15 (see Table 15.1), I suggested that nowadays we would try to avoid using the word 'wandering'. This deserves further comment here since 'wandering' appears in Table 19.1. Many reading this book will already be used to the idea that we should really talk about 'walking with a purpose'. This is not mere political correctness. There are at least two points. First, it reminds us of the broader issue which is that people living with dementia will generally do things for a purpose. It may be that their perspective on what is required or what is going on is askew as far as everyone else is concerned, but their behaviour is not necessarily aimless. The worry is that we associate dementia with aimless wandering, which may be very far from the truth. The person living with dementia may have a definite objective which they ought to be able to achieve. Assistive technology should help them, not hinder them, to succeed. Second, it is important to notice that 'wandering' includes a great variety of activities and needs to be considered in detail. Hope and Fairburn (1990) set out a typology of 'wandering' showing that it is a complex phenomenon and needs to be thought about in detail. If someone is walking in order to get home, but the person's home no longer exists, using an electronic tag to stop the person 'wandering' is not going to be helpful, except perhaps in a restrictive way. Looking at old pictures of the town may be more so; but if this does not work, at least understanding the behaviour, rather than writing it off, provides a better basis from which to help.

Patterns of practice and Margaret Strathbone

If we are looking at whether Mrs Strathbone's robot is an ethical intervention, we should look at what the practice of using this assistive technology aims at and whether the practice is coherent with this aim. The aim is to do some good and to avoid harm. The robot does seem to be a good way to achieve these aims. There is nothing incoherent in using the robot for these aims. We should exercise some caution however, because we need to consider exactly how the robot is used and Mrs Strathbone's reaction to it. Does she miss out on anything else? Does she need more real human contact from her son or from other people? What would this entail? Would it mean she would have to be taken into a long-term institution? As far as we can tell, the robot is suiting her and helping her to stay independent. Her brother's complaints about his nephew might have some validity, but we do not know the constraints on Mrs Strathbone's son's time.

What about internal intra-personal coherence? How does what we are doing in this case compare to other similar cases? Well, we would need to get into the details of the differences between cases. In another case we might consider working harder to get a home care worker to be accepted in order for them to ensure the person received her medication. But Mrs Strathbone has put up a lot of resistance to such a move, whereas she seems very happy with the robot.

Someone else living with dementia might object to the robot and may, in any case, not be able to afford it. But this solution makes sense for Mrs Strathbone and does not seem to raise significant ethical issues, except the background worry about real human contact. Perhaps it could still be suggested that a befriender pop in from time to time, in the hope this might become acceptable to Mrs Strathbone.

What about external coherence? How do we flourish as human beings in this situation? There will be a variety of ways. Dutiful visits by Mrs Strathbone's son might represent flourishing. But there are other ways too. It could be argued that practical wisdom would suggest the robot is a good way for the son to stay in touch with his mother whilst trying to ensure her independence. It can be regarded as a compassionate response, as long as the son is in regular contact with his mother and visits frequently enough. There is a sort of hopefulness about the use of the robot. If Mrs Strathbone trusts her son and if he is trustworthy, this might be a way to care for her at least for a while. The literature makes the point that what works at one stage of a person's dementia may not work when it advances. But this can be faced with realism by Mrs Strathbone's son later on. Meanwhile he must bear with fortitude the stress of caring for his mother – along with the other things he must do – and the criticism from his uncle. For now he has, with patience, persuaded the GP that the robot is the way to go.

Conclusion

Assistive technology is neither good nor bad. There is a great variety of devices available and people's circumstances are very different. Individual judgements will be required and will have to be revised over time on the basis of experience. Technology can enhance personhood and can undermine it (Hughes 2014b: 248). It is difficult to better the conclusion about technology in *Dementia: Ethical Issues*:

> Where a person with dementia lacks the capacity to decide for themselves whether to make use of a particular technology, the relative strength of a number of factors should be considered on a case-by-case basis, including:
>
> - the person's own views and concerns, past and present, for example about privacy;
> - the actual benefit which is likely to be achieved through using the device;
> - the extent to which carers' interests may be affected, for example where they would otherwise have to search for the person with dementia in the streets at night; and
> - the dangers of loss of human contact
>
> (Nuffield Council on Bioethics 2009: 100, §6.12).

20 Accepting care

Introduction

Mr Carter found it difficult to accept that others should take over tasks he could not do (Chapter 3). Mrs Smith insisted she could cope perfectly (Chapter 17). Misael Fischer was certain he could still drive safely (Chapter 18). Margaret Strathbone did not wish to have anyone helping her (Chapter 19). These are all examples of people, rightly or wrongly, refusing to accept that they needed more help. To accept care is to accept dependence and, perhaps particularly in our society which stresses individualism and autonomy, where we seemingly have the right to do as we see fit as long as we do not encroach on the similar rights of others, many find this difficult (see Chapter 8 for fuller discussion of autonomy). This is more so – and understandably so – when we do not recognize that we are having any difficulties, or where we feel others are exaggerating those difficulties.

In this chapter, I shall discuss what might be regarded as an ultimate example of accepting care, at least as far as independent community living goes, when a person has to move into an institution of some sort: residential or nursing care in the UK. What are the ethical issues at play? The main ones will be familiar from the previous chapter: safety versus freedom or independence. But there is a new spin, because we must also consider what 'home' represents and something more about society and citizenship.

There is much to say about residential and nursing care: such care and such institutions raise all sorts of issues. Luckily, I do not need to cover this material, which has been ably covered previously (Clare et al. 2008; Conn et al. 2017; Dening and Milne 2011, 2021). Instead, I shall focus on ethical issues in connection with people living with dementia where a decision has to be made about going into long-term care.

Vignette: Mrs Anand's discharge from hospital

Mrs Anand's dementia was worse than the family had thought, but this was because she had been so well looked after at home by Mr Anand, her husband. Once admitted to hospital with a sudden worsening of her confusion (a delirium) caused by an infection, it was apparent that out of her normal surroundings she found it very hard to cope because of her poor communication, recall, orientation, judgement and understanding as well as her dyspraxia. Her infection was treated but she remained quite bewildered and unable to do even the most day-to-day tasks, such as washing herself.

What the family also saw now was the extent of Mr Anand's exhaustion. He was not well himself. Staff at the hospital said Mrs Anand was incontinent of urine. Mr Anand said this had not previously been the case. He felt she would be better once she got home. The family, alternatively, felt that things had now reached a point at which they would not be able to cope, even with input from the local social services. There was an occupational health assessment in the hospital, but Mrs Anand found it hard even to make a pot of tea. She said she had not understood how the electric kettle worked, because at home they boiled water on the hob.

A multidisciplinary meeting was held. Some of the staff said it was difficult to deal with Mrs Anand, particularly at night when she had been incontinent. Mr Anand said this would not be a problem at home. His family, however, pointed out that he was not getting any younger and that he seemed quite frail now himself. Mrs Anand was not in the meeting, but staff said she had agreed to go into a home. Mr Anand doubted that she would have understood the question. The staff said the family should start to look at suitable care homes. Mr Anand said he would want a second opinion before they did anything.

Bound for a home or just home?

Making decisions about whether or not someone like Mrs Anand should be discharged to her normal home or into a care home should be seen as exceptionally difficult. The reality is that such decisions are so routine as to seem almost mundane to the multidisciplinary teams involved. Of course, to the families and to the people living with dementia these decisions are life-changing. And yet, families are more or less involved, the person living with dementia scarcely ever. What we know is that these decisions are replete with ethical issues, as well as with matters relating to human rights. Elsewhere, we have suggested the criteria which should be used to make decisions about residence capacity (Emmett et al. 2013; Hughes et al. 2015). We have also suggested that, whereas the test for capacity should be strict, judgements about best interests (when the person lacks capacity) should be made very broadly (Greener et al. 2012; and see Chapters 11 and 12 above). This is to reflect the imperative to consider the person's will, preferences, beliefs and value judgements in as much detail as possible.

There are many ethical considerations. Safety and well-being over against the person's wishes and preferences provides the most significant conflict in terms of values (Macmillan 1994; Carrese 2006; Swidler et al. 2007). The duty of beneficence and the duty to protect the person from poor decisions that might lead to harm (non-maleficence), as well as to respect autonomy, are in evidence in the literature too (Strang et al. 1998; O'Keefe 2001). Awareness that institutionalization does not always ensure physical safety or quality of life (Zuckerman 1987) has prompted some to suggest that respecting the person's autonomous wishes should be given precedence (Chadwick and Russell 1989).

We know that vulnerability increases the chances of abuse and of contravention of human rights. 'Ironically, despite the strengthening of user rights and the alleged reduction in the power of health service professionals, the risk of violating a person's rights, including their mental and physical integrity, increases with a person's vulnerability' (Cahill 2018: 102). Under the CRPD (see Chapter 9), people have a right to 'protection from torture or cruel and inhuman or degrading treatment', as well as to respect for their privacy and their ability to 'participate in cultural life, recreation and leisure' (p. 100). All of these rights and others are discussed in connection with care homes by Suzanne Cahill (2018: 99–129). Such rights can be either supported or undermined by the culture of a particular care home.

There are other issues to consider which are fundamental. For instance, we need to think a little about the nature of 'home'. Our homes are important for us emotionally, as was recognized by Mr Justice Baker in the Court of Protection when he said: 'There is, truly, no place like home, and the emotional strength and succour which an elderly person derives from being at home, surrounded by familiar reminders of past life, must not be underestimated' (*CC v KK and STCC* [2012]: para. 70).

Dekkers (2011) has dug deeper and argued that 'being human *is* to dwell' (p. 297). He cites Heidegger (see Chapter 9) and states 'that dwelling not only refers to an activity amidst a material environment, but also to the psychosocial and existential dimensions of human existence: being human *is* dwelling, that is, staying with and among things' (Dekkers 2011: 294). From this, we have concluded that being at home 'is part and parcel of what it is to be a human being in the world'; and we went on to say: 'So, assessing a person's capacity to make decisions about where to live has fundamental significance' (Hughes et al. 2015: 307). This fundamental significance suggests there is an ethical imperative to make our assessments and judgements about people going home with the utmost thought and seriousness.

It also means that care homes, whether residential or nursing, need to be homely in a deep sense. There is pressure on staff – indeed on the community which the home serves – to ensure that the home provides the appropriate psychosocial and spiritual environment. This was the aim of Kitwood and person-centred care (see Chapter 13). What people want is for homes to be places where people can feel truly at home.

In a detailed study involving family carers, staff and people living with dementia in care homes in the London area, Train et al. (2005) identified five themes: (i) people regard privacy, dignity and choice as important, which includes concerns about personal possessions, food and money; (ii) relationships are vital – and under this theme participants also discussed vulnerability, abuse, complaints and protection; (iii) people are interested in activities; (iv) the physical environment, even the smell of the floor coverings, is important; and (v) there were also expectations on the part of the family and professional carers about what they would expect if they were to live in long-term care themselves. Some family members felt it would be unbearable to live in the setting in which their relative now dwelt, which raises a question about how we – as societies and communities – can allow the conditions of some care homes to persist. Of course, we have to say that many care homes are good and many residents of the homes are happy.

In a study of care settings in Australia, Moyle et al. (2011) identified the importance of relationships with family, other people and with things, all of which could potentially contribute to (or detract from) quality of life. Residents wanted to have control over their lives and also wished to contribute to their communities, otherwise they felt useless and of limited value to society. Interestingly, staff presence was not enough, if they were simply 'doing their job' rather than emotionally engaging with residents. Being put to bed too early left little time for conversation. People were often waiting for activities or for people to visit and Moyle et al. (2011) commented poignantly: 'Residents in this situation felt that they were left waiting in anticipation' (p. 975).

Several of these themes were picked up in our own pilot study of citizenship in a care home in the north-east of England (Hughes et al. 2021b). One daughter told us of her mother's refusal to be put into her nightwear too early. Although some felt somewhat helpless in the care home – one said of citizenship: 'it's gone' – others felt that they could still participate in the community, both within the home and in society. A couple of residents felt very strongly that everyone had a duty to vote. Another resident with a diagnosis of mild cognitive impairment reflected on her role in the care home: 'I just like to help people. That's my way of being a citizen … And I love to walk up that path, though, and go into the coffee room and have a bit of a chat' (p. 12).

To take a slightly different tack, Naue (2008) has interrogated the notion of 'self-care' and considered what it might mean in dementia. Using Michel Foucault (1926–1984), the argument is made that, 'First, the conduct of the self incorporates 'others' and second, and at the same time, brings power relations into play' (p. 320). This leads to the thought that the concept of self-care pushes us, once it can be said that the person lacks self-care, into the realms of dependency. Especially in institutional settings, deficits in self-care warrant the imposition of care by others, where care must be accepted and independence is lost. There is 'a kind of vicious circle for persons with dementia and also a tightrope walk between autonomy, support and protection' (p. 323). Naue (2008) commended the 'intersubjectivity of the social' found in, for instance, Sabat and Harré (1992) and suggested 'a person is a self when he or she is connected to a world that will include and integrate this person no matter how 'confused' or forgetful he or she may be …' (Naue 2008: 323).

The impression that emerges from the literature, therefore, is that care homes have the potential to be places where relationships, individuality and citizenship can flourish. The reality for many, however, is that care is not initiated or maintained at a level that would allow true engagement and flourishing by the individual resident. For this reason, it will often be the case that a move to institutional care, especially against the person's wishes, will be detrimental, if not in terms of health and safety (although even these cannot be guaranteed), then in terms of the person's morale, dignity and mental state.

Patterns of practice and Mrs Anand

A coherent pattern of practice would involve a thorough and broad assessment. Evidence should not be ignored in order to arrive at the preferred professional or family option. Mr Anand's view should be given weight. Mrs Anand was admitted with a delirium. It might be true, therefore, that the couple could now cope with support. And she may well be more competent in her own home than she has seemed on the ward. As a matter of personal coherence, there should be no trace of ageism and no ableism (discrimination against those with disabilities such as dementia) in the assessment or decision-making around Mrs Anand's discharge.

Turning to external coherence, the question is what are the moral dispositions that need to be brought to bear in order to allow Mrs Anand to lead as good a life as possible. We shall certainly need compassion. There must also be trust in the context of good relationships: '... trust is also about the background fiduciary relationship that is often taken to exist between professional caregivers and those being cared for. ... Both trust and relationships seem key to the proper balancing of autonomy and best interests' (Greener et al. 2012: 172). Professionals will need to show fortitude and a degree of bravery in sticking up for what is right for the person and not bending to the understandable concerns of some staff and the family. Practical wisdom will also help in terms of providing support for the couple that will actually be useful whilst not rendering Mrs Anand more dependent than she needs to be at this stage.

Conclusion

Most of us will, at some stage, need care. It is not an altogether pleasing prospect. The fact that most of us feel this way should direct us towards helping others to maintain their independence for as long as possible. Prudence will mean that we must pay attention to risks. But they must be real and the freedom to take risks is one that must be treasured as one that will allow people to flourish humanly.

So, what does this mean for families and people living with dementia? As so often, the more that matters have been discussed beforehand the better. This may be in the context of a legal framework, involving (for example) powers of attorney. Or it might be informally. But if families know what the person's wishes would be under particular circumstances it can be very helpful when difficult decisions need to be made. People living with dementia should be advised to recognize the importance of making their views known. Families may well have to stick up for the rights of the person to have decisions made in a manner that fully complies with capacity legislation by, for instance, giving the person every possible opportunity to participate meaningfully in any discussion. But just as families must advocate for the people they love, so too professionals must take their responsibilities seriously.

Simon Winner (1999), a physician with great experience in this field, suggested that – when it comes to discharge from hospital – clinicians had to be 'liberal and permissive' in order to give vulnerable older people 'the benefit of the doubt'. It seems apt to end with his very wise words: 'A good clinical service is one that has a small but definite incidence of discharges that go wrong: a paternalistic service that never risks sending a doubtful prospect home should only seem desirable to the uninformed' (Winner 1999: 64–65).

21 Behaviour

Introduction

As I shall discuss, it has been difficult to decide on the title of this chapter. Basically, it is about how we should respond ethically to behaviours in the context of dementia. But it transpires that what counts as an ethical response is bound up with the names we use to describe the phenomena. I shall come back to this.

This is not a chapter on the management of behaviours that can be found challenging. There are numerous papers, chapters, books and guidelines to describe the management of such behaviours (for example: Alzheimer's Society 2011; Cohen-Mansfield 2014; James and Jackman 2017; James et al. 2020). The focus here is on ethical issues. But, as we shall see, a major ethical issue is to do with how we see such behaviours in the first place, which is why language is so important.

Vignette: Mr Thomas's aggression

Mr Thomas, who had been a steel worker for much of his life, was a 62-year-old man living with a diagnosis of the behavioural variant of frontotemporal dementia. His family had not been able to cope with his behaviour at home where he was frequently aggressive and disinhibited. He had been compulsorily admitted under the Mental Health Act 1983 for assessment of his behaviour.

The staff on the behaviour assessment unit, who were highly skilled, spent many hours getting to know Mr Thomas and his family. They worked out a formulation taking account of his life history, mental health, personality, physical health, the social environment, his cognitive abilities and medication. They tried to understand his needs and possible thoughts and looked very hard for triggers to his aggressive behaviour. Although they felt they had some rapport with him, and although they felt fond of him and recognized what a nice man he was, he was still aggressive at times. Moreover, his aggression could come out of the blue and he could suddenly be very violent to staff, other people living with dementia and their families who visited. He had punched people viciously in the face and pinned a member of staff to the wall by his throat. Some people were very scared of him and no one could feel totally relaxed, however friendly he seemed. It was thought that he was hallucinating, but his speech was hard to make out, so it was difficult to understand what he said and exactly what was going on for him.

Various psychosocial, person-centred measures had been put in place to help to support him and to make him feel as calm and as well as possible. But given the extreme nature of his aggression, the multidisciplinary team decided that a low dose of an antipsychotic medication once a day was in order.

Behaviour and ethical issues

Strikingly, despite the enormous amount that has been written about the management of behaviours that are found challenging, which can also be referred to as the behavioural and emotional expressions of needs, it is difficult to find detailed discussion of the ethical issues that arise in the management of such behaviours. The behaviours we are considering here include: many types of aggression (such as swearing, spitting, kicking and biting), repetitive shouting, pacing, urinating in inappropriate places, agitation, sexual acts in public places, constant requests for help, as well as depression, apathy and so on (James and Jackman 2017: p. 32, Table 3.1). Of course, there are individual case discussions and passing reference to ethics in connection with different types of behaviour. But there is a noticeable lack of detailed overtly ethical discussion. This may be because these cases do not actually pose much of an ethical problem in the sense that the ethical discussion seems quite clear. Of course, in practice cases like that of Mr Thomas are exceedingly difficult to deal with and can cause significant worry and upset trying to decide what the right thing to do might be. But the framework of such decisions seems somehow settled: How can we do the best for Mr Thomas (beneficence)? How do we do the least harm (non-maleficence)? What would he want (respect for autonomy)? What does his family think is best for him (best interests)? What about the other people affected by his violence (safety)? How do we maximize everyone's welfare (consequentialism)? What of our duty of care towards him and towards others (deontology)? These are relevant but standard ethical considerations (see Chapters 3 and 4) and, even if they require nuanced discussion in individual cases, perhaps they warrant neither too much textbook debate, nor too many learned papers.

There is, however, much concern about the general approach to such issues, which tends to focus on discussion of the labels that surround these behaviours. In a thoughtful study, Dupuis et al. (2012) looked at what staff said about the behaviours of people living with dementia. They found staff tended to filter behaviours 'through the lens of pathology' (p. 162). In a similar manner, the behaviours were then described as 'challenging'. Finally, the reaction to the behaviours tended to involve 'crisis management', which might involve, say, giving medication or removing the person from a place where others were upset by the behaviour. Dupuis et al. (2012) identified as a unifying concept the notion of 'pathologizing behavior' (p. 162). An implication of this is that 'staff rarely contextualized behaviors biographically or historically' (p. 170).

Dupuis and colleagues acknowledged that their work had similarities to that of Downs et al. (2006) who talks of an 'explanatory model', which tends to view 'the person as having a brain disease' and 'therefore naturally positions the person as a patient' (p. 240). This leads to 'stigmatizing and depersonalizing' effects which may be disabling. 'Furthermore, a process of diagnostic overshadowing can result where all actions and expressions are attributed to the labelled condition' (Downs et al. 2006: 240). The concern with 'diagnostic overshadowing' – in one form or another – is pervasive in the literature from Kitwood (1997a) to Sabat (2001), from Bartlett and O'Connor (2010) to Cahill (2018).

Dupuis et al. (2012) suggested that, rather than thinking of these behaviours as 'challenging', we should think in terms of 'responsive behaviors'. This would help to shift our view to see 'actions as meaningful'. (Remember, by the way, that this is the stance taken in hermeneutic ethics; see Chapter 4.) 'It means moving from a focus on dysfunction, deficit and decline, to recognizing, valuing and believing in the continued abilities of persons with dementia to express their experiences and act in purposeful, meaningful and even intentional ways' (Dupuis et al. 2012: 170). One quick thought, in a debate that can often seem quite polarized, is that it is possible and reasonable to hold both perspectives in mind. People can manifest *both* 'dysfunction, deficit and decline' *and* 'purposeful, meaningful and ... intentional' actions. The key is to retain the broad encompassing human person perspective (Hughes 2011b: 223–250). Talk of responsive behaviours should move us away from diagnostic overshadowing to consider 'the broader social and physical environment' since the meaning of actions will be located in this broader field 'beyond the individual' (Dupuis et al. 2012: 171). It certainly behoves us to take a broad view if we hope to understand the behaviours of people living with dementia (Hughes and Beatty 2013).

In what seems to counter the claim that there are few papers looking at behaviours from an ethical perspective, Grigorovich et al. (2019) considered resident-to-resident aggression and made the point that aggression is 'influenced by broader structural conditions' (p. 173). In fact, the paper does much flag-waving for a human rights approach to dementia care. There are the familiar moves (see Chapter 13) from concepts of the self and person to the idea of citizenship, which is described as 'relational' (which begs the question, what other type of citizenship is there?). But citizenship is transcended in favour of the human rights approach. In contrast to citizenship models, 'Human rights ... transcend political and/or social boundaries by virtue of their universality, albeit to be recognized and implemented at the local citizenship level' (Grigorovich et al. 2019: 177).

Of course, there is no reason to think that human rights cannot be supported and encouraged, or undermined and destroyed at every level: personal, institutional, state, national and international. Yet, human rights talk can become wishy-washy. Rights and their correlative duties need to be instantiated. In other words, by saying that someone has a right to something, we mean that someone else has a duty to ensure that right. Those who create the laws (the politicians) and enforce them (the judges and the police) have a duty to protect my right to free speech. One good question, therefore, when someone claims a right, is to question its enforceability. I might claim that everyone has a right to a garden. It would certainly be nice if everyone did have a garden. But how could this be enforced? Who has the duty to provide everyone with a garden? My claim that everyone has this right is simply vacuous.

It could be suggested that Article 5 of the *Universal Declaration of Human Rights* is relevant to the case of Mr Thomas: 'No one shall be subjected to torture or to cruel, inhuman or degrading treatment or punishment' (United Nations General Assembly 1948). But this would need to be considered quite carefully. Would the judicious use of an antipsychotic medication by trained and experienced staff in extreme circumstances and in accordance with national guidelines (National Institute for Health and Care Excellence (NICE) 2018) amount to 'cruel, inhuman or degrading treatment'? If not, then which (if any) alternative human right is applicable? Some might argue that the case of Mr Thomas does not reach the threshold for the use of medication. Some might argue that all psychiatric treatment is 'cruel, inhuman or degrading treatment'. But there would need to be concrete arguments to substantiate these claims otherwise talk of human rights seems empty.

This much is allowed: 'The minimum necessary restrictions on individual liberty should only be used as a last resort' (Grigorovich et al. 2019: 179). But there is also talk of 'the current approach of scapegoating individual residents who exhibit aggression' (p. 178). Although we know, sadly, that abuse of people with dementia takes place in care homes and elsewhere, is it true to say that there is a 'current approach of scapegoating'? Only in a bad institution would a person like Mr Thomas be 'blamed' for his behaviour; he would not normally be a scapegoat. In good institutions, the current approach is to discern, if possible, any unmet needs (which could include the need for physical treatment, say of an infection) and – given their long-term risks (Ballard et al. 2009) and the efficacy of psychosocial care (Fossey et al. 2006) – only to use antipsychotics or sedating medication as 'a last resort'.

Grigorovich et al. (2019) also contained repeated talk of 'an ethic of human flourishing'. Now, I like the idea of human flourishing because I like the idea of virtue ethics (see Chapter 3) which is where this notion mostly appears. In that context, we flourish if we live life in accordance with the virtues. But I am not sure what it means in this paper apart from something nice to be brought about by a nebulous focus on human rights. At this point we come up against the reality of Mr Thomas seriously injuring someone. The paper is absolutely correct to suggest we need to attend to 'the structural and relational underpinnings of aggression' and that there are 'ethical and legal imperatives to address them' (p. 180). It does not, however, tell us what to do about Mr Thomas today.

The literature seems more focused on castigating anyone who uses the label 'behavioural and psychological symptoms of dementia' (BPSD) to describe the behaviours with which we are concerned. I should say that I have always disliked this wording for scientific reasons (it lumps too many things together), for semantic reasons (they are mostly not symptoms but signs), for aesthetic reasons (it lacks grace) and for reasons of veracity (they may not be signs *of* dementia at all – perhaps signs *in* dementia, which is also ungainly).

In an enterprising study, Wolverson et al. (2021) asked people living with dementia what they thought about terminology. There was no overall agreement. The term 'unmet needs' had the most support (28.3 per cent), but unfortunately this is so ambiguous as to be largely unhelpful specifically because it does not mention behaviour. If I simply say Mr Thomas has unmet needs, he could merely require new batteries for his radio. Some participants did not like the word 'behaviour', but it could be retorted that the phenomena being studied amount, unfortunately, to behaviour. Only a small percentage of people disliked the term BPSD, but they were 'vociferous in the intensity of their dislike of this term, associating it with unnecessary medication and chemical restraint' (p. 1998). I learned of the term 'behavioural and emotional expressions of needs' (p. 1996) from this paper, which I think may be the best of a bad lot. The somewhat negative conclusion I draw from the study is that we are never going to get the overarching terminology correct. The simpler the better perhaps.

Just to pick up a minor point, the researchers say they took 'a human rights approach' (Wolverson et al. 2021: 1995). By this they meant they listened to the voices of the people with dementia. Given the aims of their study ('to explore the views of people with dementia') what else could they do? Again, I think we see here some flag-waving. And yet, the clarion call of the disability rights movement – 'nothing about us without us' – is relevant. Much research on dementia would be better if we had involved people with dementia and heard what they think, but it is not completely clear that research without such involvement will have transgressed human rights, even if it is less good as a result. Although the point is a minor one in Wolverson et al. (2021), it suggests a larger concern, namely that the movement towards a human rights approach to dementia has limitations.

This whole issue of terminology is deeply political. In a thoughtful piece which attempted some balance, Cunningham et al. (2019) considered the pros and cons of the movement to ban the use of BPSD. They commended 'behaviours and psychological symptoms of dementia' (p. 1112), but might change their minds once they have read Wolverson et al. (2021). The fact that there is such a movement, now spearheaded by dementia activists, shows the depths of feeling about the language we use to talk about people who live with dementia. It seems absolutely correct that their voices must be heard. So, too, must the voices of people who live with dementia who are not activists; and so, too, the voices of their family and professional carers. We need the holistic view.

Patterns of practice and Mr Thomas's aggression

There is nothing internally incoherent about following good practice guidance, as long as we are sure it is properly authoritative. But we must follow it carefully and honestly. Are there other practices which we might consider instead of resorting to a low dose of an antipsychotic? We could consider other medications. But why would we (in the absence of any evidence that they would be more effective)? We could ask that Mr Thomas be subjected to close one-to-one observations. But, first, we know this might increase his agitation; and, secondly, it would not stop him from suddenly being aggressive. Whoever was observing him would probably not be quick enough to intervene if he lashed out and may, anyway, become the object of his aggression. We could do nothing, but we worry about the safety of others and we worry that he is in some way tormented. Perhaps the low dose of medication might lessen his distress from the hallucinations we suspect he is experiencing.

What about external coherence? How can we ensure that, insofar as he is able, Mr Thomas is enjoying as much well-being as possible? Have we really shown empathy to Mr Thomas and really tried to understand him with genuine warmth? Have we reached our decisions about him with justice and prudence? Justice here does not need to mean fairness with respect to resource allocation; but rather, have we shown good judgement? In getting to know Mr Thomas, have we demonstrated real respect for him as a person? Have we been suitably humble in listening to the thoughts of others and shown the virtue that Radden and Sadler (2010: 132) call 'unselfing', which refers 'to the personally effaced yet acutely attentive and affectively attuned attitude toward the patient, the relationship, and its boundaries, adopted by the ethical and effective practitioner'? We shall use the smallest dose of medication we can for as short a time as possible. A careful judgement will have to be made about whether the medication is working and whether its effects are acceptable. We may have to accept that there is no good answer for Mr Thomas, even if we find a route we consider likely to cause the least harm.

Conclusion

The use of medication to treat behaviours such as aggression is now generally agreed to be a bad thing if it can possibly be avoided. In practice, however, difficult decisions are sometimes required. They must not be random and they should cohere with our other decisions and with the values and virtues that guide our judgements. As compassionately suggested by Treloar et al. (2010), antipsychotics could ethically be regarded as justified when used with care to treat severe distress in the context of a palliative approach.

22   Forced care

Introduction

This chapter continues, to some extent, the theme from the last. But here I shall consider a particular type of behaviour, namely where people living with dementia refuse basic care, which their carers (family members or paid staff) regard as essential and, therefore, have to provide against the person's will. This has been called 'forced care': 'restraining a resident so that personal care may be carried out, forced feeding or making people take medications' (Commission for Social Care Inspection 2007: 49). As the definition suggests, it falls under the wider label of restraint. But it is restraint for the specific purpose of providing essential treatment. The literature is sparse.

Vignette: Mrs Chen and forced care

Mrs Chen, who was in the more advanced stages of Alzheimer's disease, has been in the care home for just over two years. She has become increasingly reluctant to accept personal care. Now she is refusing altogether. The staff take to leaving her, even though she becomes malodorous, is called 'smelly' by other residents and no one sits near her. But she is now incontinent of urine and faeces. The staff decide that it is not right to leave her in this state. They make a plan, therefore, that when they have enough staff they will carry her to the bathroom to ensure she is washed properly. They try to do this swiftly, conscious of the need to protect her dignity. Her family are pleased to see her looking cleaner after she has been forcibly washed. Staff decide they will use the same procedure every time she is incontinent of faeces.

Research on forced care

Psychologists in the north-east of England, who were busy providing an individual-specific, formulation-led approach (James and Jackman 2017) to behavioural and emotional expressions of needs (that is, behaviour that was regarded as challenging), noticed an increase in referrals to their services 'where resistance to personal care interventions (such as help with using the toilet, continence and hygiene needs) was a key factor' (Sells and Howarth 2014). They carried out a survey (n=86) and found that forced care was frequently being used by staff (Howarth et al. 2014): 'The aspects of forced care practised most frequently … were those most clearly related to risk (i.e. helping someone to eat and drink and preventing someone from leaving the building) and also the most intimate (i.e. helping someone wash and go to the toilet and changing someone's pad)' (p. 769). Their concern was that the staff providing this care, in care homes or in the community, were not well acquainted with its legal basis; and whilst training was fairly readily available for person-centred care, there was not much guidance on what to do if that approach failed. Hence, they developed the Forced Care Framework (Sells and Howarth 2014; Howarth et al. 2017) to guide staff through the processes and considerations necessary for forced care to be used. They were aware that staff were confused about the circumstances under which restraint of any sort could be applied: staff showed a lack of awareness of the underpinning legislation. (Further review and advice about restraint for personal care can be found in Crooks et al. 2021.)

They also conducted a literature review but found forced care was not being discussed to any great extent, despite evidence that its use was prevalent (Sells and Howarth 2014). Guidelines tended not to be specific, for instance focusing on maintaining safety and preventing movement, rather than actually on how to provide such care. The Forced Care Framework set out to:

* provide a clear unambiguous guide
* encourage open and honest discussion
* clarify issues around restraint
* ensure that the safety and well-being of the person concerned was centre stage
* facilitate a transparent process, and
* improve the quality of the care being delivered (Sells and Howarth 2014: 32).

Very sensibly they emphasized that the Framework was not intended to give the impression that forced care was to be encouraged. It supported the use of force 'only as a last resort' (p. 34).

Other colleagues in the north-east were pointing out that the training required by staff needed to include legal training, since this is integral to care and is required 'so that the human rights of the vulnerable are protected' and so that the care delivered 'is legally (and ethically) defensible' (Jackman and Emmett 2014). Elsewhere (Jackman et al. 2014), they highlighted the relevant law, which is particularly to do with assessing whether the person lacks the capacity to make decisions about personal care (see Chapter 11), and with judgements about the person's best interests if they lacked the requisite capacity (see Chapter 12). They stressed that 'Decisions to use restrictive physical interventions in a person's best interests will have serious implications for a person's civil liberties and human rights' (p. 28). Such interventions had to be 'a necessary and proportionate response to the likelihood of harm to the person and used as the last resort' (p. 28). Raising the spectre of human rights in regard to forced care is entirely appropriate because, unless undertaken legally, it really does amount to the sort of 'cruel, inhuman or degrading treatment' envisaged by Article 5 of the *Universal Declaration of Human Rights* discussed in the previous chapter. In addition, therefore, we can specify not only rights but also duties; and the rights, if ignored, are enforceable.

Otherwise, the literature is sparse when it comes to the issue of forced care, rather than restraint more generally. A recent paper on 'forced treatment' from Norway, which was mostly concerned with prevalence, defined it as being where 'interventions of treatment and care are carried out, despite the resistance of the patient, and/or against the patient's will or knowledge' (Gjellestad et al. 2021: 373). Most (57 per cent) of the decisions to use 'forced treatment' in this study were to do with admission to a health institution; then there were medical and safety decisions (27 per cent); assistance with activities of daily living accounted for only 16 per cent of cases (p. 377). The authors highlighted the ethical importance of striking a balance between autonomy, dignity and vulnerability.

Patterns of practice and Mrs Chen's hygiene

Thinking of intra-practice internal coherence, the expression 'forced care' in certain lights can be seen as an oxymoron. Of course, it is possible to explain why it is not. But this should be a warning to us that the practice is one which needs to be considered carefully. On the face of it, care which requires force, to which the person is objecting, does not sound like care.

In casuistical vein (see Chapter 5), how does it compare to our other practices? Well, there are many other circumstances where things might be done against a person's wishes, if the person lacks capacity and it is in that person's best interests. But capacity and best interests need to be tested and judged assiduously. It is not clear that this has occurred in the case of Mrs Chen. It looks as if her lack of capacity has been assumed, which is in contravention of one of the first principles of the *Mental Capacity Act 2005*. Although the family are pleased with the outcome, it is not clear to what extent they were involved in the decision before forced treatment took place; nor were other professionals (from primary or secondary care) involved.

Perhaps more significantly, the story gives no evidence that any broader therapeutic strategy has been attempted. Has there been any attempt to understand why Mrs Chen is against help with personal hygiene? What unmet needs or emotional concerns underlie her refusal to accept help? Is there something traumatic in her life history that she is reliving in her dementia? Therefore, can we really say that forced care represents the least restrictive option (Jackman et al. 2014)? In this case, was it really the last and only resort?

What about external coherence? If done properly, in accordance with best practice guidelines, such as the Forced Care Framework (Sells and Howarth 2014) or something similar, although possibly extremely upsetting for the person living with dementia, forced care can be seen as a coherent practice, in keeping with the virtues of charity, compassion, fidelity, integrity, realism and respect for the person.

In discussing forced care elsewhere, we emphasized the virtue of practical wisdom, which involves reasoning about how to achieve the good end at which you are aiming (Hughes et al. 2021a: 128–134). We want Mrs Chen to be clean, free from smells that alienate others, less likely to suffer skin breakdown or urinary tract infections and so on. If forced care is truly the only way to achieve this – we have consulted others for advice, followed guidelines rigorously, assessed her capacity, given thorough consideration to what might be best for her – we then have to consider in detail how it will be achieved. How will staff approach her? Who will be involved? Do they have the necessary training? How will we ensure that the process is smooth, safe and swift? How will her dignity be maintained? Practical wisdom is *practical*! Forced care will not be in accordance with practical wisdom, for instance, if none of the staff is trained. The decision to use forced care is not one that can be made lightly. It should be a difficult decision.

Conclusion

Forced care, in a sense, epitomizes much that is important in caring for people who lack the capacity to make decisions for themselves. It is an extreme example. To take someone by force, against their expressed wishes, to strip them naked, put them in a shower and wash them intimately sounds as close to 'cruel, inhuman or degrading treatment' as almost anything we might be able to conceive. Such action sits near the cusp of being a human rights violation. Only if it can be justified by practices and procedures that provide its overt justification will it stay on the right side of the law. In the absence of conscientious justification, such action is an affront to human rights and human dignity. This should not frighten us from providing such care if it is necessary; but it emphasizes the great moral responsibility assumed by those who work on our behalf with some of the most vulnerable people in our societies.

23 Covert medication

Introduction

This continues themes from the last two chapters. Sometimes people living with dementia refuse to take their medication. What are the circumstances under which it might be reasonable to give them medication without them knowing? If they have the decision-making capacity to refuse medication, decisions must be honoured (see Chapter 11). If they lack the required capacity – the particular capacity to refuse this specific medication – then their carers (professional or family) must act in their best interests (see Chapter 12). Under what circumstances is it ethical to give medication covertly in order to force their compliance? Again, there are issues of trust and power, coercion and (covert) force, as well as a lack of truthfulness.

Vignette: Alexandra Chenoweth and the antihypertensives

Alexandra had in her day been a formidable music teacher. She now has Lewy body dementia. She had hallucinations early on, but since treatment with a cholinesterase inhibitor these have settled. She also has a degree of heart failure, occasional angina and essential hypertension. She stopped taking her medications because she did not want them. The staff were worried about her heart conditions and felt that they would have to hide the medication in her food. They consulted the GP first to see if there were any medications she could do without. They also discussed matters with the old age psychiatry team and with Alexandra's brother, who is her next of kin. Their worry was that if she tasted the medication and knew that they were deceiving her, she might stop eating and have no faith in them whatsoever. The old age psychiatry team helped to assess her capacity to make the decision about treatment and concluded that she lacked this particular decision-making capacity because she was unable to retain the information that she has a serious heart condition. She tended to think she was much younger than she was and that she was still teaching. Having spoken to all involved, the staff team judged that it was in her best interests for her to be treated. They knew from her brother that she was always keen to accept medical advice when she was younger and, indeed, enjoyed visiting the doctor, having been, in her brother's opinion, 'something of a hypochondriac'.

Covert medication – studies and opinions

There was quite a media stir in 2001 when the United Kingdom Central Council for Nursing, Midwifery and Health Visiting (UKCC) – which in 2002 became the

NMC – approved guidelines on covert medication (BBC News 2001). One concern was that it would encourage the use of antipsychotic drugs and sedatives in frail older people. The media reports cited research which showed that 71 per cent of care homes and inpatient units in the south-east of England were resorting to covert medication (Treloar et al. 2000). The same research showed that few institutions had formal policies to guide practice and 98 per cent of people caring for someone living with dementia in the community thought covert medication was sometimes justifiable. It was the research by Treloar et al. (2000) that had galvanized institutions and national bodies in the UK to look at the issue in the first place. The researchers made the point that the lack of transparency around the issue, where 'practices go unrecorded and unmonitored', heightened the potential for abuse (p. 410). They opined that the relevant ethical principles were autonomy and duty of care, but suggested that 'to seek consent from the incapacitated is futile' (p. 410).

As we shall see, there are broader ethical issues to consider, but this last opinion about consent can be challenged. Put simply, there is still the possibility of *assent* even if someone cannot formally consent. In Chapter 11, we saw this was proposed by Coverdale et al. (2006). It might not be futile, but it would seem nonsensical to seek consent to do something surreptitiously. Still, seeking permission before doing anything to a person, even if you suspect they will not be able to consent, is not completely absurd. Indeed, it is good practice to do so.

Haw and Stubbs (2010), in a review of the literature, albeit on the basis of few studies, found covert medication was being used in 43 to 71 per cent of nursing homes, where the proportion of the residents receiving covert medication was reported as 1.5 to 17 per cent. In a specialist centre, they found the figure was 12 per cent. Munden (2017) included figures from the Mental Welfare Commission for Scotland which showed the prevalence increasing slowly from 1.1 per cent of nursing home residents in 2010, to 1.3 per cent in 2011 and 1.6 per cent in 2012. Haw and Stubbs (2010) recorded: 'Factors associated with covert medication include more severe cognitive impairment, learning disabilities, low function in activities of daily living, agitation, aggression and being prescribed antipsychotic medication' (p. 764).

The year after their survey, Treloar et al. (2001) wrote a piece on the ethical and legal issues raised by covert medication. They mentioned a variety of possible ethical concerns: deception is wrong; trust will be broken; the least restrictive tactic should be used; there is the risk of abuse; avoiding deception may lead to harm; processes must be transparent; the patient must lack the capacity to consent; there needs to be discussion with relatives, advocates and other professionals; the practice must be recorded. They concluded: '... in exceptional circumstances, professional carers may need to administer medications covertly to undertake their duty of care to mentally incapable patients' (p. 63).

Welsh and Deahl (2002) made similar points. They noted that there is a fundamental requirement 'to respect autonomous decision-making', but then questioned whether, if the person lacks capacity, all medication should be considered 'covert'. If medication is given in the person's best interests, they asked, 'is there any difference (ethically) between a patient passively accepting medication and having it disguised in some way following refusal?' (p. 123). The ethical difference is that in one case the person refuses and in the other the person does not! The point would only make sense if it were presumed that the person's 'passive' acceptance was on a par with active refusal. They went on to highlight the principles of beneficence and non-maleficence, as well as the least restrictive principle, the need to weigh harms and benefits and 'to maximise each patient's liberty and dignity' (p. 123). In a mildly inchoate manner, they wondered whether to take a deontological or utilitarian approach, but more straightforwardly considered whether extra safeguards might help.

The useful task that McCullough et al. (2007) set themselves was to outline how to undertake a systematic review of the argument-based clinical ethics literature. Luckily for the current chapter, they decided to do this using the example of covert medication. The paper, therefore, provided at the time a useful review of the literature. On the whole, they were (justifiably) rather uncomplimentary about the ethical argumentation of the papers they considered. They were careful to point out the shortcomings of their own study. But they highlighted the need for 'a process of accountability' (p. 73). For their part, they judged that the 'ethical issues concern mainly whether concealed medication violates patient autonomy and undermines trust in the physician–patient relationship' (p. 73). They were dismissive of the argument about trust because they felt that people living with dementia 'lack the cognitive apparatus to appreciate a trusting relationship' (p. 73). Clearly, they had not read Sabat (2001), where the examples of people who had very low marks on cognitive testing but formed highly trusting relationships with Sabat are striking. McCullough et al. (2007) went on to discuss the need for beneficence, professional integrity and the need to prevent abuse 'through a system of organizational accountability' (p. 74). They concluded that when autonomy was severely compromised by a lack of decision-making capacity and where there was physical resistance to necessary medication, covert administration in accordance with 'an organizational policy of accountability' would be ethically justified. The need for clear documentation and guidance was repeated by Munden (2017).

Abdool (2017) set out the ethical dilemma in terms of the Autonomy Account (where the overriding thing is to honour the person's wishes) versus the Trust Account (where the key thing is the maintenance of trust). But Abdool (2017) rejected both accounts because she felt the justification of deception required 'a much more comprehensive account', particularly given the 'conflict among a multiplicity of values' (p. 195), which calls to mind the salience in these sorts of discussions of values-based practice (Chapter 5). Abdool (2017) highlighted the four principles of medical ethics (Chapter 3) but introduced the interesting idea of 'reliability as a form of trust' (p. 199) and argued that, even where people are deemed 'incapable', autonomy should still be considered. Her conclusion, however, was that 'there may be cases where deception is morally justifiable' (p. 201).

More recently, Guidry-Grimes et al. (2021), as well as covering the familiar territory discussed above, introduced a new dimension to the debate.

> Food and eating practices are sources of health, opportunities to exercise autonomy, ways to create valuable experiences (e.g., pleasure, cultural connections), ways to express/reinforce identity and ways of reinforcing/building connections with others. Eating is also a relational practice, one that entails significant vulnerability to and dependency on others.
>
> (p. 390)

The use of covert medication can threaten both trust in food and the trust in carers. Moreover, it threatens the very identity of the person. The authors cited a paper about people with schizophrenia in India (Srinivasan and Thara 2002) where 26 per cent of those given medication without their knowledge learned of the deception; the common reaction was anger and resentment. The threat to trust, they argued, is real. Having control of, or at least faith in, what we eat is basic to our sense of ourselves as agents. The enormity of undermining this faith must be considered before covert medication is allowed.

Pickering (2021) commented on Guidry-Grimes et al. (2021) in order to give the analysis more global relevance. The point is that, in some cultures – Pickering (2021) was particularly thinking of India – the person is seen much more as 'embedded in the collectivist family milieu' so that covert feeding may not be seen as so morally objectionable, even by the recipient. As Pickering (2021) stated: '… where individuality and identity is understood and experienced not just as the product of relationships, but also in terms of role, responsibilities to family and community, then the ethical analysis of [covert medication] may appear in rather different terms'(online).

It would be possible to extend this analysis and to argue that, even without the specific cultural angle, whether in a family or in a care institution, it might be that relational autonomy, which I argued in Chapter 8 was a more realistic way to think of autonomy, would suggest that the preferences and perceptions of individuals meld with the preferences and perceptions of those who genuinely care for them. The basis of this *is* genuine care based on authentic relationships. Under such circumstances, covert medication might seem less heinous.

Patterns of practice and covert medication

If we regard helping someone to eat as a practice of care, it is easy to see why medication hidden in food might be regarded as odious, especially given the need to respect the person's autonomy and the requirement for trust. But if this practice of care is seen in the context of other practices of care, it is easier to see some coherence. The questions are the same when providing any form of care. Can the person consent? Does the person have the capacity to consent to this particular treatment at this specific time? If not, what will be in the person's best interests (broadly conceived)? Well then, if without medication there is a serious enough risk to the person's health and well-being (and perhaps to that of others) and if it can be hidden (that is, it is unlikely to be discovered and it is pharmacologically possible to give it in the intended form), then it would seem unobjectionable to give it covertly. Of course, if the medication could be stopped, that would be even better (Baqir et al. 2014; Baqir et al. 2017)!

Care – genuine, thoughtful, beneficent, non-maleficent, loving, respectful, reliable and trustworthy care – is the context we should be dealing with in connection with covert medication. Abusive care is what we are worried about. But there is nothing obviously incoherent in saying that the nature of care requires that we consider covert medication – carefully.

Conclusion

Covert medication should only be considered by professionals: (i) when the person who refuses medication lacks the capacity to consent to its use; (ii) if it is given in accordance with authoritative best practice guidelines; and (iii) if it is the best option for this particular person under these particular conditions (Pickering 2021). Its use should be recorded and reviewed. It should be regarded as exceptional treatment and stopped when it can be. The fiduciary issues, along with the threats to the moral integrity of those who care and to the personhood of the person living with dementia, remain real. Hence, if there is evidence that covert medication is being given thoughtlessly or in a potentially abusive manner, all staff should feel able to report the matter either to their managers, or to the regulatory body that inspects institutions (currently in England this would be the Care Quality Commission (CQC)).

For families, the same issues apply: the person being cared for must lack capacity, which may or may not need to be assessed by someone with training; covert medication should be given in a sanctioned manner, which will probably mean getting professional advice because, for instance, some medications can only be given in certain ways; and giving the medication covertly must be in the person's best interests. To be certain of this last point, a conversation with the person with dementia when they had the requisite capacity would help to establish that covert medication was something that could be regarded in the future as in the person's best interests. However, family carers will often learn through experience that caring can be made much easier and less stressful all round if a particular medication is slipped into some jam or yoghurt. This will frequently be perfectly ethical, but to be more ethical still a conversation should be had with a healthcare professional to check the practice will be efficacious and safe. Finally, the consequences of the covert medication being discovered by the person, who might then refuse to eat or just become suspicious, need to be considered carefully.

24   Truth-telling

Introduction

In this chapter we are sticking with the subject of deception, but now confronting the issue, which crops up in numerous guises in dementia – from diagnosis (Marzanski 2000; Pinner 2000), to driving (see Chapter 18), to the use of robots (Martens and Hildebrand 2021), as well as in connection with covert medication (as in Chapter 23) – square on.

Vignette: Mrs Usman and the terrible truth

Mrs Usman, who lived with a diagnosis of mixed vascular and Alzheimer's dementia, lingered near the door of the care home waiting for her husband to come to take her home. Each day, she was sure he would come that afternoon. What she did not know was that the reason she was in the care home was because Mr Usman, who had been caring for his wife diligently at home, had fallen ill, been taken into hospital and had died. Her family did not wish her to be told this shocking news and the staff were colluding with the deception with varying degrees of ease. Mrs Usman would start to get distressed in the afternoon and would ask staff, with increasing agitation, when her husband would be arriving.

Truth-telling and dementia

Much has been written about the dilemma which now faces the staff looking after Mrs Usman. Ought they to tell her the truth? Or ought they to persist in deceiving her and, if so, how? By a bare-faced lie?

Cutcliffe and Milton (1996) raised the question about lying to people with dementia and discussed the issues in terms of a tension between the principles of respect for autonomy and of non-maleficence, recognizing that staff will have to give one principle more value than the other. They recognized that autonomy might well be compromised by dementia, lessening the requirement to respect it. This theme is present in Schermer (2007), who suggested that at some point 'the truth cannot contribute to a good life in any way anymore' (p. 21). For Schermer, the ethical tension is between well-being and truth. However, she stated: 'Outright lies to demented patients [sic] should be avoided if possible because they compromise the liar, as well as threaten to undermine trust in the whole practice of care' (p. 21). She also made the point that avoiding pain (by not telling the truth), is not always the best way to enhance well-being. Lying can harm staff too, but Schermer (2007) accepted that truth can also 'become a mere burden' (p. 22).

The idea that lies become less problematic in more severe dementia is repeated by Day et al. (2011). In fact, it reflects an idea that has been around since at least the time of Hugo Grotius (1583–1645), who held that lying was always wrong but that it was not possible to lie to children or (what he called) the insane, 'since infants and insane persons do not have liberty of judgement' (Grotius 1925: 614). The trouble with lying, according to Grotius, was that it offended 'liberty of judgement'; but if this was not present, then no lie had been perpetrated.

Some people take an absolute stance against lying. Feil and Altman (2004), for instance, wrote with some passion: '... we do not lie to persons with dementia, because we know that on a deeper level they will recognize it as such. ... Don't all people with dementia deserve to be treated with dignity and respect and to be listened to instead of lied to?' (pp. 77–78). They made the point that people (including those living with dementia) are capable of awareness at different levels at the same time. In terms of their absolute moral stance, Feil and Altman (2004) reflect Kant (introduced in Chapter 2): 'To be truthful (honest) in all declarations is ... a sacred and unconditionally commanding law of reason that admits of no expediency whatsoever' (Kant 1993: 65). For Kant, a lie undermined all other communications.

Nevertheless, there is quite a literature to attest to the reality of therapeutic lying to people living with dementia in a variety of settings. Wood-Mitchell et al. (2006) wished to spark the debate because of their finding that care staff were using therapeutic lies quite frequently. The team, led by the psychologist Ian James (whose work we came across in Chapter 21 in connection with behaviour), reported that 96 per cent of care staff looking after people living with dementia in a variety of settings in the north-east of England had resorted to lies (James et al. 2006). They later surveyed 76 psychiatrists (albeit the survey only had a 38 per cent response rate) and found that 69 per cent had resorted to lying where the person lacked capacity and they thought it was in the person's best interests (Culley et al. 2013). They also interviewed people living with a diagnosis of dementia and asked if they would find lying and deception acceptable (Day et al. 2011). Most would if the lie or deception were in the person's best interests; but a minority were against lying under any circumstances. The reason for and nature of the lie were important factors in determining whether the lie or deception were acceptable or not.

In a study in a general hospital, it was found that, '... participants suggested that they would prefer not to lie. However, they were equally reluctant to tell the truth' (Turner et al. 2017). The authors highlighted the tension in those who were inclined to feel that you should 'do as you would be done by' and that a lie which prevented distress and upset would be acceptable, but who also wished to hang on to their long-standing belief that lying is always wrong. Clearly the issue is one that causes moral angst to practitioners. Turner et al. (2017)

described an 'overwhelming sense of paralysis amongst staff' (p. 867) when faced by the dilemma of whether to lie to a person living with dementia.

The issue is certainly not confined to the UK. Similar tensions were found in Italy. Of 106 nurses, only a few would not lie to prevent or reduce aggressive behaviour, but only about half would lie in order to save time and avoid long explanations (Cantone et al. 2019). The authors suggested that there was a low propensity amongst the nurses to ethical reflection.

There are two further points to highlight from the work of James and his colleagues, both about language. In Elvish et al. (2010), whilst developing the 'Attitudes towards Lying to People with Dementia' questionnaire, the authors also showed that the effect of workshops was that participants tended to move in the direction of feeling that lies could be used where this was in the best interests of the person concerned. Participants 'appeared to move from a generic ethical perspective, to a more person-centred and situational one' (p. 261). The authors were admirably honest in stating that 'the workshop material was not neutral and implicitly supported the use of deception' (p. 261).

The point about language here is the contrast between 'a generic ethical perspective' and 'a more person-centred and situational one'. My inclination would always be, as in casuistry (see Chapter 5), to look at the particularities of a case. But moral theories or approaches still have to be applied. The particularities may suggest that X is not a case of lying – a stance which will still itself need some justification. The specific ethical perspective lends detail to the generic but does not necessarily vitiate it. Moreover, 'a more person-centred' perspective should not be contrasted at all with 'a generic ethical' one. The person-centred perspective might be to honour the person by not lying to them just as easily as it could be to deceive them in order to avoid distress.

In McKenzie et al. (2020), of 30 learning disability student nurses, 96 per cent admitted to using 'therapeutic untruths'. The picture was much as it is in the field of dementia. The tactic of omitting to say something was the most usual type of therapeutic untruth. As in other studies, this one suggested that more training and more research was required. But the point about language is a contrast made within the paper between 'non-therapeutic lies', which are used 'in the interests of the person providing support' (p. 1608), and 'therapeutic untruths', which are used by staff in the person's best interests. Now, according to this schema, it is not possible to lie to a resident in a care home for that person's benefit, you can only be involved in an 'untruth'; whereas, if it is for yourself, then it is a lie and is not considered therapeutic. Well, a lie for yourself could, after all, be therapeutic. But, more seriously, conflating all deceptions under the rubric of 'therapeutic untruths' could seem like a means to obfuscate the reality which is that this includes lying to people.

Even if you are prone to say that you can lie under some circumstances, it is important not to conflate a downright lie with helpfully changing the subject or not saying something that is true but hurtful. The latter may be examples of deception, but not all deceptions are lies. We do need in these debates a definition of lying. According to Sissela Bok's seminal work, a lie is 'any intentionally deceptive message which is *stated*' (Bok 1999: 13). Of course, lies can be defined in other ways, but the prohibition on lying is not meant to stop people from changing the subject in an empathic manner to lessen distress, which is a good thing to do. This is simply called humility; it is not lying. So, when Mrs Usman asks for her husband, we should not conflate, on the one hand, asking her if she is worried and then suggesting that we get a cup of tea with, on the other, stating to her that he has died. It may or may not be better to tell her (carefully, empathically) that he has died. But the lie, even if compassionately done, is very different from the act of compassion without the lie.

Some of these complexities were considered in the Mental Health Foundation's (2016) report *What is Truth?* Unfortunately, it is not possible to go into all the details contained in that report. As with many of the references in this book, if the reader is interested in pursuing this topic (or any other) it would be worthwhile to consult the original works cited, which contain a depth of discussion it is difficult to capture briefly. The Mental Health Foundation's Inquiry was established in 2014 to look at 'when people with dementia experience a reality or set of beliefs different to those around them' (Mental Health Foundation 2016: 1). For those interested, although now a little out of date, the inquiry started with a rapid review of the literature (Kartalova-O'Doherty et al. 2014).

The conclusion of the inquiry (and for the sake of transparency I should say that I was involved in it) was 'that one should always start from a point as close to whole-truth-telling as possible, and only when this is causing a person with dementia unnecessary distress, move on to a response that includes an untruth' (Mental Health Foundation 2016: 29). The Report set out a spectrum: from (a) whole-truth-telling; to (b) looking for alternative meaning; to (c) distracting; to (d) going along with; to (e) lying. 'Looking for an alternative meaning' is where the person's reality is acknowledged and explored to show empathy and perhaps to understand the person's meaning and whether there might be some unmet needs which could then be addressed. To Mrs Usman, for instance, someone might say, 'Your husband sounds like a wonderful man. I'm wondering if you could tell me about him.' In this way, there is the potential to validate and support her feelings, without the need to lie to her. Towards the other end of the spectrum, 'going along with' is where, without lying, the carer agrees and accepts all that the person living with dementia says. In a sense, this too validates their experience.

Anthony Tuckett, from Australia, has written a number of important papers in this field (for example, see Tuckett 2004). In Tuckett (2012), a four-stage communication strategy for interacting with people living with dementia in long-stay care facilities was set out. The first stage involved meeting the need directly. The second involved meeting the need being expressed by some other means. Perhaps, if the person is looking for comfort a doll might be given, but only if this would be acceptable. The third stage would be distraction. Finally, a lie might be used.

Tuckett (2012) listed some of the arguments in favour of truth-telling: it upholds autonomy, it may help with someone's physical healthcare, it could be psychologically helpful, and it is 'intrinsically good' (p. 8). The arguments against being completely truthful are that this might prevent psychological harm in the form of 'distress, anguish, depression' (p. 8). One worry Tuckett (2012) mentioned is that deceptive practices might become the norm; and there is also the concern that people with dementia can show awareness of when they are being deceived. He commended the thought that the right question, when a carer is faced with the dilemma about whether or not to lie, should be 'What is a *fitting* response?' He went on to suggest that following an ethical response based on consequentialist (it will bring about a good result) or deontological (it is the right thing to do) thinking, there is still a requirement that virtue ethics is used to give guidance in how to apply the other ethical theories (Tuckett 2012: 16–17).

The concern about deceptive practices becoming the norm was one that Bok (1999) had also voiced: 'The entire institution of medicine is threatened by practices lacking in candor, however harmless the results may appear in some individual cases' (p. 68). She also talked of '...coarsened judgment and diminished credibility...' (p. 132). I would go a little further than Tuckett (2012) in terms of virtue theory. Rather than regard it as the theory which tells you *how* to do things, I also think of it, like consequentialism and deontology, as an action-guiding theory. Hursthouse (1999) put it this way: 'Not only does each virtue generate a prescription— do what is honest, charitable, generous – but each vice a prohibition – do not do what is dishonest, uncharitable, mean' (p. 36).

I shall end by providing an adumbrated account of six papers that appeared in a special issue, on 'Truthfulness and Authenticity in Dementia Care', of the journal *Bioethics* (Byers et al. 2021). Apologetically, I have to say that each article deserves more consideration.

Carter (2021) agreed, to some extent, with Hertogh et al.'s (2004) suggestion that something is radically different about the world of people living with dementia. In this world, regarding the requirement for truth in Kantian deontological terms does not make sense. In fact, it excludes people with dementia and is in this sense unjust. So, ethical deception is acceptable inasmuch as it involves entering the subjective world of the person living with dementia. According to Carter (2021), this creates equality between the person with dementia and the carer.

I would reply that entering the world of the person with dementia will often be the right thing to do, but seeking equality in the sense suggested seems chimerical. A person with heart failure, for instance, will simply not (on the whole) be able to walk as far and fast as the person without it. This will sometimes be (and sometimes not be) a source of sadness, but it is nothing to do with justice in the sense in which it is being used. We may say it is unjust that the person with a healthy lifestyle succumbed to heart failure whereas the person with the unhealthy lifestyle did not. But if whilst out walking with someone with heart failure I hammer home that I find the person slow and weak, this is callous and unkind and yet, the inequality between us is a given. So, too, I should not hammer home to Mrs Usman that her husband is dead. If we were to regard the fact that she thinks he is alive and I know he is dead as unjust, then the just thing to do might be to inform her of the truth. But this sense of justice is simply irrelevant. What she requires is kindness, which can indeed be helped by entering her world.

Hodge (2021) gave a good account of where going along with someone else's reality was clearly the correct thing to do. The person had their own 'subjective lived narrative' (p. 868). It is still possible, however, to distinguish this from the bare-faced spoken lie. Tieu (2021) argued that diversion (which involves less than the whole truth) is a technique which can be used ethically if it meets the needs of the person living with dementia, rather than the needs of the carer. In this way, such techniques can be seen as person-centred. This seems correct, as long as there is no more honest way of being person-centred!

Honesty also comes into play in connection with the use of robots (see Chapter 19). Robot pets could be regarded as dishonest if the person living with dementia takes them to be real. Martens and Hildebrand (2021) used Gendler's (2008) notion of 'associative, automatic, and arational' mental states termed 'aliefs' (Gendler 2008: 641) to explain how a person might reasonably respond to something as if it were real despite knowing it is not. Thus, we may all experience a degree of vertigo when climbing over the top of the Sydney Harbour Bridge, even though we know we are attached with a safety harness and that the bridge is very unlikely to fall down. Similarly, once we no longer see the love for the robot pet as implying a belief in it as real, but rather as an alief, we do not have to judge the belief in terms of its truth content. This is an ingenious way of saying that there is something different about the belief state of the person living with dementia which we must be sympathetic to and which we can embrace.

MacKenzie (2021) argued that 'Within caregiving relationships, we are bound by a set of norms that often permit or require us to suspend our commitment to the truth' (p. 882). This is because within such relationships there is 'mutual concern', involving caring about the same interests and values, which allows us to assume 'hypothetical consent' (p. 877) to some deceptions within the limits of the mutual concern. Relationships characterized by mutual concern entitle 'moral allowances' (p. 879). This makes some sense, even if the argument needs to be considered more carefully – as MacKenzie (2021) makes plain – where the relationships are professional as opposed to informal.

My own position (J.C. Hughes 2021) is that we should still say that lying is objectively wrong, but it might have a good intention and the circumstances, which includes its consequences, might make it praiseworthy. So the thing we are aiming at, for example to bring some relief, need not be regarded as a deception. We can also think about the illocutionary force of saying something – that is the function of the utterance rather than the actual words – which again might be to calm or relieve frustration and not primarily to deceive.

Patterns of practice and lying

The difficulty here is that, if we wish to hold that lies are justifiable, we are prone to incoherence unless we can find some justifiable difference between the cases where we lie and those where we do not. In the papers outlined above, you can see the authors striving for this by pointing to how things are different when you enter the other person's reality, go along with them, recognize your mutual standing with them in a caring relationship, and so on.

However we decide to justify our practices internally, they must also cohere with our conceptions of what it is to live well humanly. This is why truthfulness must be a major concern. My conclusion was and remains, 'that there are concrete exigent circumstances where not to speak the truth to a person with dementia may be excusable, even if (other things being equal) telling a lie should be avoided at all costs. However, the lie must seem ineludible, not just convenient; it should stem from virtues such as charity, compassion and practical wisdom; yet it should engender a sense of unease or guilt in response to the virtuous inclination to honesty' (J.C. Hughes 2021: 848).

Conclusion

The virtue of truthfulness is central to the whole question of whether or not one ought to lie: not if you wish to flourish as a human being, the virtue ethicist would say. Because connected to the virtue of truthfulness is that of being trustworthy and that, in turn, is connected to our standing as human beings in relationship with one another: '… truth and the virtues of truth—truthfulness, sincerity, honesty—are connected with trust and the value of truth ultimately resides in what is essential for human flourishing: trustworthy relationships' (Hertogh et al. 2004: 1691). Hertogh et al. (2004) brought into the discussion the very thoughtful idea that in dementia what is increasingly lost is 'a common shared world', which (it is suggested) upsets our normal judgements in ethics and law because truth and reality no longer mean the same for everyone (p. 1692). Although I think this idea holds some water (sometimes we might have to conform to the person's reality, for instance (J.C. Hughes 2021)), I am not sure that it should be pushed too far for the simple reason that, even in severe dementia, there are still things that continue to be shared – trustworthy relationships, indeed, may provide an example.

We spoke of communicative ethics in Chapter 4 and, not surprisingly, Moody (1992a) argued in favour of 'a presumption in favour of truth telling'; he added that communicative ethics 'can settle for nothing less' (p. 53). He continued:

> But it is a rebuttable presumption, and the claims of relationship, of love and respect, are prior to abstract rights like truth telling. The normative ideal of open communication must take account of the 'concrete other', which is to say that the ethics of truth telling is less a matter of individual rights than of social relationship.
>
> (p. 53)

25 Sexuality and intimacy

Introduction

Sexuality in old age is not a new thing. And people have been studying it for years now (Berezin 1969). More and more research has been carried out looking at the frequency and nature of sexual activity in older people, sexual dysfunction and its management in old age, sexual health in old age, the effects of dementia on sexual expression, how to communicate about sexuality and intimacy with older people, and so on (Lightbody 2014; Stratford 2017; Hinchliff and Fileborn 2021; Albert et al. 2022). This chapter will focus on the ethical issues around sex and sexuality in connection with dementia.

In previous publications, as is common, we have used vignettes based around people living with dementia in care homes (Hughes et al. 2014: 232–236; Hughes et al. 2021a: 149–159). These have included: discussion of sexual disinhibition; the problem of the person with dementia who is in a longstanding relationship but in the care home seems to forget this and establishes a relationship with someone else; homosexual and lesbian relationships in care homes; and the need for privacy to allow sexual behaviour.

Most of the ethics literature focuses on the problems associated with sexuality and intimacy in care homes. Familiar themes then emerge about ageist, ableist and sexist discrimination, as well as the need for staff training. The ethics focus in the literature used to be heavily biased towards worries about capacity and consent as a way to respect autonomy, but has slowly swung towards a more holistic approach with recognition of the importance of sexuality and intimacy in terms of quality of life, dignity and integrity (Benbow and Beeston 2012; Gove et al. 2021; Albert et al. 2022).

In this chapter, however, the vignette concerns a couple living in their own home. The importance of the broader, more holistic approach becomes obvious.

Vignette: Major and Mrs Trotter

Mrs Trotter, who had been living with a diagnosis of Alzheimer's disease for about 12 years, was a regular attender at the local dementia café. Major Trotter always brought her and sometimes stayed with her. In recent months, the staff were becoming more concerned by Mrs Trotter's marked deterioration. Her speech had become very difficult to understand and she was now quite dyspraxic, finding it difficult to know what was expected of her when she was invited to sit down on a chair or to drink a cup of tea. Major Trotter was also having greater difficulty getting her out of the car, because she did not seem to understand his instructions to her. She remained in good spirits, even when he shouted quite loudly at her to try to get her to follow his commands. He would swivel her around on the back seat and then pull her out of the car by her legs until he let them naturally fall to the ground, at which point she supported herself. He remained upbeat during all of these manoeuvres, never seeming to lose his patience with her or his sense of humour.

Staff wondered how he was coping at home, since the Trotters received a fairly meagre package of care. They tentatively suggested that he might start to think about long-term care for Mrs Trotter. He abruptly dismissed the idea, saying he had promised to care for her and that was what he would do. He said they had a good time together. Meanwhile, at the dementia café it was noticed that Mrs Trotter was becoming quite amorous with the male helpers and, indeed, with the men generally. When Major Trotter was present, he would guide her away from other men and say things like, 'You need to keep your powder dry until we get home,' after which he would laugh uproariously. Between themselves, the helpers at the dementia café started to wonder what was going on at home. There were some ribald jokes, but Mrs Trotter's social worker thought that this should be taken more seriously and decided to ask Major Trotter about their sexual relationship at home.

This was done in the context of a longer conversation about how he was coping. When asked directly about sex, Major Trotter said only that they lived a full married life and that there were no problems, before diverting the conversation to how awful the weather had been recently and how muddy they got when they went for their daily walks. Feeling concerned about Mrs Trotter's dignity and safety, the social worker made a referral to the local old age psychiatry team for assessment of her capacity to have sexual relationships.

Sex and intimacy in dementia

One way to focus attention on issues around sex in later life is to ask whether it is right for a resident in a care home to be allowed to hire a prostitute to visit the home in order to provide sex (Laurance 2004). Our reactions can be prudish or permissive, but they are often conflicted: some may be opposed to prostitution generally; others may feel that the resident in the home should be able to exercise some autonomy and should not be blocked by bureaucracy (Jacobson 2004). This tension, between a legalistic and bureaucratic reaction on the one hand and a libertarian and catholic one on the other, is in sharper focus when it comes to dementia. This can be seen in the reactions to incidents of sexual expression where studies of the attitudes of nurses, for example, have shown that 'the prevailing view of persons with dementia expressing their sexuality is generally conservative and negative' (Nilsson et al. 2022). Reactions of insecurity, distress and embarrassment are mixed with expressions concerning 'the importance of protecting the integrity of the person with dementia and consequently their right to sexual expressions' (Nilsson et al. 2022).

The 2021 Alzheimer Europe report on sex, gender and sexuality provided a refreshingly broad approach to a variety of relevant issues (Gove et al. 2021). Amongst many things, it recommended, for instance, that we should 'protect the rights, promote the well-being and provide support to people with dementia and their partners, families and friends of all gender identities and sexual orientations at the end of life and during the bereavement process' (p. 21). It laid heavy emphasis on the need to 'provide opportunities and, if necessary, practical, emotional and administrative support for LGBT* people with dementia to manage effectively their gender identities' (p. 21). ('LGB refers to people who are lesbian, gay or bisexual and the T* refers to people who are transgender, transsexual, transvestite, genderqueer, gender fluid, non-binary, genderless, agender, non-gender, third gender, two spirit and bi-gender' (p. 51)). The report acknowledged how dementia can have an impact on sexual relations and leave those concerned (either the people with dementia or their partners) feeling lonely at the diminution of important relationships. There are particular problems that can face those in the LGBT* community, who are sometimes neither recognized as the main carers nor as the legitimate partners of those with whom they have lived in long-term relationships (p. 23).

The report also highlighted the 'greater tendency to view male sexuality as pathological and female sexuality in terms of vulnerability and abuse when involving people with dementia' (p. 28). Male transgressions are more likely to be met by punishment, such as discharge from a care home, whereas reactions to females tend to be more protective.

A standard response when sexuality emerges involving people living with dementia is to ask about capacity. This then leads to questions about the criteria for saying that someone lacks the capacity to engage in sexual relations (Tarzia et al. 2012; Lightbody 2014). Commentators have looked back to Lichtenberg and Strzepek (1990) and to work in the field of intellectual disability (Murphy and O'Callaghan 2004) in order to find appropriate criteria. In my view, it can be argued that these criteria set the bar too high so that many people who do not have cognitive impairment would fail to meet them. Lichtenberg and Strzepek (1990) include questions such as: 'Does patient [sic] realize that this relationship may be time limited …?' and 'Can the patient describe how they will react when the relationship ends?' (p. 119). It is not unreasonable to say that many people (young people especially perhaps) may not answer these questions correctly (but how would we know?). Should they be told they lack capacity to have sexual relations? Murphy and O'Callaghan (2004) mention 'the ability to recognize potentially abusive situations' (p. 1349) as a criterion for capacity. This is obviously an important point, but, again, many people do not recognize the 'potentially abusive situations' into which they put themselves. Perhaps people with cognitive impairment will be worse in this regard. But plenty of people at a younger age do not seem to recognize the possibility of abuse. Should sex be prohibited for them too?

There are legal criteria in the UK derived from case law (*IM v LM, AB and Liverpool City Council* [2014] EWCA Civ 37). To have capacity to consent to sexual relations the person must be able to (i) describe the nature of the act,

(ii) understand its possible consequences, including the risk of sexually trans-mitted diseases, (iii) recognize that the person has a choice and the right to refuse sex, and (iv) understand the possibility of pregnancy (Dunn and Holland 2019: 85–86). If there is the possibility that the person simply is not educated enough to understand these factors, 'the expectation should be that the person would be supported to gain the necessary information' (Dunn and Holland 2019: 86). This takes us back to the importance of value judgements in connec-tion with assessments of capacity (see Chapter 11): how strict should we be in applying these tests of capacity?

There are also human rights to be considered. Article 8 of the *European Convention on Human Rights* protects the rights of people to have respect for privacy and family life (and thus to respect autonomy) (Council of Europe 1950). But this 'does not confer an *absolute* right for individuals to do as they please' (Hughes et al. 2021a: 154). The rights and interests of others need to be considered and 'health and morals' must also be protected. The worry is that there may be too many ways to circumvent the rights of people with dementia.

> The right to a sexual life where there is true consent and mutual desire has been acknowledged by the courts as a 'fundamental human right'. ... How-ever, proper enjoyment of the rights to sexuality of persons with dementia has been prevented by a range of ageist and mentalist stereotypes
> (Peisah et al. 2021: 1022).

Peisah et al. (2021:1024) argued that the capacity to engage in sexual activ-ity was not a binary state, but could be regarded as 'dimensional', which they felt would allow supported decision-making and be consistent with Article 12 of the CRPD (see Chapter 9, Box 9.2). They highlighted the importance of con-sidering the person's will and preferences. People can be supported to enjoy sex safely, with appropriate attention to dignity and privacy. This might, said Peisah et al. (2021: 1024), also include helping residents in long-term care to buy any clothes or paraphernalia they require, including the opportunity to seek support from sex workers.

On the basis of their research with care staff, Schouten et al. (2021) sug-gested that the conversation should be reframed, away from the language of needs and rights, to focus on intimate touch, well-being and care of the whole person. This alternative approach 'contextualises relationship, intimacy and sexuality as part of an overall person-centred approach which focuses on well-being, strengths, resilience and quality of life of an individual' (online). Albert et al. (2022), in their systematic review, found very few studies that included the views of people with dementia. But in those that did, there was a wish 'to be acknowledged and considered desirable as sexual partners, despite the illness. The importance of intimacy and sexuality for maintaining one's subjectivity' (online) was also identified.

Director (2019) considered whether giving prior consent might be a way to get around any lack of valid consent once a person has dementia. His argument is almost convincing, though few people are likely to accept this legalistic approach to what they might see as a basic human instinct and intrinsic to the nature of relationships.

In a number of highly thoughtful articles, Mahieu and Gastmans have shifted the emphasis away from considerations of autonomy and formal consent and towards a greater understanding of the philosophy of care, which is otherwise lacking in the literature (Mahieu and Gastmans 2012). Moving away from the principles approach (discussed in Chapter 3), they encouraged a more holistic vision, with emphasis on, for instance, human embodiment. They also emphasized how we are contextualized, or situated, and cannot free ourselves of our cultural and personal characteristics (Mahieu et al. 2014: 379). Our embodied nature establishes the centrality of intimacy and sex to our lives (p. 381). They made this point, which contains a caution: 'Having a body means that we as human beings can meet the eye of our fellow human beings. It is through our corporeality that we relate to the world and to others. Being embodied, however, also makes us susceptible to objectification by other persons' (p. 384). Ultimately, it is their view of the human person which guides their approach to sexuality and intimacy. The person is a 'decentred self' (we never have full control over our destiny), an embodied being (with bodily agency based sometimes on tacit knowledge, but also making us vulnerable), a being-with-others (from which stem our moral obligations), and a being-in-the-world (which provides a network of relationships) (Mahieu et al. 2017: 57). Much of this is redolent of our discussion of personhood in Chapter 13.

Patterns of practice and Major and Mrs Trotter

For the sake of internal coherence, I must think about Mrs Trotter's capacity to consent to sex with her husband and I should do this in the same way that I assess other types of capacity. The question, however, is to what extent I allow value judgements to enter into my assessments of capacity? And if someone lacks capacity, to what extent do I allow evaluative judgements to colour my estimations of the person's best interests?

One thing is sure, the nature of the consent required from a university graduate at the age of 32 years having orthopaedic surgery for a knee injury is quite different from the nature of consent from an 82-year-old living with dementia and making a decision about whether to have sex with a partner with whom they have lived for 50 years. The information that the 32-year-old requires is factually much more straightforward (the success rate of the operation, the possible side effects, the infection rate, the long-term prognosis and so on), whereas the information required by the 82-year-old is much less certain, more evaluative. For a start, what sort of sex will it be? It is perhaps less likely to be penetrative sex. What have been their sexual habits previously? Was it a happy marriage? Does the person need to know about the risk of pregnancy (it could be an 82-year-old having sex with someone of 50)? And what if the person no longer speaks? Should they on this ground alone be denied intimacy?

Then, thinking of external coherence, how do we allow people to flourish and how do we flourish as human beings assessing Mrs Trotter? We should beware of the presumption that Major Trotter is a brute, a charming sociopath set on taking advantage of his vulnerable wife. But he could be a brute and she is vulnerable. We can ask Mrs Trotter a bunch of questions that she will not be able to answer and then declare that she lacks the requisite capacity. But this may be to trample on her rights.

Actually, we need to do something much more nuanced. It will be difficult to assess what goes on behind closed doors. But we can get to know the Trotters; we can observe them over time; we can form a therapeutic relationship with them; we can listen to what staff and other relevant people say. Do they have children and are they expressing concerns? A host of virtues will be required: humility, charity, practical wisdom, sincerity, fidelity, trustworthiness, gender-sensitivity, respect and integrity.

As Tarzia et al. (2012) suggested, we should not be rushing for our capacity assessments. They cite Appel (2010), who said that in the context of people who cannot talk, a 'rule of reasonability, derived from overt social cues, should guide caregivers in determining … acceptable conduct … A simple smile might be enough to betoken consent' (p. 153). Tarzia et al. (2012) commented that, of course, 'a smile does not *necessarily* mean consent; however, the point is that body language and non-verbal cues can provide a good first indication of whether a relationship or behaviour is welcome' (p. 612). What is required is a holistic approach to the situation, with attention to the multiple ways in which those involved act and interact as situated persons.

Conclusions

We must approach each case uniquely with close attention to the values that might be at play (Hughes et al. 2014). As always, it will be useful if couples have discussed at an early stage the issue of continuing intimacy, if one of them has a diagnosis of dementia, so that the partner without dementia might feel on safer ground later when initiating sexual contact. Even then, however, the fact that someone has in the past said that they would wish to have continuing sexual relations does not mean that they would consent in the present. There is a good deal of nuance to these decisions, which is why professionals who are asked to judge matters from the outside need to understand the couple's narrative and relationship in some detail, which itself suggests the need for good therapeutic relationships. Of course, anyone – a home care worker or relative – who suspects abuse should report their concerns, which may be to a particular professional who is already involved (for example, a GP or social worker), to a line manager, or to the local safeguarding team or some similar statutory body.

As with so many issues in dementia, whether or not someone is allowed to have sexual relations is a matter of great importance. To allow sexual abuse of any kind is anathema to good practice and to the idea of human flourishing. And yet, to deny someone sexual relations and intimacy (in the absence of distress or offence) when these might give them solace and comfort, to infantilize them and to disrespect their dignity, really is to trample on, not only their rights, but also their standing as persons in the world.

26 Admissions and transfers

Introduction

In this chapter, I take a slightly different approach. I wish to discuss briefly two separate but related issues: first, admitting someone with severe dementia from a care home to a hospital; and, secondly, relocating someone living with advanced dementia from one care home to another. Rather than use vignettes, and in the absence of a significant literature specifically aimed at the ethical issues, I shall focus on only a couple of studies.

Hospital admission

It is commonplace to say that acute hospitals do not offer the right environment for people living with marked cognitive impairment. They are noisy, busy, frightening and bewildering places. In addition, we know that people living with advanced dementia, when admitted to acute hospitals, are subjected to inappropriate interventions and inadequate treatment (Sampson 2010: 118). The more appropriate approach to people with advanced dementia is the palliative one, which is described in Hughes et al. (2020) and the breadth of which – it should not be equated simply with end-of-life care – has been defined elsewhere (van der Steen et al. 2014). Nevertheless, when someone with advanced dementia falls ill in a care home, it can be a very difficult decision not to admit them to hospital. Typically, it is families that are keener on pursuing curative treatments, but this might change when appropriate conversations have been had with staff (Moe and Schroll 1997). The decision not to admit someone has often only been made when the person is very close to death (Lamberg et al. 2005).

My focus here is on the study by Sampson et al. (2009). In brief, this was a six-month, prospective, longitudinal cohort study. During the course of the six months, 617 people over 70 years of age were admitted to a London hospital. Seventy-five of these people died during their admission. Of those who died, only 7.9 per cent had no dementia. Over three times as many people died who had a diagnosis of dementia (this was 18 per cent of them). In those who had severe cognitive impairment, 24 per cent died, which was five times as high as for those who did not have any evidence of dementia. The association of cognitive impairment and death was strong even after correcting for age and the severity of the acute illness. So, the study shows that people with dementia who are admitted to an acute hospital are more likely to die than those who do not have dementia. The authors felt they could not judge

> ... whether these admissions were necessary, but the high short-term mortality risk in people with dementia suggests that this intervention did not prolong life for a meaningful length of time. Individuals may have received better-quality care in a familiar environment if more support [were] available in the community.
>
> (Sampson et al. 2009: 65).

Ignoring all of the practical matters that could be raised (for example concerning the use of electronic advance care plans so that a person's recorded wishes might be known even out-of-hours by all concerned), there is an ethical question about the right thing to do. I think it can be put in terms of patterns of practice. Is your pattern of practice, when it comes to caring for people living with advanced dementia, to pursue a palliative or a curative approach?

Under some circumstances, a significant fracture, for example, it would be best to pursue a curative approach. Not to do so would be internally incoherent because elsewhere, when a condition can be cured, it would be; and it would be a derogation from the duty of care not to treat a treatable condition (unless the person had, with capacity, refused to consent to the treatment). But, equally, not to pursue a palliative approach in the knowledge that death is inevitable and where comfort could be given would be an incoherent practice. Optimal palliative care for people living with dementia has been defined for some years (van der Steen et al. 2014). To ignore good practice in favour of something less optimal would immediately suggest incoherent practices.

Forced transfers

Occasionally, care homes shut, or regulators close them down. I have also worked in a service where a hospital long-stay ward had to be changed into a behavioural unit, so that families who had thought their relative had a home for life were told they had to be moved on. Forcing frail elderly people to be transferred to another care environment, especially against the wishes of family, is stressful, not least because of the worries about consequent morbidity and mortality. In a very helpful review, Holder and Jolley (2012) confirmed that mortality rates have ranged from zero to 45.8 per cent following such transfers. Their conclusion was as follows:

> The recent evidence suggests that ill-planned or casually implemented closure and relocation is stressful and linked to adverse outcomes in terms of symptoms, health and survival, and that careful, respectful, person-centred planning and implementation of closure and relocation moderates the likelihood of adverse outcomes.
>
> (p. 314)

Some unpredictable transfers quickly become inevitable. However, where transfers can be anticipated and planned, internal coherence can be maintained, once again, by following good (clinical, ethical and legal) practice (Jolley et al. 2011; Holder and Jolley 2012).

Conclusion

In concluding, I wish to focus on the external coherence of the relevant patterns of practice to do with admitting to hospital or transferring to alternative care facilities frail older people living with marked dementia. There really has to be a sense of what is being aimed at and of how this will be achieved. In other words, practical wisdom is essential. But these moves also require a good deal of humility: humility in the face of the anxieties of relatives and staff and humility in the face of the evidence in favour of what counts as best practice. Practitioners require honesty and integrity too: to recognize openly the difficulties and the adversities that might follow any particular decision. Courage and fortitude are required to face the deaths that will inevitably follow. Finally, fidelity: if all concerned feel that those making decisions are trustworthy, will be faithful to those in their care and can be relied upon, then the difficult decisions that are required are more likely to be accepted.

27 Ethics in the time of pandemic

Introduction

If it took great courage – which it surely did – to work in a medical intensive care unit (ICU) during the COVID-19 pandemic, something more than courage was required to work in care homes for people with dementia. Whereas workers in the ICU were fairly quickly provided with personal protective equipment (PPE) and, in the UK, had the support of staff from other departments, in care homes PPE was slow to arrive, chronic understaffing was exacerbated, transmission of the virus seemed inevitable and death rates were high. The importance of supporting the NHS was in sharp juxtaposition to the initial lack of interest in supporting social care, which came on top of years of neglect. The courage shown by workers in care homes was physical, psychological, spiritual and moral.

What we now know is that people living with dementia had an enhanced risk from COVID-19 both in terms of the severity of the illness and in terms of mortality (Hariyanto et al. 2021; Wang et al. 2021). Furthermore, in many countries, including in the UK, people living with dementia endured decreased social interaction (that is, loneliness), decreased support, problems accessing and using technology that might have helped, which included difficulties in dealing with remote consultations with their GPs, emotional suffering, decreased cognitive and physical health, decreased carer wellbeing, difficulties in understanding the restrictions imposed on them and general deconditioning (Di Lorito, Masud, et al. 2021; Giebel et al. 2021; Tuijt et al. 2021; Daley et al. 2022; Giebel et al. 2022). The problems experienced by people living with dementia were mirrored by the experiences of their families. We also now know of the profound impact of the pandemic on the personal and professional wellbeing of staff, especially on those who provided prolonged and intimate care (Nestor et al. 2021). Indeed, the impact of the public health measures taken in response to COVID-19, at least in the UK (but elsewhere too), have been significant in the longer term for people living with dementia and for their unpaid carers, especially because of the lack of support (Hanna et al. 2022).

In this chapter, I shall start by discussing justice and resource allocation in a little more detail. I shall discuss the ethical issues that have arisen in the COVID-19 pandemic in the UK in the context of patterns of practice, which will finally bring us back to think about the virtue of justice.

Justice and resource allocation

According to Pellegrino and Thomasma (1993), 'The virtue of justice is the strict habit of rendering what is due to others' (p. 92). At least three types of justice can be picked out: *distributive justice* is to do with giving things (beneficial or burdensome) from the common stock to others according to their due; *commutative justice* is to do with the exchange of goods and paying what is due to another; *retributive justice* (about which I shall say no more) concerns the appropriateness of punishment. In connection with pandemics, distributive justice seems most relevant (at least at first blush). In a situation where people need treatment, equipment, help and support but there is not enough to go around, or not immediately, how should resources be allocated?

In Chapter 3 (see Table 3.1), we came across the notion of justice as fairness, derived from Rawls (1971). His idea was that it is rational to choose in favour of the worst-off in society. Those who are better off should not be favoured by the system of resource allocation. This approach emphasizes people's needs. However laudable it might initially seem, it is not clear that this idea is helpful in a crisis where everyone has needs and for many the needs are extreme.

Daniels (1988) used Rawls (1971) in a manner that overtly favours the young as opposed to the old. This is said not to be ageist: it does not discriminate between people. Given that we all expect to be young and then old, according to Daniels (1998) it would be prudent for me to favour treatment for my younger self rather than for my older self. If I (imprudently) plump for treatment to my older self and then fall mortally ill when young, I shall not reach old age. Similarly, Callahan (1987) suggested that after a natural life span, say about 80 years, people should not receive aggressive therapies. In other words, the idea was that there is such a thing – to use a metaphor from cricket – as a fair innings: you have enjoyed your time batting, now others should have a go!

Such theories, if accepted, gain a purchase in times of relative calmness. Should we devote money to neonatal care or to chemotherapy for the very old? Here the ideas of Daniels (1988) and Callahan (1987) come into play. Nevertheless, such ideas have been criticized as ageist (see Rivlin (2012) and Wagland (2012a and 2012b)). During a pandemic, however, things may not be so clear-cut. First, prognoses may not be known. It could be that young people have a much greater chance of survival and, therefore, are less in need of expensive interventions. But perhaps younger people are less likely to survive. Secondly, things are certainly not clear-cut when decisions are being made about funding to health services as opposed to social services, where both services look after older people. Should we spend our money on the 80-year-old lucky enough to get into a hospital who requires ventilation, which is available, or on the similar person in the care home where ventilation is not available?

One alternative to needs theory, to answer such questions about resource allocation, is to use cost-effectiveness analysis; and a specific example of this involves Quality-Adjusted Life Years (QALYs) (see Box 27.1).

> **Box 27.1 Definition of Quality-Adjusted Life Years (QALYs)**
>
> A QALY is a measure which combines the length of life with the quality of that life. Different states of health can be given a score from one, which indicates perfect health, to less than one, which indicates poorer health (and zero would indicate death). The key thing then is to find out what score would or should be given, say, to a year of life with mild dementia or a year of life with severe dementia. Different states of health (and the costs of their treatment) can then be compared.

Resource allocation is a big topic to which I cannot give sufficient attention; there are also alternatives to QALYS to be considered, such as Disability-Adjusted Life Years (DALYs). (See Hope et al. (2003: 177–191) for a clear succinct account; and Lesser 1999 and 2012 for fuller discussion). QALYs encourage us to look at the quality of life that will result from an intervention and then to compare QALYs between different interventions in order to judge cost-effectiveness. But, it has been argued, QALYs are intrinsically ageist because the older person can expect fewer QALYs than the younger person (Harris 1987). I tend to agree with John Harris (1987), who has argued 'that a society, through its public institutions, is not entitled to discriminate between individuals in ways that mean life or death for them on grounds which count the lives or fundamental interests of some as worth less than those of others' (p. 121).

Patterns of practice in the time of pandemic

The first question is: does a pattern of practice make sense within itself: does it have intra-practice internal coherence? One of the claims of the British government during the COVID-19 pandemic, especially during the first wave in 2020, was that it was 'following the science'. This makes some sense, except that it leaves out the important point that we also need to consider ethics and evaluative judgements (see Chapter 5). We can question, therefore, whether a practice of 'following the science' makes sense. Which science is being followed? Do not scientists have different opinions? How has it been decided to use this particular scientific model? Does following the science conflict with other values? Should policies of isolating those infected and social distancing mean that an elderly wife cannot sit with her dying husband?

The second question is whether there is intra-personal internal coherence: what do we do in other situations? Well, we do undertake triage and we do instigate infection control. But we might then ask how do we do these things? We saw during COVID-19 that there were questions about how PPE was issued and accessed within hospitals (Shelton et al. 2021). A greater inequality was that when NHS units had been issued PPE, many care homes were struggling to acquire it. In some countries, triage also took place, for instance when ICU beds were not available, to the detriment of older people (Faggioni et al. 2021).

The underlying values and principles for such policies should be made overt (Teles Sarmento et al. 2021). Whilst triage can be regarded as a just approach under some circumstances, 'chronological age cannot in itself be a valid ground for assuming without further investigation that … treatment cannot do any good' (Lesser (2012b: 180)).

Finally, we must ask about external coherence, where we should look for coherence between our patterns of practice and the moral norms that define and constitute the good life for human beings. Actually, was there justice for people living with dementia during the COVID-19 pandemic?

We might wish to answer 'yes' on the grounds that safety was a high priority and the vaccines were distributed in many countries according to need, with vulnerable older people receiving their vaccinations sooner. Distributive justice is said to reflect the common good (Pellegrino and Thomasma 1993: 92–93) and there are a number of ways in which what was given as due to older people was in line with the common good. Of course, richer countries had better access to the vaccines, so distributive justice between countries was not so evident. But here we might wish to return to the notion of commutative justice, which is to do with individual good and 'the altruism of agapeistic ethics' (Pellegrino and Thomasma 1993: 93).

The real concern has been to do with care homes. In particular, there is a concern that human rights have been over-ridden in institutions where they were not given high priority in the best of times. Evidence from 21 countries that 46 per cent of all COVID-19 deaths were residents in long-term residential care has reinforced the feeling that 'the segregation and unilateral sequestering of people living with dementia away from their familiar communities highlights profound stigma-related inequities that undermine the principles of a just, caring, and inclusive society' (Kontos et al. 2021a: 1396). We should be careful to distinguish between denigrating some and all care homes. Is it that some, perhaps many, are not up to the mark, or is it that, in principle, no care homes would ever satisfy humane and just standards of care?

Commentators have not hesitated to suggest that long-term care institutions have been found wanting during the pandemic partly because they were unacceptable to start with.

> The default option of segregating older persons has exposed the heightened vulnerability of congregated settings … It also re-emphasized the fact that despite attempts to transform the institutional landscape of residential care for older persons, it still lacks a true, human rights-based culture.
> (Peisah et al. 2020: 1200)

These authors cite work from Australia suggesting 'congregation, separation and confinement of people living with dementia by the care home built environment constitute "segregation"'; and that such segregation unjustly contravenes the rights established in the United Nations CRPD 'to non-discrimination (Article 5), liberty and security of the person (Article 14), equality before the law (Article 12), accessibility (Article 9), and independent living and community inclusion (Article 19)' (Steele et al. 2019: online).

In the UK, the High Court found that the Secretary of State for Health and Social Care, as well as Public Health England, had acted unlawfully in their policies to do with discharge from hospitals to care homes in March and April 2020, which were found to be 'irrational in failing to advise that where an asymptomatic patient (other than one who had tested negative) was admitted to a care home, he or she should, so far as practicable, be kept apart from other residents for 14 days' (*R on the application of Gardner and another v Secretary of State for Health and Social Care and others* [2022] EWHC 967 (Admin): §298). In the same ruling, however, the judges did not find that there had been a breach of the *Human Rights Act 1988*. In particular, they considered Article 2 of the *European Convention on Human Rights* (Council of Europe 1950) concerning the right to life, as well as Article 8, the right to respect for private and family life. To understand why these rights were not considered to have been transgressed, we must keep in mind that to every right there is a correlative duty. In this case, the court did not think the duty of the government to protect life caused by an epidemic or pandemic extended to 'as broad and undefined a sector of the population as residents of care homes for the elderly' (§252).

In judging the external coherence of this pattern of practice I have resorted to the virtue of justice. Were older people living with dementia treated with justice? I do not think we can give a definitive overall answer. Some were and some were not. But it is undoubtedly true that some of the cruellest stories during the worst of the COVID-19 pandemic involved people living and dying in care homes with little human contact and no contact with family. This was made worse by the lack of support for beleaguered staff working in these environments and by the initial attitude that seemed to overlook the needs and rights of all those involved with social care.

What we know, however, is that many staff in care homes put themselves in jeopardy, showing great courage, fortitude and charity. From my own perspective, as someone who spent much of my working life visiting care homes, I must say that these virtues have been apparent to me in abundance, even if I have also witnessed poor care and misery. Individual acts of charity are often secret. And we must remember that 'the root of justice lies in the individual's good, not only in the common good, in commutative as well as distributive justice' (Pellegrino and Thomasma 1993: 93).

Conclusion

When I reflect on what happened in care homes during the COVID-19 pandemic, I am often left with feelings of paradox. We wanted residents to be kept safe, but did we want them to be totally secluded? We applauded staff, but realized they might be spreading the disease. We recognized the need for family solidarity, but not if it compromised others.

There are three reflections which are perhaps helpful. First, there is the matter of scale. Extreme measures are called for under extreme circumstances.

Previously, an outbreak of diarrhoea in a care home was enough to mean that it was shut for a few days unless visits were essential. A pandemic with high mortality, morbidity and transmission rates necessitated a draconian response. Secondly, the importance of the virtues must not be ignored in favour of, say, the utilitarian requirement that welfare be maximized. For it is *how* things are done that is important. It is to do with personal (commutative) exchanges as well as with distribution of goods to the population. Practical wisdom should allow innovative approaches and the occasional breaking of rules on the grounds of thoughtful compassion (see Hughes 2012 and 2020b). And, as Murray (1994) has written, 'In practice, justice comes not from the inflexible application of moral or legal rules, but from equitable judgements in which rules are interpreted in the light of particular circumstances' (p. 98). Thirdly, where and how we care for people living with dementia, especially when this is in the advanced stages, needs careful consideration. But whatever the physical environment and however care is organized, it must be humane and full of love. If your relative is in a place that you know to be a loving environment, you will find it easier to trust the staff to do the right thing. 'Love generates and transmutes justice' (Pellegrino and Thomasma 1993: 94).

28 Food and drink

Introduction

There is a variety of problems that can emerge in the course of dementia to do with food and drink. For instance, there are stories of people with strong views about food, for example vegetarians or people with religious beliefs, who seem to have forgotten their previous lifelong habits and beliefs. Should family or staff in care institutions stop the vegetarian from eating meat if doing so seems to be giving the person pleasure? This brings into view questions about how to decide on a person's best interests (Chapter 12), as well as the debate about critical interests (the *then*-self) and experiential interests (the *now*-self) (Chapters 12 and 13). Similarly, questions are asked about a healthy diet and whether food low in salt and sugar should be foisted upon people in their best interests. In this chapter, the focus is purely on the ethical issue of what to do when the person can no longer swallow or is having difficulty swallowing.

In a sense, when it comes to artificial nutrition and hydration for people living with advanced dementia, little has changed since the review paper by Finucane et al. (1999). From the ethical perspective, little has changed since the reflections of Muriel Gillick (2000). One important change, however, is that we are now more inclined to speak of 'food and drink' rather than 'nutrition and hydration'. This simply reflects a move away from the medicalization of something that is a day-to-day human experience. Talk of 'feeding' people with dementia can also strike the wrong chord if it reminds people of feeding animals which might, thus, seem derogatory. However, we readily talk of ourselves being fed well, for example if we have been to friends or family for a meal. It is difficult to get around some locutions which inevitably suggest dependency. We do sometimes need to be fed. This does not mean that we should always resort to the language of feeding if we can avoid it. But sometimes we cannot.

Tube feeding involves tubes being placed either through the nose and down the throat (a nasogastric tube – NGT), or directly into the stomach via a percutaneous endoscopic gastrostomy (PEG) tube, which involves a hole through the abdominal wall. Finucane et al. (1999) found no good evidence that tube feeding increased survival, prevented aspiration pneumonia, reduced the risk of pressure sores or helped functionally or palliatively. Gillick (2000) used this type of evidence to argue convincingly (I think) that, because gastrostomy tubes are not effective, 'there is neither a secular nor a religious ethical imperative to use them. In addition, they are not necessary to prevent suffering' (p. 208).

We now have more evidence, albeit still of low quality. In a Cochrane systematic review, N. Davies et al. (2021) found:

> ... no evidence that tube feeding improves survival; improves quality of life; reduces pain; reduces mortality; decreases behavioural and psychological symptoms of dementia; leads to better nourishment; improves family or carer outcomes such as depression, anxiety, carer burden, or satisfaction with care; ...
>
> (p. 2).

Although they found no evidence of harm from tube feeding, they found clinically significant evidence of a risk of pressure ulcers (p. 2), all of which makes the ethical case against the use of tube feeding even more compelling. It is worth clarifying a few facts.

The prevalence of swallowing problems (dysphagia) depends on the population being studied. In older people living independently (mean age 76 years), Roy et al. (2007) found a lifetime prevalence of 38 per cent and a current prevalence of 33 per cent. The prevalence of dysphagia in those with moderate to severe Alzheimer's disease, across several studies, which included videofluoroscopy, ranged from 84 to 93 per cent (Boccardi et al. 2016). (Videofluoroscopy is the gold standard when it comes to investigating dysphagia. It involves using a small camera being placed in the larynx to visualize the mechanisms of swallowing in real time.) Although dysphagia and its consequences (such as aspiration with the potential to cause pneumonia) are typically regarded as late and often terminal events in dementia, changes in cerebral control of swallowing and in swallowing itself have been demonstrated (again using videofluoroscopy) early in the disease (Priefer and Robbins 1997; Humbert et al. 2010). Of course, that dysphagia can be detected early does not support, as some have suggested (Regnard 2010), the idea that tube feeding should be commenced sooner rather than later. Nutritional support may be required but also may not (Hoffer 2006). In any case, as we shall see shortly, there is evidence that some people living with dementia are against tube feeding.

Those providing care to people living with dementia need to be educated about how swallowing difficulties change as the disease progresses, from cognitive difficulties early on to physical challenges later; and the aims of care can also change from ensuring adequate nutrition to providing comfort (Barrado-Martín et al. 2022). The same research group undertook interviews with people living with mild dementia to explore their understanding of possible future eating and drinking problems and to seek their perspectives (Anantapong et al. 2021). Interestingly, people with dementia preferred to leave discussions and decisions about feeding issues until they occurred and in the hands of family and professionals. In addition, 'For participants, the ability to eat and drink represented quality of life, sense of identity and agency. ... There was general opposition to [artificial nutrition and hydration] as they perceived that it was unnatural and would not bring them enjoyment and quality of life' (p. 1823). They wished to protect their sense of identity and agency for as long as possible. The authors suggested: 'The main purpose of eating and drinking for people living with dementia may not be to maintain weight and have optimal nutrition, but to benefit from the psychosocial aspects of eating and drinking that retain their identity, autonomy and quality of life' (Anantapong et al. 2021: 1827).

Vignette: Mr Garcia's eating problems

Mr Garcia is in the severe stage of dementia with Lewy bodies and has been in a nursing home for nine months. He is totally dependent on staff for help with all of his basic activities. His wife visits every day and helps to look after him. The time he takes to eat has become gradually longer. He has had some episodes of choking and a mild chest infection. His wife does not mind feeding him slowly and carefully, but staff have started to question whether he needs some form of tube-feeding.

Some ethical reflections on eating and drinking in dementia

In the European Association for Palliative Care's white paper, which defined optimal palliative care in older people with dementia for the first time, the items around feeding and drinking were contentious, only achieving moderate consensus (van der Steen et al. 2014). Subcutaneous hydration was thought appropriate for infections, where the person was likely to get better, but was felt inappropriate when the person was dying (§6.4). Permanent tube feeding was deemed on the whole not to be beneficial and recommended to be avoided in people with dementia, whereas 'skilful hand feeding is preferred' (§6.5). Some years before we had followed a similar tack:

> Being fed brings personal attention and care and may, for this reason, be of value to the person with dementia. Hence, many would wish to opt for conservative methods of feeding, using good positioning, with small amounts of food of the correct consistency.
>
> (Hughes and Baldwin 2006: 112)

The aim of helping someone to eat in this way is to prevent, or at least minimize, the risk that the person will aspirate (that is, that food will go into the lungs with the risk of pneumonia) and yet still maintain the benefits of human interaction.

On the whole, however, the ethics literature contains relatively little that is specifically about eating and drinking in dementia (as opposed to more general discussions about withholding and withdrawing treatments, especially in the context of a persistent vegetative state). The treatment of the ethical issues in the literature on tube feeding in dementia tends to be perfunctory, for instance simply making brief reference to the four principles of medical ethics (for example, Chen et al. 2011).

Barrado-Martín et al. (2021) included a section on ethical concerns and highlighted decision-making, capacity and communication. They found the research literature recorded staff reflecting on dilemmas around harm reduction, autonomy and the preservation of life. There was the worry that withholding tube feeding was akin to killing the person or giving up on basic care. But even in those who felt that tube feeding was futile, there was still the feeling they should be doing something. It might have been helpful for those concerned to reflect that: 'We seem to have forgotten the difference between people who die because they stop taking in food and water, and people who stop taking in food and water because of the natural dying process' (Brody et al. 2011: 1056). Barrado-Martín et al. (2021) also recorded the tension felt by nursing home staff who had to balance 'what they were expected to do with what they thought was right' (p. 675). For instance, they had to balance respecting a person's wish not to eat with the feeling that they should keep on enticing them to do so.

Brody et al. (2011) presented a good account of the evolution of the tension between, on the one hand, regarding artificial feeding as basic care and, on the other, seeing it as an extraordinary means of treatment, one which palliative care would tend not to use. (This gestures at the doctrine of ordinary and extraordinary means, which I shall pursue further in the next two chapters.) Brody et al. (2011) made the point that this is not simply a case of 'consent for a technical procedure' (p. 1056). They went on to say: 'Patient preferences are not safeguarded through blanket statutory mandates and exceptions, but rather are best protected by those who know and, ideally, care about the now-incompetent patient' (p. 1057).

Further evidence of moral tension for those who provide care was presented in Bryon et al. (2012), who looked at the experience of Flemish nurses. The nurses found themselves in conflict with physicians over whether or not tube-feeding should be employed. The nurses felt that a raft of ethical values was ignored by decisions to pursue artificial feeding: 'respect for autonomy, mercy, beneficence, non-maleficence, quality of life, and human dignity' (p. 290). According to the nurses, 'the patient's vulnerability was not respected; on the contrary, the patient was wronged' (Bryon et al. 2012: 290). These authors felt that all the actors involved in decisions about feeding (doctors, nurses, family, but we should add speech and language specialists, psychologists and so on, as well as people with dementia insofar as they are able) should be engaged in the deliberations: 'It is in the middle of this complex tangle of strong and conflicting attitudes, intuitions, and arguments that the right decision for the patient has to be made' (p. 293). In order to navigate the tussles between the demand for aggressive care and comfort care, a consensus-building decision-making process is required that will respect values and preferences as well as the person's dignity (Dimech et al. 2021).

Just to pull some of these threads together, what we see is a real possibility of moral distress in those who look after people living with advanced dementia like Mr Garcia, who are starting to develop dysphagia. Carers, whether professionals or family and friends, wish neither to over- nor under-treat the person. They recognize that to use tube feeding might be to do harm (both physical and psychological), but not to use it might also cause (physical and psychological) harm. So even when they are doing the right thing, they can feel bad about it. There is a mixture of conflicting values, which calls for some of the insights of values-based practice (see Chapter 5). Certainly, whether to place a feeding tube is not simply a technical question. What is required is real care and close knowledge of the person, with proper recognition of the person's vulnerability and dignity.

Patterns of practice and Mr Garcia

It would seem radically incoherent to encourage a practice that involved providing a treatment to someone that was known to be futile, unnecessary and potentially harmful (Hoffer 2006; Harwood 2014; N. Davies et al. 2021) when otherwise one would never think of doing such a thing. As people enter the palliative phase of their lives, palliative measures are much more appropriate. This is not to say that artificial means of feeding and providing fluids should never be used in advanced dementia. I once looked after someone who developed macroglossia (a large tongue) and could take no food by mouth. The cause of the macroglossia was never established, but the swelling went down after several months. During this time she was fed by a tube, which was then removed when she could swallow again normally.

From the perspective of external coherence, careful hand-feeding fits in with a form of life that values nurture and human contact. Food and drink are all about the person's engagement with the world. Honesty, openness, fidelity and self-effacement are some of the virtues a clinician will require in order to navigate the difficult conversations and decisions that can arise in connection with eating and drinking in advanced dementia.

Mr Garcia is unlikely to benefit from PEG tube-feeding and he may suffer harm. His wife will need to have these realities carefully explained, along with her husband's likely prognosis; and she and the staff must be properly instructed on how best to feed Mr Garcia. His decreased requirements for food and fluid should be recognized. Mrs Garcia should be encouraged by the thought that her presence is likely to be reassuring and a comfort to her husband.

Conclusion

Iris Murdoch wrote this in *The Sovereignty of Good*: 'I have used the word 'attention' … to express the idea of a just and loving gaze directed upon an individual reality. I believe this to be the characteristic and proper mark of the active moral agent' (Murdoch 1970: 34). It is too easy to think of moral dilemmas as solved by the dispassionate and disengaged application of principles or theories. But this is not how things feel in the real world; or not how they should feel if our dilemmas are true. Rather, when we are truly attentive to the nature of the reality that confronts us, this will involve looking justly (with balance and right judgement) and with love, which means not mere sentimentality, but genuine warmth and solicitude.

Antibiotics and infections

Introduction

Where artificial means would have to be used continuously to keep someone fed and watered, the argument in favour of using such means usually emphasizes the importance of life itself, so that not to use tube feeding seems to involve aiming at the death of the person and is repudiated on that basis. This argument can be countered if it is accepted that the person is naturally dying and that aggressive treatment would be disproportionate to the reality of the situation. It is sometimes implied that all religious belief entails that everything should always be done to keep people alive. Faith traditions often emphasize the intrinsic importance of life as such; but in most there are arguments about how this insistence on preserving life can be lessened in certain circumstances. For example, the Catholic doctrine of ordinary and extraordinary means allows treatment to be stopped or not started under certain circumstances. I shall return to this doctrine in the next chapter, but it is instructive to note how Pope (now Saint) John Paul II (1995) saw matters. He said that the moral obligation to take care of yourself or to accept care 'must take account of concrete circumstances'. He went on:

> It needs to be determined whether the means of treatment available are objectively proportionate to the prospects for improvement. To forego extraordinary or disproportionate means ... expresses acceptance of the human condition in the face of death
>
> (§65).

The talk here of 'concrete circumstances' and 'the human condition in the face of death' is pertinent to the position of the person living with advanced dementia and relevant to ethical dilemmas around eating and drinking, as discussed in the last chapter, to issues around the use of antibiotics and the treatment of infections, the topic of this chapter, and to resuscitation, which will be discussed in the next. What is perhaps striking about antibiotics and infections in severe dementia is that there is a greater reliance on clinical judgement than there needs to be in the case of artificial food and fluid or CPR.

Vignette: Mr Bhatia's infection

The Bhatia family have all along been keen to look after Mr Bhatia at home, despite his dementia worsening. They have been able to do so although he is now bed-ridden. He has, however, developed a fever and has clearly become very ill. With patience and care, his family can encourage him to take small amounts of fluid. It is thought he is likely to have a urinary tract infection. The family GP thinks he probably requires intravenous antibiotics, for which he should be admitted to hospital. But the family are adamantly against this. They want him to be kept at home and given antibiotics by mouth.

Antibiotics and infections in advanced dementia

In a seminal paper, Fabiszewski et al. (1990) showed that there was no difference in terms of survival between a group of people with Alzheimer's disease who received antibiotics for fevers and those who only received comfort care (such as antipyretics, analgesics, oxygen, oral hydration and general hospice nursing care). Antibiotic treatment did not alter the outcome and most people with fevers survived in any case. The people developing fevers tended to have more advanced dementia. This lent some support to the idea that antibiotics could be withheld in the treatment of people with advanced dementia as part of palliative management.

However, van der Steen et al. (2002a) demonstrated that pneumonia in people with advanced dementia was not a benign condition (it was not, as suggested by William Osler (1849–1919), 'the friend of the aged' (Osler 1892)). It was associated with significant discomfort and, moreover, the discomfort was worse in those where antibiotics were withheld and in those who died. Van der Steen and her colleagues have confirmed this finding: pneumonia seemed to cause great suffering in people living with dementia, whereas antibiotic use before death decreased discomfort (van der Steen et al. 2009a). In a later study – which involved Ladislav Volicer, who was the inspiration behind the Fabiszewski et al. (1990) paper and, indeed, the inspiration behind the whole movement of palliative care for people living with dementia (see Volicer et al. 1986) – of male nursing home residents with advanced dementia and pneumonias, antibiotics did prolong life, but mostly only for a matter of days (van der Steen et al. 2012). The worry, then, is that antibiotics might simply prolong the dying process.

Subsequently, however, a further study of suffering in pneumonia in people with dementia seemed to suggest that symptomatic treatment of the pneumonia itself, for instance with oxygen, analgesia, antipyretics and corticosteroids, was enough to decrease distress and suffering without the use of antibiotics (van der Maaden et al. 2016). Maybe better treatment of the symptoms of pneumonia, where such treatments tend to take effect more quickly than antibiotics, would be the rational approach; or maybe both antibiotic treatment and symptomatic treatment are required. In a summary of the state of play, Parsons and van der Steen (2017) made this comment:

> A decision to treat a patient with signs and symptoms suggestive of infection may not necessarily require the prescribing of antibiotic therapy. Such a decision may ... be revisited as a patient is offered symptomatic relief and supportive care, including pain management, skin care and hydration.
>
> (p. 436)

Before leaving this brief review of the evidence, it is worth going back to an earlier observational cohort study in nursing homes in the Netherlands, to see that the clinical judgements being made reflected particular conditions and distinctions. In van der Steen et al. (2002b), antibiotics were withheld in 23 per cent of the residents with pneumonias; they were used with palliative intent in 8 per cent and with curative intent in 69 per cent of cases. Antibiotics were withheld in those with more severe dementia, who had more severe pneumonia, lower food and fluid intake and were more frequently dehydrated. In other words, these people were especially frail. The use of antibiotics palliatively might seem counterintuitive, except that elsewhere in palliative care antibiotics have been used to help with infected bronchial secretions (Clayton et al. 2003). At least in the Netherlands, there is evidence that doctors are making judgements about prognosis and withholding antibiotics when they feel the person is very close to death (van der Steen et al. 2009b).

Patterns of practice: Mr Bhatia's infection and clinical judgement

Several judgments must be made by Mr Bhatia's doctor. Does Mr Bhatia actually have a urinary tract infection? In someone with advanced dementia it can be hard to be certain. Could it be an infection elsewhere and perhaps an asymptomatic bacteriuria (Woodford 2010: 231–237)? Would oral antibiotics be effective? Does he really need hospital admission? The doctor will have certain patterns of practice when it comes to this sort of situation.

The point I wish to pursue here is that the judgements required will be part of these patterns of practice. At a basic level, for the sake of internal coherence, the practice must include taking a history, examining Mr Bhatia and performing any investigations or special tests (which will be rather limited in these circumstances). Forming a clinical judgement about the diagnosis will emerge from this pattern of practice; so too will the judgement about what treatment to recommend, which will include a recommendation about where treatment should take place and exactly what the doctor should say to the family (and how it should be said).

For the sake of external coherence, the doctor must be diligent, charitable and honest, while showing fidelity, practical wisdom and humble propriety, that is, 'internalized patterns of attention, care and sensitivity to the effects on others of one's behavior and words' (Radden and Sadler 2010: 112–113).

Clinical judgements, I wish to say, will emanate from the patterns of practice. So it is worth thinking about clinical judgements because, in a sense, they are the whole ethical deal. It is these judgements that are either right or wrong, good or bad. How do we ensure that they are right and good? Well, the answer must be that we need to get the practices right, which is why they need to show both internal and external coherence. If the practices are right (in the sense of coherent) the judgements that come from them will also be right. We can gain some insight into all of this by looking at clinical judgements in a little more detail.

The way to see the importance of clinical judgements is to ask whether they could be made by a machine. Could they be operationalized? The answer is that artificial intelligence is indeed being used to make diagnoses, to aid treatment decisions and so on (Hamet and Tremblay 2017; Secinaro et al. 2021). But is there something about clinical judgments made by human beings that could not in principle be pinned down by machine processes? I wish to say that there is something ineffable about clinical judgement. Hence, I wish to highlight some of the work on tacit knowledge.

To get there, it is worth reiterating a mantra from Chapter 6, that our actions can be regarded as, *at one and the same time* ethical and practical. Clinical judgements, therefore, must also be regarded as ethical. The normativity of clinical judgements – the fact that there are criteria of correctness surrounding clinical judgements (not just any judgement will do!) – is inherent: it is in the nature of such judgements. As such, we can say that the normativity of clinical judgements is inherent to the practices. (This argument is spelt out in more detail in Hughes and Ramplin 2012.)

The key thing is that a practice is not an algorithm. Clinical judgements can be described algorithmically, but algorithms cannot completely capture everything of relevance because there will always be particular circumstances in need of interpretation, which will, moreover, be changeable. We might think that a sophisticated enough algorithm could be set up to capture all of the variables, even those that vary. But this is where tacit knowledge comes in: '… we cannot articulate the background framework according to which we make the interpretations that culminate in clinical or ethical judgements' (Hughes and Ramplin 2012: 232). We can articulate certain backgrounds, but what are the backgrounds to these backgrounds? Eventually this regress must end at something which is accepted as a given, without interpretation, which we simply show by the way we carry on and engage with the world. There is an ineffable background to the interpretation of the changeable and particular circumstances of any case which has to be grasped correctly. Thornton (2007) put it this way: 'Even when a form of judgement can be codified as the application of a principle or rule, the application of the rule still depends on an element of uncodified skill' (p. 222). This, in turn, reflects much thought to be found in Wittgenstein's philosophy, some of which can be summarized thus: 'What determines our judgement, our concepts and reactions, is not what *one* man is doing *now*, but the whole hurly-burly of human actions, the background against which we see any action' (Wittgenstein 1981: §567). That is, we need to see the whole.

To return to the case of Mr Bhatia. The doctor needs to consider, amongst many things (and note that the host of considerations comes in part from the sort of work undertaken by van der Steen and colleagues on pneumonia, even though we think Mr Bhatia has a urinary tract infection): the type and severity of Mr Bhatia's dementia; his current health and frailty as shown by the particular symptoms which he now exhibits; the history given by the family and the results of the examination and investigations; the responses of Mr Bhatia; whether and how things are changing; whether Mr Bhatia is distressed; what the doctor knows of Mr Bhatia from the past including any sense there might be of Mr Bhatia's beliefs and preferences; his estimation of the prognosis; the views and values of the family; their resources to cope; whether there is any-one with differing opinions; anyone with a relevant power of attorney; what realistic treatment options exist; and so on.

Conclusion

Infections in people with advanced dementia may well require the use of anti-biotics, but this is not inevitable. Instead, practitioners are required to make nuanced clinical judgements, which will be more or less ethical depending on the skill with which a whole picture has been understood and interpreted. Meanwhile, families and people living with dementia might help with these later decisions if they have discussed matters much earlier when the capacity to make decisions was not in doubt. If there are worries or uncertainties about religious beliefs, it can be highly useful to bring in others of the same religion to talk through issues. Professionals facing religious insistence that treatment should not be stopped can also seek the advice of appropriate religious leaders. Again, having conversations frankly and early is probably for the best. The ethical issue here is to do with honouring and respecting the person as a whole, as a person situated as an embodied agent in a network of relationships.

30 Resuscitation

Introduction

In this chapter I shall briefly review some of the literature around cardiopulmonary resuscitation (CPR) in people living with dementia. There are three worries about the use of CPR in very frail older people. First, chest compressions can cause fractured ribs; secondly, it is an undignified process; thirdly, the person may end up in a worse state than they were in before, for example if the brain is starved of oxygen. CPR does not include other forms of resuscitation, such as treating someone with septic shock with fluid and antibiotics. In other words, even if I have stated that I do not wish to have CPR, I may still wish to be resuscitated in other ways for other conditions. Finally, I shall pursue a little further the doctrine of ordinary and extraordinary means, which has already been mentioned in the preceding two chapters.

Vignette: Mrs Doyle and the Do Not Resuscitate decision

Her family realized that as soon as Mrs Doyle was admitted to hospital they would be asked to decide on whether she should be for CPR. Having lived in a care home for four years, Mrs Doyle had fallen and fractured her hip. It was felt that surgery had to be performed, but she was very frail and had been in the advanced stages of mixed vascular and Alzheimer's dementia for some while. It was agreed she lacked the capacity to make any complex treatment decisions. The family struggled to know how they would answer a question about resuscitation.

Resuscitation in people living with dementia

Doyal and Wilsher (1994) stated that many people with advanced dementia were lacking minimal personal identity.

> When such patients reach the stage at which they no longer have any consistent sense of their past, present, or future, their 'biographical' life has ended. In such circumstances clinicians do not have a moral obligation to attempt to prolong lives that have little more than a physical dimension.
>
> (p. 1691)

I think this is a bad reason not to resuscitate because of the arguments presented in Chapter 13. Chiefly, it disqualifies people from treatment on the grounds of a very limited view of personal identity. Talk of 'little more than a physical dimension' is far too dismissive of the notion of embodied selfhood (Kontos 2005).

On the other hand, there are also bad reasons to resuscitate. Some years ago, it became the default position in the UK, as elsewhere, that everyone should be resuscitated unless it was documented that they were not for resuscitation. There were good reasons for this policy (mainly to do with paternalistic decisions not to resuscitate with no regard to the person's autonomy), but it did not always have good effects. For instance, some families found themselves frequently being asked to confirm the decision not to resuscitate, which was upsetting for them. In addition, legal cases have confirmed that the person must be consulted about decisions not to resuscitate (*R (David Tracey) v Cambridge University Hospitals NHS Foundation Trust & Ors.* 2014. EWCA Civ 822) and that relatives and carers of people who lack capacity must be consulted (*Winspear v City Hospitals Sunderland NHS Foundation Trust.* 2015. EWHC 3250 (QB)). Both rulings, again, can be seen to be motivated by good reasons, but their effects have not always been to the benefit of the people concerned (MacCormick et al. 2018). They also raise broader issues to do with the juridification of clinical practice, that is, where the law intrudes on matters of practice which are better left to those who must make decisions on the ground (Montgomery and Montgomery 2016).

It has been known for a long time that older people, even when frail, are content to discuss resuscitation (Kellogg et al. 1992; Bruce-Jones et al. 1996). It has frequently been found that family carers are keener on aggressive treatment than professionals and, indeed, than older people themselves (Harrison et al. 1995; Coetzee et al. 2003). Views might change with discussion and education; but, even so, these decisions remain difficult for carers who must accept the responsibility of making surrogate decisions despite facing the existential issues raised by the prospect of death (Albinsson and Strang 2003).

What we know is that CPR tends to be less effective in older people (Murphy et al. 1989); its chances of success were poor even when physicians were to hand in a long-term-care facility with an intermediate and 'skilled' care unit (Awoke et al. 1992); indeed, the chances of survival seem to be about the same as they are for people with metastatic cancer (Ebell et al. 1998); and, apart from being unsuccessful in most people in care homes and community hospitals, it can cause harm (see above) and seems inappropriate in such settings (Conroy et al. 2006).

For these sorts of reasons, many faith traditions allow that CPR is not compulsory when it is likely to be futile (Gordon 2006; Chamsi-Pasha and Albar 2018). In the Jewish tradition, a distinction is sometimes made between a person who is a *goses*, that is moribund and actively dying, and one who is a *treifah*, where the person is incurable and will die but not immediately (Gillick 2001). If someone is a *goses* you should not stop them from dying. More nuanced decisions will be required for the person who is a *treifah*. In the Catholic faith, as we saw at the start of Chapter 29, the Pope was against aggressive medical treatments 'which no longer correspond to the real situation of the patient' and were 'disproportionate' to any expected outcomes (Pope John Paul II. 1995: §65).

Ordinary and extraordinary means

This was, in fact, a statement by the Pope of the doctrine of ordinary and extraordinary means. There is no moral obligation to undertake an investigation or treatment which can be regarded as extraordinary, where this means that it would be unlikely to work and would be a burden. When we think of CPR in people with advanced dementia, we can say that it is unlikely to be effective and is likely to cause the person actual harm (from fractured ribs to undignified dying). So, resuscitation is not morally obligatory even if it is carried out for some other reason (for example, to allow time for a relative to attend the bedside of the dying person). Ordinary care, which is likely to be effective and is non-burdensome, is morally required.

Unfortunately, some commentators have missed the point of the doctrine by becoming confused about the definition of the words 'ordinary' and 'extraordinary' and by a focus on the autonomous wishes of the people involved (Glover 1977: 195–196; John 2007: 269–272). Gillon (1986), a clinician, perceived a consensus around 'an approach which it is widely agreed requires that medical attempts to preserve people's lives should be regarded as an extremely important good, which it is morally important to pursue except when to do so is either futile or causes disproportionate harm' (p. 146). It has certainly been my experience that, when explained to relatives of people with advanced dementia in these terms – that this type of resuscitation is unlikely to work and is likely to be burdensome, that is, harmful – they almost always agree that it would not be right to inflict such treatment on their loved ones. Importantly, it can be seen that the implied criticism is of the treatment in these particular circumstances; it is not a comment on the person's quality of life or identity.

Conclusion

Is there internal coherence to such a practice? The same considerations can apply to all other investigations and treatments, so this is a coherent pattern of practice. From the external perspective, the pattern of practice coheres with important, relevant virtues, such as the need for charity, for integrity, for honesty and transparency. It can also be regarded as a matter of medical temperance, avoiding the overuse or underuse of medical technology; Pellegrino and Thomasma (1993) suggested it could be termed '"therapeutic parsimony" – using only those interventions that may result in a reasonable ordering of effectiveness, benefit, and burdens' (p. 122).

31 Death and dying

Introduction

In a sense, one way or another, the last three chapters have all been about death and dying but this chapter more firmly focuses on the end of life. First, I shall consider what has been written about the termination of treatment, including life-supporting treatment in the context of dementia. Secondly, I shall move to the topics of euthanasia and physician-assisted suicide. Thirdly, I shall discuss palliative care. In connection with these topics, the doctrine of ordinary and extraordinary means, discussed in the preceding chapters, rears its head; but, before concluding, I shall also touch upon the doctrine of double effect.

Termination of treatments

Issues around withholding and withdrawing treatment are pertinent to dementia, as we have seen with respect to artificial feeding, the use of antibiotics and CPR. But there are many other circumstances where relevant issues arise. If someone living with severe dementia becomes anaemic, how far should this be investigated? Similarly with excessive weight loss: what would count as ordinary investigations (the sort we ought to do – according to the doctrine of ordinary and extraordinary means – because they are not burdensome and are likely to lead to efficacious therapy which is itself unlikely to cause harm) and what, in the particular circumstances that hold, would be extraordinary (because burdensome and essentially futile)? Is it worth offering bone protection to older people with dementia and, if so, with what type of regime and for how long? Are there medications we could discontinue once the person is living with advanced dementia (Baqir et al. 2014)? Is surgery necessary in severe dementia, for example, for a squamous cell carcinoma, for a fracture in someone who is immobile, or for an aortic aneurysm found by chance? And so on. In each case, depending on the details, our answer might be yes or no. We must apply the sort of ethical analysis already advertised throughout this book.

Such ethical issues in the context of advanced dementia have been around for a long while. Levinson (1981), for instance, discussed life support for older people at some length and emphasized that the person's expressed wishes should be of primary concern. The task when the person lacks capacity is to figure out, if possible, what their wishes would have been; in other words, this is to encourage substituted judgements (discussed in Chapter 12). Levinson (1981) saw no ethical difference between withholding and withdrawing a treatment, albeit we know that withdrawing is always psychologically harder than not starting in the first place. Instead, Levinson (1981) stressed the importance of the intention behind the action, but went on summarily to dismiss as 'semantic quibbling' (p. 84) the doctrine of double effect (to which I shall return). Levinson (1981) ended by saying that killing is permissible, 'but only when death is the best life has to offer' (p. 84) and only when the person concerned or those acting for the person have reached this conclusion. This raises a number of issues, to which we shall come.

The problem of knowing what the person would have wanted, in the absence of any advance care planning, is potentially solved by recognizing the extent to which the mental life of someone living with dementia 'can be viewed as extended and embodied by her supportive social environment' (Muramoto 2011: 339). This reflects the broader notion of personhood I discussed in Chapter 13, according to which the person is a situated embodied agent (Hughes 2001 and 2011b). The importance of our situatedness or embeddedness in our families and communities (amongst many other things) is very relevant to the person nearing death. Muramoto (2011) used such ideas to encourage the thought that medical decision-making for people living with dementia 'can be construed as a temporally and socially extended practice' (p. 339). In other words, accepting advance directives (sometimes called 'living wills' – see Chapter 12 and Figure 12.1 in particular – which might be very informal values statements or, under the MCA governing England and Wales, legally binding advance decisions to refuse treatment) and taking close note of the views of family and those who know the individual well, must be the ethical way to proceed if we are to show respect for the person. Hence the importance of people living with dementia and their families or close carers discussing these issues at a stage when this is still possible.

The importance of our interconnectedness is brought out very well in May's (2012) talk of the enduring covenant that characterizes the relationship of a professional to someone who is dying. Such covenants suggest the virtues of integrity, discernment and fidelity. What is required in looking after someone who is dying, particularly when the person has advanced dementia, is that the complexity of the situation should be seen, which entails seeing the nexus of relationships which surround us all. Approaching decision-making at the end of life with awareness of such complexity will make us less prone to think that decisions about investigations and treatments can be simply made. As we have seen in the preceding chapters, sometimes artificial feeding will be required (even if rarely), we might need to use antibiotics palliatively and in extreme circumstances resuscitation might be warranted. May (2012) encouraged clinicians to look at the full clinical reality: '(1) not only the empirical imminence of death but also (2) the powerful ambivalence of human beings toward death and (3) the bonds between human beings that make death what it is' (p. 48).

Callahan (1995) opined that public opinion would set great store by good nursing and palliative care but would give a 'much lower priority to the use of expensive medicine to prolong life' in people living with dementia (p. 29).

He went on to suggest criteria for treatment termination in those living with the advanced stages of dementia:

1 People should not 'have to live longer in the advanced stages of dementia' than they would have done 'in a pre-technological era' (p. 29).
2 Given the deterioration there is likely to be in the late stages of dementia, there should be a shift towards stopping rather than continuing treatments.
3 The obligation 'to prevent a lingering, painful, or degrading death' (p. 30) is as great as that of supporting healthy life.

These criteria are entirely in keeping with the tenets of palliative care, where it is taken as axiomatic that such care aims neither to hasten nor to postpone death. The third criterion, however, impels us towards discussion of euthanasia and physician-assisted suicide if there is no other way to prevent 'a lingering, painful, or degrading death'. Perhaps the egregious term here is 'degrading'. For we might say a lingering death is only shocking if it is also (for instance) painful; and pain should be treatable, at least in theory. 'Degrading' suggests a loss of dignity, which takes us back to the discussion in Chapter 10.

It also gestures to the Dutch concept of *ontluistering*. Some years ago, there was a difference of opinion between the Royal Dutch Medical Association (KNMG) and the Dutch Association of Nursing Home Physicians (NVVA). The former felt that assisted suicide could be justified in the early stages of dementia because a person might fear 'the prospect of an inevitable loss of human dignity or *ontluistering*' (Berghmans 1999: 93). Whereas, the nursing home physicians (who work more closely with people living with dementia) disagreed. They felt that 'the now demented patient [sic] cannot experience the *ontluistering* that the previously competent former self of the patient has expressed as a condition for life termination' (p. 93). One question this raises is whether the idea of loss of human dignity is best conceived as subjective or as objective. If people think that their human dignity has been tarnished or lost, is this enough to make it so, or can an outside observer disagree? There is the suggestion from Chapter 10 that, in any case, human dignity can never be lost if it is inherent or inflorescent. But the broader issue is to do with whether there can be grounds for saying that 'death is the best life has to offer' (Levinson 1981: 84), to which I now turn.

Physician-assisted suicide and euthanasia

In Chapter 10 we came across the notion of *Menschenwürde*, which suggests the inherent dignity of all human beings. Gastmans and de Lepeleire (2010) described 'the dignity of the human person as the foundation of all other values' (p. 82) and stated, if this fundamental dignity (*Menschenwürde*) cannot be lost, then 'loss of dignity cannot be used as an argument for euthanasia in persons with severe dementia' (p. 84). They also suggested that '*care* constitutes the essence of human life' (p. 85). This is likely to reflect the sort of analysis provided by Heidegger, which I considered in Chapter 9. Accordingly, Gastmans and de Lepeleire (2010) went on to suggest that care for people living with dementia should be thought of as a moral duty, 'which is performed in an individual and societal way' (p. 85). We could draw on Heidegger again to speak of 'solicitude' – the sort of care or concern that characterizes authentic human interactions; and mention of 'societal' duties should remind us of the standing of people with dementia as citizens, discussed in Chapter 13.

Another philosopher we have already come across on several occasions – in connection with deontology (Chapter 3), autonomy (Chapter 8) and lying (Chapter 24) – is Kant. There are certainly grounds upon which Kant condemns suicide, but Cooley (2007) set out a number of examples of Kant allowing or even approving of suicide. For instance, a man bitten by a rabid dog is said to have a duty to kill himself before he loses his reason and inflicts harm on others. But Cooley (2007) went further and argued that Kant's arguments in favour of death by suicide can be extended to include people living with dementia. In a nutshell, Cooley's argument goes like this: as a moral agent there could be a duty to kill yourself under certain circumstances if it became clear that you were about to lose your moral life and dignity as a person; if you have to choose between your physical life and your moral life, better to lose your physical life and retain your standing as a person (as a moral agent) right up until the end.

The obvious problem with this argument is that it ignores the broader views of personhood discussed previously in Chapter 13 and encouraged throughout this book. In discussing Cooley's (2007) paper, Sharp (2012) said he was '... not convinced that a person with less rationality is inherently less deserving of being considered human and thus less deserving of being treated morally' (p. 235). Sharp concluded that the claim that we have a duty to commit suicide if we have dementia is too prone to abuse and '... opens the door to euthanasia arguments that depend almost solely on a belief that without full rationality, life is not worth living for human beings' (Sharp 2012: 235).

More critically, Cholbi (2015) argued that Cooley (2007) had simply made a category mistake in comparing people who should (according to the Kantian argument) commit suicide to avoid acting immorally as moral agents and those (living with dementia) who should kill themselves in order not to lose that moral agency. Cholbi (2015) suggested there is 'no moral dishonour in losing one's moral agency to the mental deterioration of dementia' (p. 610). Nevertheless, Cholbi (2015) seemed to accept that people with dementia will be 'non-persons' who are 'non-dignified', which I do not think is required when it is more straightforward to say (contra-Kant) that rationality is not the whole deal anyway!

Another philosopher, who regarded suicide as weak mindedness, to be recruited to the discussion of euthanasia in dementia is Baruch Spinoza (1632–1677). Alvargonzález (2012) noted that 'memory and abstract reasoning cannot be taken as the sole criterion to evaluate personhood, but must be considered alongside the ability to form and hold relationships with others ...' (p. 381).

Alvargonzález (2012) drew on Spinoza to emphasize the virtue of strength of character, *fortitudo*, which is a mixture of firmness (*animositas*) towards oneself and generosity (*generositas*) towards others. As a person's capacities lessen through dementia those around should try 'to sustain and resuscitate the remaining abilities' (p. 381). This is, according to Alvargonzález (2012: 381), the mandate set down by Spinoza's 'virtue of generosity: 'to support the diagnosed person's efforts to persist'. Alvargonzález (2012) was cautious about societal and political rhetoric used to justify euthanasia. He gestured towards a background of implicit fear that society will be burdened by the numbers of (politically costly) people with dementia. Instead, we should pursue, as a matter of firmness and generosity, proper palliative care for those who are dying.

Kant and Spinoza would have approved of this summary by Post (1990: 717) that killing people living with severe dementia is wrong:

> ... because we cannot assert that they have biographically ceased to exist, because an ethical society has a compelling interest in maintaining the general prohibition against killing, and because destroying the severely demented sends a negative message to all those older persons who are dependent on others.

Once again, the language – talk of the 'severely demented' – now seems out of place, but Post's inclination to place the person first (and not the disease) is elsewhere clear. Later Post (1997) wrote that he regarded euthanasia as undesirable because of worries about abuse and because, '... according to medical tradition, ... it confuses the art of healing and comforting with the practice of killing' (p. 649). Instead, Post (1997 and 2000) has encouraged a hospice-type of approach for people living with dementia. He also wrote: 'Assisted suicide in the context of terminal illness is not best understood purely in terms of an individual's right to die. Rather, it must be placed in a communitarian context in which responsibilities for the common good as well as rights have moral importance' (Post 2000: 122).

At this point it would be useful to summarize quite generally the arguments for and against euthanasia and physician-assisted suicide. These are emotive issues and, as will be known, the laws governing euthanasia and physician-assisted suicide differ in different countries. Some countries and states, such the Netherlands and Oregon in the USA, have legalized these practices, but most have not. Space does not allow for a full treatment of the issues. In Table 31.1, however, I have set out the main arguments, derived loosely from Graham and Hughes (2014). Not every argument is covered. There are a number of books which present many of these arguments in more depth (Keown 1995; Dworkin et al. 1998; Tulloch 2005; Keown 2002; Woods 2007).

Rather than linger over the details of the general arguments set out in Table 31.1, I shall now cover three more specific areas that relate to dementia, assisted suicide and euthanasia. These are: advance euthanasia directives, the assessment of capacity, stigma and mental health.

I should perhaps say, in connection with my discussion and with Table 31.1, that my position is steadfastly against assisted suicide and euthanasia.

Table 31.1 A summary of main arguments about assisted suicide and euthanasia

Arguments in favour	Rebuttals
Autonomy: If it is possible for someone to choose when and how to die the person should be able to do so. People should have control over their lives and over their deaths.	**Relational autonomy:** Autonomy should be seen through the network of our relationships, so the effects of our choices on others, especially those at risk of discrimination, need to be taken into account.
Unbearable suffering: No one should be forced to suffer if there is no need, especially if treatment is not working; this might also include mental suffering from, for instance, loss of dignity. On the grounds of autonomy, a person should be free to decide whether to suffer or die.	**Palliative care:** Pain and suffering should be treatable with the right type of approach and given the right expertise; the right approach would include attention to the person's dignity. In extreme cases of suffering, palliative sedation might be a suitable solution. Palliative care needs to be tried first, but needs more funding and research.

Arguments against	Rebuttals
Prohibition against killing: As Lord Walton (1994) put it: the prohibition of intentional killing 'is the cornerstone of law and of social relationships'.	**Intentional killing is tolerated:** We allow soldiers to kill; but in the case of assisted suicide and euthanasia, the people being killed would have asked to die.
Slippery slope and dangers: There is a conceptual argument that, once killing is allowed for certain reasons, there will be no line to stop killing for other reasons: for instance, if it is allowed for unbearable suffering, then why should this be restricted only to those very near the end of life (and who will judge)? There are empirical arguments too: that countries which have allowed assisted suicide and euthanasia have seen a steady increase in the indications that warrant such deaths.	**Safeguards:** There is no reason why safeguards cannot be put in place to restrict the circumstances under which physician-assisted suicide and euthanasia are allowed; and the degree to which there has in fact been slippage in those countries which have allowed assisted suicide and euthanasia is disputed, or the expansion of criteria where such deaths are allowable is considered to be justifiable and reflect a basic right to have one's autonomous decisions respected.

I am aware that the terminology I have been using – 'assisted suicide' rather than 'assisted dying' – will be considered obtuse by those who hold different views to mine. But I cannot see such deaths as anything other than suicide and, moreover, 'assisted dying' is what hospice and palliative care have been providing for many years. We should not obfuscate the issue by using quasi-prudish language.

Vignette: The true case of Mrs A's advance euthanasia directive

Mrs A was a Dutch woman in her 70s living with a diagnosis of Alzheimer's disease. She had witnessed a relative die from dementia and she said to her family that she would rather undergo euthanasia than be placed in a nursing home. Shortly after her diagnosis she wrote an advance euthanasia directive saying that she would wish to be euthanized if she were not able to live at home with her husband. More than 3 years after her diagnosis (a year before she died) she re-wrote her directive to say she wanted 'to undergo euthanasia whenever I think the time is right...' (Wall 2019: 77). Mrs A was subsequently moved into a nursing home. Miller et al. (2019) provided details: she was sometimes unhappy in the home, but when asked if she wanted to die she replied '... not just now'; the geriatrician determined that her suffering was unbearable and that euthanasia was appropriate; this opinion was confirmed (as required by Dutch law) by two physicians; in the presence of her family, but without telling her, a sedative was given; whilst she was subsequently being given an injection of thiopental she tried to get up; her family helped to restrain her whilst the rest of the injection was given and she died.

Miller et al. (2019) raised doubts about her capacity to make her directives and suggested that there had been little evidence of her having weighed up her decision adequately. They also noted the lack of adequate protection for someone who was vulnerable. The case prompted much debate (for example, Jongsma et al. 2019; Kim et al. 2019; Menzel 2019; Asscher and van de Vathorst 2020; J.A. Hughes 2021). Between them, the required Regional Review Committee and a medical disciplinary tribunal found that the advance euthanasia directive lacked clarity and suggested that no assent was given. However, a subsequent hearing in a criminal court disagreed and acquitted the doctor of wrongdoing (J.A. Hughes 2021).

Advance euthanasia directives

Gómez-Vírseda and Gastmans (2021: online) set out the complexity that needs to inform decisions to implement advance euthanasia directives (AEDs), with an emphasis on dignity and vulnerability:

> ... 'blind' adherence to AEDs is not a care practice that provides an adequate response to the vulnerabilities experienced by persons with dementia, their relatives and healthcare professionals. An interpretative dialogue that respects the multilayered vulnerability of the different stakeholders is necessary to achieve what can be considered as good care.

These authors commend the need for a broad view of dignity, the relevance of relational autonomy and the importance of palliative care as a way to promote dignity.

Van Delden (2004) felt that advance directives for euthanasia were neither feasible nor ethically justifiable. For: 'At the moment precedent autonomy is invoked, the patient involved will no longer be able to deliberate or choose. As soon as the advance directive becomes relevant, it is this directive that determines what needs to be done, not the patient' (p. 450). Because in advanced dementia it is not possible to discuss with people the thoughts and conceptions that led them to make the advance directive, nor what it will entail, the sort of dialogical interaction, commended by Gómez-Vírseda and Gastmans (2021), is not possible. Others have also agreed with van Delden (2004). Thus Hertogh et al. (2007: 54), '– for both clinical and ethical reasons – the condition of advanced dementia can never be a reason to perform euthanasia based on an AED'. Kouwenhoven et al. (2015) also found that physicians were reluctant to do without conversations to verify a person's advance euthanasia directive and to test the extent of 'unbearable suffering'. For most of the physicians in their study, 'Performing euthanasia in a case where the presence of unbearable suffering and voluntariness of the request cannot be directly confirmed by the patient is a bridge too far…' (Kouwenhoven et al. 2015: online).

Hertogh et al. (2007) wondered why there had not been a greater use of physician-assisted suicide in people living with milder dementia where the problem of doubtful interactions would not be such an issue. Perhaps the life instinct is just too great. Meanwhile, Bolt et al. (2015) found that, whilst most Dutch physicians could conceive of undertaking euthanasia or assisted suicide for those with cancer or other physical diseases, this was not so clearcut for other conditions: only 34 per cent thought it conceivable for psychiatric disease; for early dementia the figure was 40 per cent, but it was only 29 per cent for those with advanced dementia, a written AED and in the absence of comorbidities; and the figure was only 18 per cent for those tired of living but without medical grounds for suffering (Bolt et al. 2015). Undoubtedly this shows increased uncertainty where evaluative decisions become more complicated.

On the whole, therefore, it seems there are significant ethical challenges recognized in connection with advance euthanasia directives. In the main this is because respect for autonomy can be called into question more readily in dementia; and, as we have seen in Table 31.1, autonomy is one of the main arguments in support of euthanasia and physician-assisted suicide.

Capacity

In Chapter 11, I reached the conclusion that the notion of capacity involves complexity. It is also much more evaluative than might be thought at first blush and needs – in the intricacies of real-life decision-making – to be put into effect with considerable care. All of this remains very relevant when thinking about advance euthanasia directives and about euthanasia and physician-assisted suicide in general. For instance, Hotopf et al. (2011a) asked: 'When would a patient with depression, who believes that their life is not worth living, that they should stop being a burden to their family, and should thus receive assisted suicide, be making an incapacitous decision?' (p. 84). They also pointed out that clinicians should support people to make decisions, but that it is necessary to pay attention to the seriousness and irreversible nature of decisions to end one's life. Hence, we have to ask how high should '… the mental capacity bar …

be set to end one's life by suicide' (p. 84)? Subsequently they suggested, with seeming irony, that they suspected that mental capacity assessments for assisted dying 'are unlikely to be value neutral' (Hotopf 2011b).

We also need to consider that the ideal of the autonomous agent making competent decisions in the context of knowledge that they have a deteriorating condition such as one of the dementias can seem unrealistic. 'The image of an independent, capable and voluntary person is an ideal, and not easily found in the context of the usual care for the dying geriatric patient' (Kissane 1999: 459). This is not to say that people living with dementia cannot make rational decisions. However, (a) mental capacity is often slipping by the time a diagnosis has been made (which is, after all, a reason to make earlier diagnoses) and capacity assessments are not necessarily easy in those living with mild to severe dementia (Kim et al. 2021c); (b) the possibility of strong emotions (those of the person concerned and of the family) upsetting a person's judgements are not illusory; and (c) preconceived ideas about what dementia might mean need to be faced and discussed. In other words, for many people, to be fully capacitous requires more support than they are likely to receive.

We could regard this as a matter of disability rights which supports the United Nations CRPD's call for 'legal capacity on an equal basis with others in all aspects of life' (United Nations General Assembly (2006); see Box 9.2). But the real-world application of criteria for decision-making capacity remains problematic. In connection with Dutch practice around euthanasia and assisted suicide, Kim et al. (2021c: online) state the following: '… the practice of assessing capacity … is difficult to reconcile with a strict application of the functional model of capacity. Understanding the practice in terms of a functional model would require a low threshold for capacity but no generally accepted justification for such a threshold exists.'

Stigma and mental health

In the fascinating study of metaphor, to which I have already alluded in the discussion of stigma in Chapter 7, Johnstone (2011) looked at how metaphor has been used in a problematic fashion to influence public debates about Alzheimer's disease and euthanasia. Metaphor undermines informed thinking about dementia by presenting it as the worst thing that could possibly happen to a person – as an existential threat – and it has done this in a way that reinforces the stigma, shame and secrecy associated with dementia. People then look for a reprieve or a remedy to this threat. Language becomes morally loaded. People are thought of as 'non-persons' and dementia as a 'living death'. And then, 'Once de-humanized it is but a short step to regarding such persons as being of only limited moral worth – literally *de-moralized* … And … it is but a short step to deeming such entities as "life unworthy of life" and "better off dead"' (Johnstone 2011: 388). The suggestion is that the euthanasia and physician-assisted suicide debate has been – through dramatic metaphor – 'Alzheimerized', so that suicide is felt to be a rational response to the stigma and terror of Alzheimer's disease. This might link to the trend, according to Jones (2022), of increasing numbers of non-assisted suicides in countries where assisted suicide and euthanasia have been legalized. Perhaps we are witnessing a culture that 'fails to see death properly and therefore has misguided ideas of control and dignity' (Pope 2017: 72); and perhaps the culture of legalized euthanasia and assisted suicide reflects 'a profound fear of aging and dying rooted in seeing ourselves as individual selves, separate from the collective' (Pope 2017: 72).

As Foot (1977) has argued in her scholarly discussion of euthanasia,

> ... it may be of the very greatest importance to keep a psychological barrier up against killing. ... As things are, people do, by and large, expect to be looked after if they are old or ill. This is one of the good things that we have, but we might lose it ....
>
> (p. 112)

A question arises about the extent to which people do actually say they wish to die. One concern about euthanasia and physician-assisted suicide is that people who say they wish to die may change their minds. Proponents of legalizing assisted suicide or euthanasia will often build into their proposed legislation a pause between the expression of a wish to die and the actual event. But, typically, such a pause is measured in weeks. Is this enough?

In an important study, Briggs et al. (2021) investigated the 'wish to die' in community-dwelling older people. They found that the wish to die 'is frequently transient and is strongly linked with the course of depressive symptoms and loneliness' (p. 1321). One in 29 older people said they had wished to die in the previous month. Of these, 60 per cent were depressed and almost 75 per cent were lonely. But 2 years later, 72 per cent no longer reported a wish to die; associated with this was a decrease in depression and loneliness. So, people do change their minds, but it can take a while. A change of mind would be encouraged by better support and attention to depression and loneliness. This study was not of people living with dementia, but the message that better support, more human contact and appropriate treatment of depression and other treatable conditions would lower the demand for assisted suicide and euthanasia is an important one and surely relevant to people living with dementia too. And this leads us on to the topic of palliative care.

Palliative care

The ethical points are simple. First, given the ethical worries about euthanasia and physician-assisted suicide, it would seem much more sensible to devote more attention and resources to palliative care. If palliative care, properly funded and researched, worked for people who would otherwise wish their lives to be actively terminated, would this not be a better option? Secondly, as a safeguard, proper palliative care ought to be offered to people requesting active termination of their lives, because it would be wrong for someone to be unnecessarily killed. We can support this claim by saying that, if someone benefits from palliative care, then health, welfare and pleasure will be maximized, whereas death precludes this. Or we could point to a duty to care and not to kill. Or, we might invoke the virtues and say that in caring for someone we show compassion, which cannot be shown in the same way by killing them or by helping them to kill themselves. It could be objected that it might be compassionate to kill someone if they were in misery, but the point of palliative care is to test whether the misery is necessary. In any case, to test out the claim, we could ask what do we become by caring for someone as opposed to killing them? It seems to me plausible to argue that caring makes us more compassionate, whereas killing them is more likely to coarsen our outlook on life and, as such, is not in keeping with the flourishing of the virtues.

This is not the place to discuss the details of palliative care for people living with dementia (Hughes et al. 2020). It will have to be different, in some ways, from the palliative care provided to people with, say, cancer. But we now have some idea about what would constitute optimal palliative care for people living with dementia (van der Steen et al. 2014). We also have good evidence of what is required to enable good end-of-life care for people with dementia (Bamford et al. 2018). The evidence base for palliative care for people living with dementia is overall still poor, but there is evidence that, for instance, 'Advance care planning interventions, compared to usual care, probably increase the documentation of advance directives and the occurrence of discussions about goals of care, and may also increase concordance with goals of care' (S.C. Walsh et al. 2021: 2). The ethical imperative must be to encourage more research into particular aspects of palliative care for people with dementia.

But a final ethical issue I shall discuss connected to palliative care is that of the doctrine of double effect. This is often misunderstood. You will recall Levinson (1981: 84) dismissed it as 'semantic quibbling'. It is based on a distinction between 'foreseeing' and 'intending', which is why it can seem semantic. It states that if your aim (or intention) in doing something is to bring about a good, even if there might be bad consequences which you can foresee, it is morally licit to do whatever it is. Philosophers sometimes quibble about this (Uniacke 2007). But for most clinicians it is bread and butter. I give someone an antibiotic knowing it might cause diarrhoea, but my intention was a good one: to cure the infection. (Of course, caveats must be in place: did they need an antibiotic and was there a better antibiotic less prone to such side effects?) A course of chemotherapy is given for cancer knowing it will probably cause hair loss. This side effect is foreseen. But it is not intended. This is straightforward and not semantic quibbling.

The usual scenario in which this doctrine is used is where opioids (for example morphine) have been given at the end of life and the person dies. It can then be said that the intention was to relieve pain and, if respiratory depression resulted and the person died, although this was a foreseen side effect, the intention was still good. The objection is that I might actually intend to kill the patient even if I make a little speech to myself about intending to relieve the pain.

This is true. There are two responses. One is to agree with the objection. As Anscombe (1979) wrote: 'The idea that one can determine one's intentions by making ... a little speech to oneself is obvious bosh' (p. 42). The second is to say that the scenario is, in any case, misconceived. For if opioids are used for pain and are correctly titrated, respiratory depression is not a worry. It is only incorrect use of opioids that will have this effect.

According to Anscombe (1979), to determine someone's actual intention you have to ask why the thing was done. And then you should consider that an action can have an intentional nature, so that we can speak of the intention embodied in the action. The intention embodied in the action of giving a small dose of morphine for pain is to relieve pain. The intentional nature of a large injection of potassium chloride must be to kill the person – there is no other possible reason for doing it.

But we need not be detained further by this doctrine. It may be relevant in the case of someone living with dementia who, for instance, is very agitated and is acting dangerously where behavioural techniques and good non-pharmacological approaches have not worked. We might wish to consider using a sedating drug, foreseeing the risks of falls and so forth, but intending that the person should feel calmer. Or we might use an antidepressant hoping to alleviate someone's mood, but foreseeing that it might sedate them or make them gain weight. The intention with which a treatment is used, or an investigation undertaken, is of considerable moral importance. It must, of course, be the genuine intention, which is not solely determined by what is going on in my head, but by the nature of the action undertaken.

Conclusion

Death is the end of a life. There is every reason to hope that our endings will be dignified and in keeping with the lives we have led – if these have been themselves authentic and true. But, as with birth, there is much that can go wrong. We must have the practical wherewithal in place to deal with death successfully (not that we can always succeed) and hence the importance of palliative care. But we must also have the correct moral frameworks in place to ensure, so far as is possible, that the decisions we make are in keeping with our judgements elsewhere and reflect the characteristic flourishing we seek by showing justice, compassion, wisdom and integrity.

Part **5**

Conclusion

32 Putting it all together: so what?

Introduction

A challenge, alluded to in Chapter 1, put to all the authors in this book series is to answer the question 'So what?'. What does all that has appeared in this book mean for people living with dementia, their families, people working in dementia care, policymakers, professionals, community activists and so on? In Chapter 1, I said that ethical questions are ethically imperative and that we should be ethically and morally energetic.

Part of me wishes to reject the 'So what?' question: if someone cannot see that an ethical response is required by the realities of dementia and dementia care – a response that takes seriously questions about what is morally right or wrong, good or bad – it would be like trying to play tennis with someone who simply did not recognize the rules of tennis. It should be obvious that we need thoughtful answers to questions such as: Does everyone need to be told their diagnosis? Should people with dementia drive? Would it be right to use robots to care for people living with dementia? Shall we use a feeding tube for this person with advanced dementia who now chokes when eating?

Still, it is useful to ask, 'So what?'. For one thing, as I suggested in connection with the discussion of patterns of practice in Chapter 6, most practitioners simply get on with the job without the ethical issues ever becoming obvious, although they lurk beneath the surface of practice. To put it another way, the questions to which thoughtful answers are required are often not even asked.

Throughout the book I have suggested ways in which the discussion has been relevant to the different groups involved in dementia care, including families and people living with dementia themselves. I now suggest that the implications of a book that reconsiders ethics in dementia care can be further considered at three levels: first, there are the implications for ethics itself; secondly, there are the implications for people living with dementia and for their families and (informal and formal) carers; thirdly, there are implications for the *polis*, the body politic, mentioned in Chapter 13, which would include policymakers, those who provide services and activists.

Implications for ethics

The implications for ethics are general and specific. The general implication stems from the vulnerabilities associated with dementia. This includes the cognitive vulnerabilities, but the physical and emotional vulnerabilities too. (Incidentally, Behuniak (2010: 238) argued that dementia care requires a 'theory of vulnerable persons'.) In particular, it is the implication that stems from dependence.

Traditionally in clinical ethics and bioethics, dependence would be seen as the antithesis of autonomy and the loss of autonomy would be seen as potentially catastrophic for the person living with dementia. As we saw in Chapter 8, however, our autonomy is always dependent on outside support. If this is more so in dementia, it is a matter of degree and it does not change in any fundamental way how we should see and treat people with dementia. To re-quote Agich: 'The concept of autonomy properly understood requires that individuals be seen in essential interrelationship with others and the world' (Agich 2003: 174). The general implication when we reconsider ethics and dementia is that respect for autonomy as a principle needs to be replaced by respect for relational autonomy. The person living with dementia must always be seen in a context of relationships, but interdependence and interrelationships are what characterize us all as human beings. Our judgements – of any sort, but chiefly here our ethical and moral judgements – about people living with dementia should be as judgements about anyone: they should seek to understand the perspective of the person most concerned, where this perspective will involve that individual's historical, societal, cultural and personal viewpoint.

The more specific implication for ethics to emerge from this book concerns the notion of patterns of practice. The value of this approach needs to be considered in more detail, with a more critical eye. But these pages have at least confirmed that there is some merit in pursuing its explanatory and determinative functions. It reflects – it explains – real life ethical decision-making, whereby we decide reflexively in line with the patterns of practice that instinctively shape our lives. It can also be used to determine how we think about ethical issues, how we determine what is right or wrong, good or bad, by focussing our attention on the requirement that our actions, decisions and thoughts should show internal and external coherence.

Internal coherence was conceived as meaning both within-practice coherence and coherence within the individual's practice. But I suggested this was akin to casuistry (Chapter 3); and, similarly, I suggested that external coherence was akin to virtue ethics (Chapter 5). Neither of these alignments was random. The immersion in the particularities of the case and subsequent interpretation required by casuistry (Murray 1994: 96–99) in order to judge whether or to what extent the current case is similar to some sentient case is of a piece with the demand for internal coherence. The sentient case will be drawn from the person's own collection of cases, which opens up the possibility of self-deception. I may think that the way I do things is right, but I may be way off the mark. Hence there is also the requirement for external coherence in line with virtue ethics.

Why virtue ethics? Well, there are established arguments against both utilitarianism and deontology, the other major contenders, even if they have their uses in certain circumstances (Williams 1972: 96–112; Raphael 1981: 43–66; MacIntyre 1985: 43–47, 70–71, 198–199; Hursthouse 1999: 52–55). About utilitarianism, for instance, Raphael (1981) wrote: 'Where utilitarianism goes wrong is in fastening upon the estimation of amount of happiness as such, instead of viewing the concept of happiness as subordinate to that of a person. Happiness is important for ethics because it is the chief aim of persons' (p. 54). Beauchamp and Childress (2001: 354–355) record three problematic areas for Kantian deontology: first, there is a significant difficulty where obligations conflict (if you have a duty to provide healthcare to two people who are indistinguishable from the point of view of their illnesses, but you can only attend to one of them, how do you decide between them?); secondly, Kantianism seems to overemphasize the law and underplays the importance of relationships, which are so relevant to dementia care; and thirdly, Kant's view of the moral life is too abstract and formal, without practicability.

Of course, criticisms are also levelled at virtue ethics (Hope et al. 2003: 10; Oakley 2007: 90–91; Bloch and Green 2021: 5). But it is difficult to dispute the idea that we should aim to become the best that we can possibly be. Why should we not? This is not to say that we should all be saints. It may be that I am quite limited by a variety of genetic and social factors in terms of what I can achieve, but does this mean that it is good for me to aim to be bad and to do the wrong thing? How do we know what it is to be good and to do the right thing? Well, the virtue words tell us. Who would wish to be mean, hubristic, imprudent, treacherous and so forth? Aristotle used the word *eudaimonia* to describe the good at which human beings should aim. This has been translated as 'happiness' but is better understood as 'human flourishing' and it is cashed out in terms of the virtues. As MacIntyre (1985: 148) has said:

> Human beings ... have a specific nature; ... they have certain aims and goals, such that they move by nature towards a specific *telos*. ... The virtues are precisely those qualities the possession of which will enable an individual to achieve and the lack of which will frustrate his movement toward that *telos*.

It seems commonplace, therefore, to suggest that our patterns of practice should cohere with the natural aims and goals of human beings, which is to say that there should be coherence with the virtues. In my view, virtue ethics has enough resilience to deal with conflicting virtues, to justify particular courses of action and to allow a rational account of our decisions (Hursthouse 1999).

Patterns of practice allow us to describe and explain our decisions, actions and thoughts. A feature of such descriptions and explanations, however, which is another implication of this book (derived from the ethical approaches discussed in Chapter 4), is that frequent reference will be made to the narratives of those involved, that caring and solicitude will have prominence, that there will be 'the active creation and recreation of meaning and identity' along with 'the negotiation of empowerment' (Lyman 1998: 55) and that authentic dialogue will characterize the interactions of all those concerned.

Implications for people living with dementia and for those who care for them

Perhaps shockingly, I have little to say about the implications for all those concerned with dementia care. Also shocking, perhaps, is that I have lumped together under this heading both people living with dementia and professionals, such as psychiatrists and neurologists, along with all those other formal and informal carers, including families. Is this not a mistake? Are not the implications for people living with dementia very different from those that affect the specialist physician?

Of course, all of these people face different challenges and tasks. Struggling to make a cup of tea and struggling to make a diagnosis of dementia with Lewy bodies are very different things. But they are both important struggles and my suggestion is that they have something of crucial importance in common. The thing of importance is the implication of these pages that I would wish to present to all these varied groups of people. The implication, however, is by no means new. It is straight from Kitwood (1997a): 'the person comes first'.

I take seriously the wise warning issued by Baldwin and Capstick (2007: 273): 'For all we owe to Kitwood's work (and the debt is considerable) it may, in some ways, be time to come out from his shadow'. We can criticize Kitwood – as I have done (Hughes 2019) – and there is certainly no need to feel hidebound by his work. His work was wide-ranging in many ways, but there was a definite focus on the inner psychology of the person, despite the social spin. Talk of citizenship and human rights, of power relations and politics, indeed of the important socio-cultural context within which dementia care takes place, is (except tangentially or in passing) absent from Kitwood's work (Baldwin and Capstick 2007: 184–186). For instance, Baldwin and Capstick (2007) suggest that 'because personhood is essentially an apolitical concept it does not provide the language for discussing people's situation in terms of power relations' (p. 184). They also say: 'the challenge will be to move beyond personhood while simultaneously retaining a focus on it' (p. 186).

I think this is spot on. Well, almost! My quibble is that I see no reason to 'move beyond' personhood, partly because, for instance, stubbornly I see no reason to regard personhood as 'essentially an apolitical concept'. If we return to the notion of the person as a situated embodied agent (Hughes 2001), why would the person not be situated in the *polis*? How can I, qua person, avoid being political, even if only in the minimal sense that I live in a state that is governed? Even if I were stateless, as many people are, this is itself a political issue.

In this book I have stressed that even mundane decisions in health and social care have an ethical component. In Chapter 2, I argued that politics is ethics writ large: it is the public expression of our private ethical beliefs. For the concept of personhood to be apolitical it would also have to lack all moral content. But it does not. For we are inherently ethically situated. Part of what it is for us to be the persons that we are is that we care about things, we have values, there are things of importance to us. In saying this I am reflecting the work of Charles Taylor (1989: 34): 'What I am as a self, my identity, is essentially defined by the way things have a significance for me. ...we are only selves insofar as we move in a certain space of questions, as we seek and find an orientation to the good'. Or, as Schneewind (1991: 422) wrote in reviewing *Sources of the Self*, 'The self, on Taylor's view, is not an objectively given entity like a star or a bacillus. Its identity is constituted largely by its values'.

My point is that we should not 'move beyond' personhood but expand it. Or rather, see that it is an expansive notion. We need a broad view of personhood, what I have referred to as 'the uncircumscribable human-person-perspective' (Hughes 2011b: 241–249). Then the point is, not that this remains a detached theoretical construct, but that it is a reality in all of our dealings with persons, including with persons living with dementia. This individual in front of me in this care home is someone of value, who also has values, who may to a greater or lesser extent be able to signal what is of personal significance, concerning whom our judgements now about whether or not to start a medication are inherently ethical in nature, and probably arise because of economic decisions by the management of the chain of care homes concerning levels of staffing, but whose placement in this home reflects a socio-cultural crisis in the family, which in turn stems from political decisions about the provision of care in the community. And so on.

To be the person that I am is for me to have a history, but it is also for me to have (amongst many others) moral and political orientations, even if these are sordid and ignominious; and even if they are unrecognized by me. The notion of personhood, therefore, is deeply rich. But so too are real people. One of the great privileges of being a clinician or carer of any sort is to learn so much about the personal lives of the people we serve and care for: to see into their histories, into the dramas of their lives and families. Reflection should also help us to see that we stand in relationship to the person as part of a bigger socio-cultural and political framework. But these larger frameworks and discussions within the broader perspectives relevant to personhood are always, at root, about a particular person or persons. In the UK, when the Prime Minister announces a new grand scheme to revitalize the country, how often does the Leader of the Opposition retort by pointing to the deprivation that will still be suffered by a particular constituent? Politics seems to be about the big picture, but in reality it is about individual lives and people.

The person, therefore, still comes first (Kitwood 2019). Kitwood's conception of personhood was profoundly experiential and relational, it was about psychological well-being and about embodiment, but it was also social and organizational. If he did not pursue some of these topics far enough and if he did not go beyond them to offer a picture of the person as a citizen and as a bearer of rights, so be it. But this does not mean that personhood itself is confined. To think so would indeed be to live under Kitwood's shadow and to be hidebound by his work.

The person living with dementia may wish to demand a right to be heard; the family member may wish to advocate for the person whose communication is impaired; the carer in the nursing home may wish to spend some time brushing the resident's hair; the social worker may wish to work harder to find funding; the GP may wish to take some time to listen to what the person living with dementia is saying; and the psychiatrist may wish to encourage a psychosocial approach to the management of the behaviours that some are finding challenging. These are all the sorts of ethical responses that, I hope, would emerge from understanding the lines of reasoning suggested in this book. But they are all based on the implication that *the person comes first*. Arguments about citizenship and rights are only of value because they are, first and foremost, arguments about real people who, *as persons*, are citizens and human beings embedded in the *polis*.

Implications for the polis

So, what are the implications of this book for those who make up the body politic, for the activists, the policymakers and politicians? In Chapter 13, there was an implicit movement from personhood to citizenship and then to rights. All of this is to the good. What I have said above, however, may seem contradictory. Because now I wish to suggest that we also need to move back to person-centred care. Or, at least, back to the idea that personhood and the person come first.

My point is this: that citizenship is a function of personhood and that rights reflect the ethical standing of persons. The person comes first.

It is perhaps useful to turn our attention to the whole question of rights, since the cutting edge of theorizing about dementia encourages a rights-based approach. As we saw in Chapter 21, there is the suggestion that in contrast to citizenship models, 'Human rights … transcend political and/or social boundaries by virtue of their universality, albeit to be recognized and implemented at the local citizenship level' (Grigorovich et al. 2019: 177). I had the temerity to suggest that there was some flag-waving here in favour of human rights. For one thing, it is noteworthy that human rights have to be 'implemented at the local citizenship level'. Just so; and at the 'citizenship level' they have to be implemented by individuals, person to person. The global proclamation of a right is a glorious thing, but empty without personal endeavour. My belief (expressed in Chapter 9) is that fundamental human rights do reflect something radical about how we should engage with each other in the world. Once rights are established, the person has protection (at least in theory) under the law; and United Nations conventions, such as the CRPD, help to encourage support for those who claim rights. As I suggested in Chapter 13, the assertion of rights for people with dementia seems crucial and certainly relevant in connection with forced care (Chapter 22), sexuality and intimacy (Chapter 23) and in the time of pandemic (Chapter 27). Nevertheless, in Chapter 13, I also suggested there are conceptual limitations to claims about rights.

We might wish to argue that there are no such things as human rights. A right can be defined as 'the capacity to exercise a certain choice with institutional impunity' (Pettit 1980: 77). If you have a right to freedom of expression, no one can stop you from saying or writing or in any other way expressing yourself. However, according to a thinker as formidable as MacIntyre (1985), '… there are no such rights, and belief in them is one with belief in witches and in unicorns' (p. 69). He is not talking about rights given to certain specified groups by law or custom, but of so-called 'natural' or 'human' rights: '… those rights which are alleged to belong to human beings as such and which are cited as a reason for holding that people ought not to be interfered with in their pursuit of life, liberty and happiness' (pp. 68–69).

Nevertheless, laws – such as the *Human Rights Act 1988* (Home Office 1998) – can establish rights, even if they cannot be given further metaphysical underpinnings. If by custom and practice we elect to say that every innocent person has the right to life, then they do, even if that right cannot be proven to exist other than by its instantiation in law. (MacIntyre (1985: 69,) denies that the assertion of such a right cannot be shown to be self-evidently true, for instance.) Exactly what such a right entails, who counts as an 'innocent person' for instance, will be established by argument and precedent in the courts.

What I take from this is that there are legally established rights to which we can appeal, and we can argue about exactly what might count as falling under the description of such rights, but we should be chary of waving the rights flag willy-nilly. Instead, the person comes first. Mostly, I should be treated respectfully and courteously because I am a person. I do not have a right to respect and courteousness as such. Simone Weil (1909–1943) wrote that the notion of obligations (or duties) was prior to that of rights. It is only once the obligation is recognized that the right becomes effectual. Hence, she wrote: 'An obligation which goes unrecognized by anybody loses none of the full force of its existence. A right which goes unrecognized by anybody is not worth very much' (Weil 2002: 3).

She went on to say (using the gendered language of her day): 'A man left alone in the universe would have no rights whatever, but he would have obligations' (p. 4). Persons, as such, have duties even to themselves; but these are not rights. The duties, to ourselves or to others, stem from our nature as persons. It might not be the most sensible thing to place more weight on rights than they can withstand.

In an interesting article on social policy and human rights, Boyle (2010: 511) started by asserting that 'Autonomy is a fundamental human right, essential for equality'. Ignoring the possibility that my right to autonomy might conflict with yours, from an ethical perspective it is certainly true that people have obligations (or duties) to respect the wish for self-determination of people living with disabilities. These can be established by thinking about what it is to be a person (to be innately interrelated and interdependent) and how we flourish as people, which we do by demonstrating the virtues of, for example, compassion, justice and respect. So, social care emanates from the standing of the person as such, not from a right as such. To assert one has rights is the obverse of such duties. To do so is a political act, but one that is empty without the ethical obligations of friendship and love which stem from personhood

I note that Butchard and Kinderman (2019) were keen to push the idea of identity, which they linked to personhood. They suggested that preserving identity might enhance human rights. But if we can preserve identity, is that not enough? What do rights add to that? It makes more sense to argue that rights might preserve identity, but not without other things being in place which do not, after all, require rights. They said, 'There is no obligation to carry out person-centered care other than knowing that it is the right thing to do' (p. 165); but what greater reason is there to do something other than knowing it is the right thing to do? As they reasonably argue, once something has a legal basis and framework, people will be more inclined to do it. At which point I am inclined to ask how a right to person-centred care and indeed a right to personal identity (which they commend at the end of their paper) would be translated into an enforceable law? Simone Weil, in any case, might well argue that there is an obligation to be person-centred; it comes from the nature of our personhood (Heidegger's *being-with* perhaps). Strikingly, Kitwood himself espoused a similar line to that of Weil when writing of the criteria for a model or theory of personhood. One criterion was that '… it must view the person as a social being, not as a monad… That is why a moral theory that speaks of persons and obligations is more powerful than one which merely speaks of individuals and their "rights"' (Kitwood 1997b, cited in Baldwin and Capstick 2007: 236).

Hence, my suggestion is that the implication for reconsidering ethics in dementia care at the level of the *polis* is not to do with rights as such, nor even with our obligations, but is to do with grasping and encouraging as broad a view of the person as possible. This means including people living with dementia in every way possible, not as a matter of rights (although their rights should be respected), not because they are citizens (although they are), but because of their personhood and all that this entails (see Chapter 13). Inclusion should be at every level possible, from within the family and community to social and political involvement. This is where the importance of activists is seen; this is where it is important to involve people living with dementia in research in a meaningful way; this is where the will and preference of people living with dementia should be honoured; this is where people with dementia should be at liberty to pursue their legitimate goals in a manner that suits them best.

Conclusion

The broad view also suggests something much more. In an article published in the year of Kitwood's death, there are a series of fascinating statements right at the end, where he wrote that the 'ethic of context' cannot be ignored (Kitwood 1998: 33). He noted that interactions which either maintain or undermine personhood fall within the category of practical morality, but that these interactions also have 'an aesthetic dimension' (p. 33), which is not merely contingent. Drawing from the idea of authentic acting, Kitwood emphasized the requirement for 'total sincerity, on being set free from the limitations imposed by ego, and drawing freely and fluently on one's emotional resources' (p. 33). He suggested that philosophers drew too heavily on the Apollonian mode rather than the Dionysian. In other words, he accused them of being too rational and not emotional and instinctive enough.

Whether or not this is wholly fair to philosophers, interest in aesthetics and dementia is a flourishing business (Hughes 2014c). Zeilig et al. (2015) suggested that an arts-based approach might be a way to engage with staff in care homes and empower them to recognize their skills and to focus on person-centred care. Pia Kontos and John Killick have been using the arts to enable people with dementia to flourish and to reduce stigma for some years (Killick and Cordonnier 2000; Killick 2013; Kontos and Grigorovich 2018; Kontos et al. 2021b). Through co-creation, which means inclusion, people living with dementia can be as involved in an artistic process as are the professionals (Zeilig et al. 2018). Our own work has connected art, authenticity and citizenship (Hughes et al. 2021b). The links between aesthetics and dementia are wide and deep (Hughes forthcoming). But the point is that an aesthetic approach to the person – seeing the person through this lens – reflects and encourages the broad perspective of personhood, from which obligations flow. Personhood and aesthetics are intimately linked, not necessarily by human rights (*pace* Kontos et al. 2021a), but necessarily.

In the end, we need authentic solicitude which reflects our ethical and aesthetic standing as human beings in the world with all that this involves. If we could achieve this, the world would be a better place, including for people living with dementia. As Kitwood (1998: 34) wrote: 'The excellent caregiver is, so to speak, a moral artist, and sets an example to all of us as we search for the right and the good'.

References

Abdool, R. (2017) Deception in caregiving: unpacking several ethical considerations in covert medication, *Journal of Law, Medicine & Ethics*, 45: 193–203.

Afshar, P.F., Wiig, E.H., Malakouti, S.K., et al. (2021) Reliability and validity of a quick test of cognitive speed (AQT) in screening for mild cognitive impairment and dementia, *BMC Geriatrics*, 21: 693. Available at: https://doi.org/10.1186/s12877-021-02621-z (accessed 31 December 2021).

Agich, G.J. (2003) *Dependence and Autonomy in Old Age: An Ethical Framework for Long-Term Care*. Cambridge: Cambridge University Press.

Albert, S.C., Martinelli, J.E. and Pessoa, M.S.C. (2022) Dementia and its impacts on the intimate, sexual couple relationship: a systematic review of qualitative research studies, *Dementia*, 0: 1–18. Available at: https://doi.org/10.1177/14713012211073205 (accessed 20 April 2022).

Albinsson, L. and Strang, P. (2003) Existential concerns of families of late-stage dementia patients: questions of freedom, choices, isolation, death, and meaning, *Journal of Palliative Medicine*, 6: 225–235.

Alderson, P. and Goodey, C. (1998) Theories of consent, *British Medical Journal*, 317: 1313–1315.

Alexander, G.C., Emerson, S. and Kesselheim, A.S. (2021) Evaluation of aducanumab for Alzheimer disease: scientific evidence and regulatory review involving efficacy, safety, and futility, *Journal of the American Medical Association*, 325: 1717–1718.

Alghrani, A., Case, P., Fanning, J. (2016). The Mental Capacity Act 2005 – ten years on, *Medical Law Review*, 24: 311–317.

Alpinar-Sencan, Z., Schicktanz, S., Ulitsa, N., et al. (2021) Moral motivation regarding dementia risk testing among affected persons in Germany and Israel, *Journal of Medical Ethics*. Available at: http://dx.doi.org/10.1136/medethics-2020-106990 (accessed on 9 March 2022).

Alvargonzález, D. (2012) Alzheimer's disease and euthanasia, *Journal of Aging Studies*, 26: 377–385.

Alzheimer's Research UK (2021) Government's missed opportunity on research funding leaves dementia community disappointed (28 October 2021). Available at: https://www.alzheimersresearchuk.org/blog/governments-missed-opportunity-on-research-funding-leaves-dementia-community-disappointed/ (accessed 25 January 2022).

Alzheimer's Society (2011) *Optimising Treatment and Care for People with Behavioural and Psychological Symptoms of Dementia: A Best Practice Guide for Health and Social Care Professionals*. London: Alzheimer's Society. Available at: https://www.alzheimers.org.uk/sites/default/files/2018-08/Optimising%20treatment%20and%20care%20-%20best%20practice%20guide.pdf?downloadID=609 (accessed 6 April 2022).

Alzheimer's Society (2018) *A Practical Guide Representing Dementia in the Arts, Culture and Popular Discourse*. London: Alzheimer's Society. Available at: https://www.alzheimers.org.uk/sites/default/files/2018-09/Dementia%20Friendly%20Media%20and%20Broadcast%20Guide.pdf (accessed 24 October 2022).

American Psychiatric Association (2013) *Diagnostic and Statistical Manual of Mental Disorders*, 5th ed. (DSM-5). Washington DC: American Psychiatric Publishing.

Ames, D., O'Brien, J.T. and Burns, A. (eds) (2017) *Dementia*, 5th edn. Boca Raton: CRC Press, Taylor & Francis Group.

Anantapong, K., Barrado-Martín, Y., Nair, P., et al. (2021) How do people living with dementia perceive eating and drinking difficulties? A qualitative study, *Age and Ageing*, 50: 1820–1828.

Anscombe, G.E.M. (1958) Modern moral philosophy, *Philosophy*, 33: 1–19.

Anscombe, G.E.M. (1979) *Intention*. Oxford: Blackwell.

Appel, J.M. (2010) Sex rights for the disabled? *Journal of Medical Ethics*, 36: 152–154.

Aquilina, C. and Hughes, J.C. (2006) The return of the living dead: agency lost and found? in J.C. Hughes, S.J. Louw and S.R. Sabat (eds) *Dementia: Mind, Meaning, and the Person*. Oxford: Oxford University Press.

Aquinas, T. (1990) *Summa Theologiae, Volume 23 (1a2ae. 55–67): Virtue* (translated by W.D. Hughes OP). Cambridge: Cambridge University Press.

Arapakis, K., Brunner, E., French, E., et al. (2021) Dementia and disadvantage in the USA and England: population-based comparative study, *BMJ Open*, 11: e045186. Available at: http://dx.doi.org/10.1136/bmjopen-2020-045186 (accessed 22 January 2022).

Aristotle (1980) *The Nicomachean Ethics* (translated by D. Ross, revised by J.L. Ackrill and J.O. Urmson). Oxford: Oxford University Press.

Ashcroft, R.E., Dawson, A., Draper, H. and McMillan, J.R. (2007). *Principles of Health Care Ethics*, 2nd edn. Chichester: John Wiley & Sons.

Asscher, E.C.A., van de Vathorst, S. (2020) First prosecution of a Dutch doctor since the euthanasia act of 2002: what does the verdict mean? *Journal of Medical Ethics*, 46: 71–75.

Aumann, G.M-E., Cole, T.R. (1991) In whose voice? Composing a lifesong collaboratively, *The Journal of Clinical Ethics*, 2: 45–49.

Awoke, S., Mouton, C.P. and Parrott, M. (1992) Outcomes of skilled cardiopulmonary resuscitation in a long-term-care facility: futile therapy? *Journal of American Geriatric Society*, 40: 593–595.

Bach, M. and Kerzner, L. (2010) *A New Paradigm for Protecting Autonomy and the Right to Legal Capacity*. Toronto: Law Commission of Ontario.

Baier, A. (1986) Trust and antitrust, *Ethics*, 96: 231–260.

Bailey, A., Dening, T. and Harvey, K. (2021) Battles and breakthroughs: representations of dementia in the British press, *Ageing & Society*, 41: 362–376.

Bailey, C., Clarke, C.L., Gibb, C. et al. (2013) Risky and resilient life with dementia: review of and reflections on the literature, *Health, Risk & Society*, 15: 390–401.

Baldwin, C. (2008) Family carers, ethics and dementia: an empirical study, in G. Widdershoven, J. McMillan, T. Hope and L. van der Scheer (eds) *Empirical Ethics in Psychiatry*. Oxford: Oxford University Press.

Baldwin, C. (2010) Narrative, supportive care, and dementia: a preliminary exploration, in J.C. Hughes, M. Lloyd-Williams and G.A. Sachs (eds) *Supportive Care for the Person with Dementia*. Oxford: Oxford University Press.

Baldwin, C. and Capstick, A. (eds) (2007) *Tom Kitwood on Dementia: A Reader and Critical Commentary*. Maidenhead: Open University Press.

Baldwin, C., Hope, T., Hughes, J., Jacoby, R. and Ziebland, S. (2004) Ethics and dementia: the experience of family carers, *Progress in Neurology and Psychiatry*, 8: 24–28.

Baldwin, C., Hope, T., Hughes, J., Jacoby, R. and Ziebland, S. (2005). *Making Difficult Decisions: The Experience of Caring for Someone with Dementia*. London: Alzheimer's Society.

Baldwin, C., Hughes, J., Hope, T., et al. (2003). Ethics and dementia: mapping the literature by bibliometric analysis, *International Journal of Geriatric Psychiatry*, 18: 41–54.

Ballard, C., Hanney, M.L., Theodoulou, M., et al. (2009) The dementia antipsychotic withdrawal trial (DART-AD): long-term follow-up of a randomised placebo-controlled trial, *Lancet Neurology*, 8: 151–157.

Bamford, C., Lamont, S., Eccles, M., et al. (2004) Disclosing a diagnosis of dementia: a systematic review, *International Journal of Geriatric Psychiatry*, 19: 151–169.

Bamford, C., Lee, R., McLellan, E., et al. (2018) What enables good end of life care for people with dementia? A multi-method qualitative study with key stakeholders, *BMC Geriatrics*, 18: 302. Accessed via: https://doi.org/10.1186/s12877-018-0983-0 (accessed 3 June 2022).

Bamford, S-M., Holley-Moore, G. and Watson, J. (2014) *A Compendium of Essays: New Perspectives and Approaches to Understanding Dementia and Stigma*. London: The International Longevity Centre-UK.

Baqir, W., Barrett, S., Desai, N., et al. (2014) A clinico-ethical framework for multidisciplinary review of medication in nursing homes, *BMJ Quality Improvement Reports*, 3(1): u203261.w2538. Available at: https://doi.org/10.1136/bmjquality.u203261.w2538 (accessed 14 April 2022).

Baqir, W., Hughes, J., Jones, T., et al. (2017) Impact of medication review, within a shared decision-making framework, on deprescribing in people living in care homes, *European Journal of Hospital Pharmacy*, 24: 30–33.

Barrado-Martín, Y., Hatter, L., Moore, K.J., et al. (2021) Nutrition and hydration for people living with dementia near the end of life: a qualitative systematic review, *Journal of Advanced Nursing*, 77: 664–680.

Barrado-Martín, Y., Nair, P., Anantapong, K., et al. (2022) Family caregivers' and professionals' experiences of supporting people living with dementia's nutrition and hydration needs towards the end of life, *Health and Social Care in the Community*, 30: 307–318.

Bartlett, P. (2012) The United Nations Convention on the Rights of Persons with Disabilities and mental health law, *Modern Law Review*, 75: 752–758.

Bartlett, R. (2016) Scanning the conceptual horizons of citizenship, *Dementia*, 15: 453–461.

Bartlett, R. (2021) Inclusive (social) citizenship and persons with dementia, *Disability & Society*, available at: https://doi.org/10.1080/09687599.2021.1877115 (accessed 28 February 2022).

Bartlett, R. and O'Connor, D. (2007) From personhood to citizenship: broadening the lens for dementia practice and research, *Journal of Aging Studies*, 21: 107–118.

Bartlett, R. and O'Connor, D. (2010) *Broadening the Dementia Debate*. Bristol UK, Portland OR: Policy Press.

Bartley, M. (2009) Medical Classics: *The Moral Challenge of Alzheimer Disease: Ethical Issues from Diagnosis to Dying* by Stephen G Post, first published 1995, *British Medical Journal*, 339: 1205.

BBC News (2001) Rules on 'hidden' medication, BBC. Available at: http://news.bbc.co.uk/1/hi/health/1525381.stm (accessed 12 April 2022).

Beauchamp, T.L. and Childress, J.F. (2001) *Principles of Biomedical Ethics*, 5th edn. New York: Oxford University Press. [There is now an 8th edition, published in 2019.]

Behuniak, S.M. (2010) Toward a political model of dementia: power as compassionate care, *Journal of Aging Studies*, 24: 231–240.

Benbow, S.M. and Beeston, D. (2012) Sexuality, aging, and dementia, *International Psychogeriatrics*, 24: 1026–1033.

Bentham, J. (1789) *An Introduction to the Principles of Morals and Legislation*, in M. Warnock (ed.) (1962) *Utilitarianism, On Liberty, Essay on Bentham, together with selected writings of Jeremy Bentham and John Austin*. Glasgow: William Collins, Fount.

Berezin, M.A. (1969) Sex and old age: a review of the literature, *Journal of Geriatric Psychiatry*, 2: 131–149.

Berghmans, R.L.P. (1999) Ethics of end-of-life decisions in cases of dementia: views of the Royal Dutch Medical Association with some critical comments, *Alzheimer Disease and Associated Disorders*, 13: 91–95.

Berlin, I. (1967) Two concepts of liberty, in A. Quinton (ed.) *Political Philosophy*. Oxford: Oxford University Press.

Binstock, R.H., Post, S.G. and Whitehouse, P.J. (eds) (1992) *Dementia and Aging: Ethics, Values and Policy Choices*. Baltimore: The Johns Hopkins University Press.

Bitenc, R.A. (2020) *Reconsidering Dementia Narratives: Empathy, Identity and Care*. London and New York: Routledge.

Black, B.S. and Rabins, P.V. (2017) Quality of life in dementia: conceptual and practical issues, in D. Ames, J.T. O'Brien and A. Burns (eds) *Dementia*, 5th edn. Boca Raton, FL: CRC Press, Taylor & Francis Group.

Blennow, K. and Skoog, I. (1999) Genetic testing for Alzheimer's disease: how close to reality? *Current Opinion in Psychiatry*, 12: 487–493.

Bloch, S. and Green, S.A. (2021) The scope of psychiatric ethics, in S. Bloch and S.A. Green (eds) *Psychiatric Ethics*, 5th edn. Oxford: Oxford University Press.

Boccardi, V., Ruggiero, C., Patriti, A. and Marano, L. (2016) Diagnostic assessment and management of dysphagia in patients with Alzheimer's disease, *Journal of Alzheimer's Disease*, 50: 947–955.

Bok, S. (1999) *Lying: Moral choice in public and private life*. New York: Vintage Books.

Bolt, E.E., Snijdewind, M.C., Willems, D.L. et al. (2015) Can physicians conceive of performing euthanasia in case of psychiatric disease, dementia or being tired of living? *Journal of Medical Ethics*, 41: 592–598.

Bond, J. (1999) Quality of life for people with dementia: approaches to the challenge of measurement, *Ageing and Society*, 19: 561–579.

Boyle, G. (2010) Social policy for people with dementia in England: promoting human rights? *Health and Social Care in the Community*, 18: 511–519.

Boyle, G. (2014) Recognising the agency of people with dementia, *Disability & Society*, 29: 1130–1144.

Bravo, G., Sene, M. and Arcand, M. (2018) Making medical decisions for an incompetent older adult when both a proxy and an advance directive are available: which is more likely to reflect the older adult's preferences? *Journal of Medical Ethics*, 44: 498–503.

Brayne, C. and Kelly, S. (2019) Against the stream: early diagnosis of dementia, is it desirable? *British Journal of Psychiatry Bulletin*, 43: 123–125.

Briggs, R., Ward, M. and Kenny, R.A. (2021) The 'Wish to Die' in later life: prevalence, longitudinal course and mortality. Data from TILDA, *Age and Ageing*, 50: 1321–1328.

Brindle, N. and Holmes, J. (2005) Capacity and coercion: dilemmas in the discharge of older people with dementia from general hospital settings, *Age and Ageing*, 34: 16–20.

Brini, S., Hodkinson, A., Davies, A. et al. (2021) In-home dementia caregiving is associated with greater psychological burden and poorer mental health than out-of-home caregiving: a cross-sectional study, *Aging & Mental Health*. Available at: https://doi.org/10.1080/13607863.2021.1881758 (accessed 11 January 2022).

Brock, D.W. (1988) Justice and the severely demented elderly, *The Journal of Medicine and Philosophy*, 13: 73–99.

Brock, D.W. (2009) Medical decisions at the end of life, in H. Kuhse and P. Singer (eds) *A Companion to Bioethics*, 2nd edn. Malden MA: Blackwell.

Brody, H. (2007) Narrative ethics, in R.E. Ashcroft, A. Dawson, H. Draper and J.R. McMillan (eds) *Principles of Health Care Ethics*, 2nd edn. Chichester: John Wiley & Sons.

Brody, H., Hermer, L.D., Scott, L.D., et al. (2011) Artificial nutrition and hydration: the evolution of ethics, evidence, and policy, *Journal of General Internal Medicine*, 26: 1053–1058.

Brooker, D. (2004) What is person-centred care in dementia? *Reviews in Clinical Gerontology*, 13: 215–222.

Brooker, D., La Fontaine, J., Evans, S., Bray, J. and Saad, K. (2014) Public health guidance to facilitate timely diagnosis of dementia: ALzheimer's COoperative Valuation in Europe (ALCOVE) recommendations, *International Journal of Geriatric Psychiatry*, 29: 682–693.

Brooker, D. (2019) Personhood maintained: commentary, in T. Kitwood, *Dementia Reconsidered, Revisited: The Person Still Comes First* (D. Brooker (ed.)). London: Open University Press.

Brooker, D. and Latham, I. (2016) *Person-Centred Dementia Care: Making Services Better with the VIPS Framework*, 2nd edn. London and Philadelphia: Jessica Kingsley.

Broström, L., Johansson, M. and Nielsen, M.K. (2007) 'What the patient would have decided': a fundamental problem with the substituted judgment standard, *Medicine, Health Care and Philosophy*, 10: 265–278.

Bruce-Jones, P., Roberts, H., Bowker, L. and Cooney, V. (1996) Resuscitating the elderly: what do the patients want? *Journal of Medical Ethics*, 22: 154–159.

Dryon, E., de Casterlé, B.D. and Gastmans, C. (2012) 'Because we see them naked' – nurses' experiences in caring for hospitalized patients with dementia: considering artificial nutrition and hydration (ANH), *Bioethics*, 26: 285–295.

Buber, M. (1937) *I and Thou* (trans. R. Gregor Smith). Edinburgh: Clark.

Buchanan, A. (1988) Advance directives and the personal identity problem, *Philosophy and Public Affairs*, 17: 277–302.

Buchanan, A.E. and Brock, D.W. (1989) *Deciding for Others: The Ethics of Surrogate Decision Making*. Cambridge: Cambridge University Press.

Budak, K.B., Atefi, G., Hoel, V., et al. (2021) Can technology impact loneliness in dementia? A scoping review on the role of assistive technologies in delivering psychosocial interventions in long-term care, *Disability and Rehabilitation: Assistive Technology*. Available at: https://doi.org/10.1080/17483107.2021.1984594 (accessed 1 April 2022).

Buller, T. (2015a) Advance consent, critical interests and dementia research, *Journal of Medical Ethics*, 41: 701–707.

Buller, T. (2015b) Response to commentaries by Karin Rolanda Jongsma and Suzanne van de Vathorst, and Oliver Hallich, *Journal of Medical Ethics*, 41: 711.

Bunnik, E.M., Richard, E., Milne, R. and M.H.N. Schermer (2018) On the personal utility of Alzheimer's disease-related biomarker testing in the research context, *Journal of Medical Ethics*, 44: 830–834.

Burgess, M.M. (1994) Ethical issues in genetic testing for Alzheimer's disease: lessons from Huntington's disease, *Alzheimer Disease and Associated Disorders*, 8: 71–78.

Butchard, S. and Kinderman, P. (2019) Human rights, dementia, and identity, *European Psychologist*, 24: 159–168.

Byers, P., Matthews, S. and Kennett, J. (2021) Truthfulness in dementia care, *Bioethics*, 35: 839–841.

Caddell, L.S. and Clare, L. (2010) The impact of dementia on self and identity: A systematic review, *Clinical Psychology Review*, 30: 113–126.

Caddell, L.S. and Clare, L. (2011) I'm still the same person: the impact of early-stage dementia on identity, *Dementia*, 10: 379–398.

Cahill, S. (2018) *Dementia and Human Rights*. Bristol UK and Chicago IL: Policy Press.

Callahan, D. (1987) *Setting Limits: Medical Goals in an Aging Society*. New York: Simon and Schuster.

Callahan, D. (1995) Terminating life-sustaining treatment of the demented, *Hastings Center Report*, 6: 25–31.

Cantone, D., Attena, F., Cerrone, S., et al. (2019) Lying to patients with dementia: attitudes versus behaviours in nurses, *Nursing Ethics*, 26: 984–992.

Carmel, S. and Mutran, E.J. (1999) Stability of elderly persons' expressed preferences regarding the use of life-sustaining treatments, *Social Science and Medicine*, 49: 303–311.

Carrese, J.A. (2006) Refusal of care: patients' well-being and physicians' ethical obligations: but doctor, I want to go home, *Journal of the American Medical Association*, 296: 691–695.

Carter, M. (2021) Grief, trauma and mistaken identity: ethically deceiving people living with dementia in complex cases, *Bioethics*, 35: 850–856.

Cassel, C.K. (1998) Genetic testing and Alzheimer disease: ethical issues for providers and families, *Alzheimer Disease and Associated Disorders*, 12 (Supplement 3): S16–S20.

Chadwick, R. and Russell, J. (1989) Hospital discharge of frail elderly people: social and ethical considerations in the discharge decision-making process, *Ageing and Society*, 9: 277–295.

Chamsi-Pasha, H. and Albar, M.A. (2018) Do-Not-Resuscitate Orders: Islamic viewpoint, *International Journal of Human and Health Sciences*, 2: 8–12.

Chandra, M., Harbishettar, V., Sawhney, H. and Amanullah, S. (2021) Ethical issues in dementia research, *Indian Journal of Psychological Medicine*, 43: 25S–30S.

Charland, L.C. (1998) Is Mr. Spock mentally competent? Competence to consent and emotion, *Philosophy, Psychiatry, & Psychology*, 5: 67–81.

Charland, L.C. (2001) Mental competence and value: the problem of normativity in the assessment of decision making capacity, *Psychiatry, Psychology and Law*, 8: 135–145.

Chen, H-L., Shih, S-C., Bair, M-J., et al. (2011) Percutaneous endoscopic gastrostomy in the enteral feeding of the elderly, *International Journal of Gerontology*, 5: 135–138.

Chochinov, H.M. (2007) Dignity and the essence of medicine: the A, B, C, and D of dignity conserving care, *British Medical Journal*, 335: 184–187.

Cholbi, M. (2015) Kant on euthanasia and the duty to die: clearing the air, *Journal of Medical Ethics*, 41: 607–610.

Chopra, S.S. (2003) Industry funding of clinical trials: benefit or bias? *Journal of the American Medical Association*, 290: 113–114.

Christensen, K.D., Roberts, J.S., Uhlmann, W.R., and Green, R.C. (2011) Changes to perceptions of the pros and cons of genetic susceptibility testing after APOE genotyping for Alzheimer disease risk, *Genetics in Medicine*, 13: 409–414.

Clafferty, R.A., Brown, K.W. and McCabe, E. (1998) Under half of psychiatrists tell patients their diagnosis of Alzheimer's disease, *British Medical Journal*, 317: 603.

Clare, L., Rowlands, J., Bruce, E., et al. (2008) The experience of living with dementia in residential care: an interpretative phenomenological analysis, *The Gerontologist*, 48: 711–720.

Clayton, J., Fardell, B., Hutton-Potts, J., et al. (2003) Parenteral antibiotics in a palliative care unit: prospective analysis of current practice. *Palliative Medicine*, 17: 44–48.

Coetzee, R.H., Leask, S.J. and Jones, R.G. (2003) The attitudes of carers and old age psychiatrists towards the treatment of potentially fatal events in end-stage dementia, *International Journal of Geriatric Psychiatry*, 18: 169–173.

Cohen-Mansfield, J. (2014) Understanding behaviour, in M. Downs and B. Bowers (eds) in *Excellence in Dementia Care: Research into Practice* 2nd edn. Maidenhead and New York: Open University Press.

Collopy, B.J. (1988) Autonomy in long term care: some crucial distinctions, *The Gerontologist*, 28 (Suppl.): 10–17.

Commission for Social Care Inspection (2007) *Rights, Risks and Restraints: An Exploration into the Use of Restraint in the Care of Older People*. CSCI: Newcastle. Available at: https://www.equalityhumanrights.com/sites/default/files/restraint.pdf (accessed 8 April 2022).

Comstock, G. (2013) *Research Ethics: A Philosophical Guide to the Responsible Conduct of Research*. Cambridge: Cambridge University Press.

Conn, D., Snowdon, J. and Purandare, N. (2017) Residential care for people with dementia, in D. Ames, J.T. O'Brien and A. Burns (eds) *Dementia*, 5th edn. Boca Raton, FL: CRC Press, Taylor & Francis Group.

Conroy, S.P., Luxton, T., Dingwall, R., et al. (2006) Cardiopulmonary resuscitation in continuing care settings: time for a rethink? *British Medical Journal*, 332: 479–482.

Cooley, D. (2007) A Kantian moral duty for the soon-to-be demented to commit suicide, *American Journal of Bioethics*, 7: 37–44.

Corner, L. and Bond, J. (2006) The impact of the label of mild cognitive impairment on the individual's sense of self, *Philosophy, Psychiatry, & Psychology*, 13: 3–12.

Corner, L. and Hughes, J.C. (2006) Quality of life for people with dementia, in J. Hughes (ed.) *Palliative Care in Severe Dementia*. London: Quay Books.

Corrigan, P.W., Kerr, A. and Knudsen, L. (2005) The stigma of mental illness: explanatory models and methods for change, *Applied and Preventive Psychology*, 11: 179–190.

Corrigan, P.W. and Watson, A.C. (2002) Understanding the impact of stigma on people with mental illness, *World Psychiatry*, 1: 16–20.

Cotrell, V. and Schulz, R. (1993) The perspective of the patient with Alzheimer's disease: a neglected dimension of dementia research, *The Gerontologist*, 33: 205–211.

Council of Europe. (1950) *European Convention for the Protection of Human Rights and Fundamental Freedoms*, as amended, 4 November 1950, Rome: ETS 5. Available at: https://www.echr.coe.int/Documents/Convention_ENG.pdf (accessed 28 February 2022).

Coverdale, J., McCullough, L.B., Molinari, V. and Workman, R. (2006) Ethically justified clinical strategies for promoting geriatric assent, *International Journal of Geriatric Psychiatry*, 21: 151–157.

Cowley, C. (2018) Dementia, identity and the role of friends, *Medicine, Health Care and Philosophy*, 21: 255–264.

Craigie, J. (2015) A fine balance: reconsidering patient autonomy in light of the UN Convention on the Rights of Persons with Disabilities, *Bioethics*, 29: 398–405.

Crooks, M., Wakenshaw, K., Young, J., et al. (2021) Restraints and restrictive interventions during essential personal care in elderly people living with dementia in care homes, *International Neuropsychiatric Disease Journal*, 15: 26–38.

Crutch, S.J., Yong, K.X., Peters, A., et al. (2018) Contributions of patient and citizen researchers to 'Am I the right way up?' study of balance in posterior cortical atrophy and typical Alzheimer's disease, *Dementia*, 17: 1011–1022.

Culley, H., Barber, R., Hope, A., and James, I. (2013) Therapeutic lying in dementia care, *Nursing Standard*, 28: 35–39.

Cunningham, C., Macfarlane, S. and Brodaty, H. (2019) Language paradigms when behaviour changes with dementia: #BanBPSD, *International Journal of Geriatric Psychiatry*, 34: 1109–1113.

Cutcliffe, J. and Milton, J. (1996) In defence of telling lies to cognitively impaired elderly patients, *International Journal of Geriatric Psychiatry*, 11: 1117–1118.

Daley, S., Akarsu, N., Armsby, E., et al. (2022) What factors have influenced quality of life in people with dementia and their family carers during the COVID-19 pandemic: a qualitative study, *BMJ Open*, 12: e053563. Available at: http://dx.doi.org/10.1136/bmjopen-2021-053563 (accessed 14 May 2022).

Daniels, N. (1988) *Am I My Parents' Keeper? An Essay on Justice Between the Young and the Old*. Oxford: Oxford University Press.

Danis, M., Garrett, J., Harris, R. and Patrick, D.L. (1994) Stability of choices about life-sustaining treatments, *Annals of Internal Medicine*, 120: 567–573.

Davies, N., Barrado-Martín, Y., Vickerstaff, V., et al. (2021) Enteral tube feeding for people with severe dementia. *Cochrane Database of Systematic Reviews 2021*, Issue 8. Art. No.: CD013503. Available at: https://doi.org/10.1002/14651858.CD013503.pub2. (accessed 26 April 2022).

Davies, T., Houston, A., Gordon, H., et al. (2021) Dementia enquirers: pioneering approaches to dementia research in UK, *Disability & Society*. Available at: https://doi.org/10.1080/09687599.2021.1916887 (accessed 31 October 2022).

Davis, D.H.J. (2004) Dementia: sociological and philosophical constructions, *Social Science & Medicine*, 58: 369–378.

Davis, D.S. (2014) Alzheimer disease and pre-emptive suicide, *Journal of Medical Ethics*, 40: 543–549.

Day, A.M., James, I.A., Meyer, T.D. and Lee, D.R. (2011) Do people with dementia find lies and deception in dementia care acceptable? *Aging & Mental Health*, 15: 822–829.

DEEP (Dementia Engagement and Empowerment Project) (2014) *Dementia Words Matter: Guidelines on Language About Dementia*. Available at: http://dementiavoices.org.uk/wp-content/uploads/2015/03/DEEP-Guide-Language.pdf (accessed 24 October 2022).

DEEP (Dementia Engagement and Empowerment Project) (2020) *The DEEP-Ethics Gold Standards for Dementia Research*. Exeter: Innovations in Dementia. Available at: https://www.dementiavoices.org.uk/wp-content/uploads/2020/07/The-DEEP-Ethics-Gold-Standards-for-Dementia-Research.pdf (accessed 10 March 2022).

Dekkers, W. (2011) Dwelling, house and home: towards a home-led perspective on dementia care, *Medicine, Health Care and Philosophy*, 14: 291–300.

Dening, T. and Milne, A. (2011) *Mental Health and Care Homes*. Oxford: Oxford University Press.

Dening, T. and Milne, A. (2021) Care homes for older people, in T. Dening, A. Thomas, R. Stewart and J-P. Taylor (eds) *Oxford Textbook of Old Age Psychiatry*, 3rd edn. Oxford: Oxford University Press.

Department for Constitutional Affairs. (2007) *Mental Capacity Act 2005: Code of Practice*. Norwich: The Stationery Office.

Department of Health. (2010) *'Nothing Ventured, Nothing Gained: Risk Guidance for People with Dementia*. London: Department of Health. Available at: https://www.gov.uk/government/publications/nothing-ventured-nothing-gained-risk-guidance-for-people-with-dementia (accessed 29 March 2022).

Department of Health and Welsh Office. (1999) *Code of Practice. Mental Health Act 1983*, 3rd edn. London: The Stationery Office.

Di Lorito, C., Duff, C., Rogers, C., et al. (2021) Tele-rehabilitation for people with dementia during the Covid-19 pandemic: a case-study from England, *International Journal of Environmental Research and Public Health*, 18: 1717. Available at: https://doi.org/10.3390/ijerph18041717 (accessed 12 May 2022).

Di Lorito, C., Masud, T., Gladman, J., et al. (2021) Deconditioning in people living with dementia during the COVID-19 pandemic: qualitative study from the Promoting Activity, Independence and Stability in Early Dementia (PrAISED) process evaluation, *BMC Geriatrics*, 21: 529. Available at: https://doi.org/10.1186/s12877-021-02451-z (accessed 14 May 2022).

Dimech, J., Agius, E., Hughes, J.C. and Bartolo, P. (2021) Challenges faced by patients, relatives and clinicians in end-stage dementia decision-making: a qualitative study of swallowing problems, *Journal of Medical Ethics*, 47: e39. Available at: http://dx.doi.org/10.1136/medethics-2020-106222 (accessed 29 April 2022).

Director, S. (2019) Consent's dominion: dementia and prior consent to sexual relations, *Bioethics*, 33: 1065–1071.

Donnelly, M. (2014) A legal overview, in C. Foster, J. Herring, and I. Doron (eds) *The Law and Ethics of Dementia*. Oxford and Portland, Oregon: Hart Publishing.

Donnelly, M. (2016) Best interests in the Mental Capacity Act: time to say goodbye? *Medical Law Review*, 24: 318–332.

Dowlen, R., Keady, J., Milligan, C. et al. (2018) The personal benefits of musicking for people living with dementia: a thematic synthesis of the qualitative literature, *Arts and Health*, 10: 197–212.

Downs, M. and Bowers, B. (2008) Caring for people with dementia, *British Medical Journal*, 336: 225–226.

Downs, M., Clare, L. and Mackenzie, J. (2006) Understandings of dementia: explanatory models and their implications for the person with dementia and therapeutic effort, in J.C. Hughes, S.J. Louw and S.R. Sabat (eds) *Dementia: Mind, Meaning, and the Person*. Oxford: Oxford University Press.

Doyal, L. and Wilsher, D. (1994) Withholding and withdrawing life sustaining treatment from elderly people: towards formal guidelines, *British Medical Journal*, 308: 1689–1692.

Draper, B., Peisah, C., Snowdon, J. and Brodaty, H. (2010) Early dementia diagnosis and the risk of suicide and euthanasia, *Alzheimer's & Dementia*, 6: 75–82.

Dresser, R. (1995) Dworkin on dementia: elegant theory, questionable policy, *Hastings Center Report*, 25: 32–38.

Dresser, R. (2014) Pre-emptive suicide, precedent autonomy and preclinical Alzheimer's disease, *Journal of Medical Ethics*, 40: 550–551.

Drickamer, M.A. and Lachs, M.S. (1992) Should patients with Alzheimer's disease be told their diagnosis? *New England Journal of Medicine*, 326: 947–951.

Driver and Vehicle Licensing Agency (2022) *Assessing Fitness to Drive: A Guide for Medical Professionals*. Swansea: DVLA. Available at: https://www.gov.uk/guidance/assessing-fitness-to-drive-a-guide-for-medical-professionals#full-publication-update-history (accessed 23 January 2023).

Dubinsky, R.M., Stein, A.C. and Lyons, K. (2000) Practice parameter: risk of driving and Alzheimer's disease (an evidence-based review): report of the Quality Standards Subcommittee of the American Academy of Neurology, *Neurology*, 54: 2205–2211.

Dunn, M. and Foster, C. (2010) Autonomy and welfare as *amici curiae*, *Medical Law Review*, 18: 86–95.

Dunn, M. and Holland, A. (2019) Mental Capacity Act application: social care settings, in *Mental Capacity Legislation: Principles and Practice*, 2nd edn. Cambridge: Cambridge University Press.

Dunn, M., Fulford, K.W.M., Herring, J. and Handa, A. (2019) Between the reasonable and the particular: deflating autonomy in the legal regulation of informed consent to medical treatment, *Health Care Analysis*, 27: 110–127.

Dupuis, S.L., Kontos, P., Mitchell, G., Jonas-Simpson, C. and Gray, J. (2016) Re-claiming citizenship through the arts, *Dementia*, 15: 358–380.

Dupuis, S.L., Wiersma, E. and Loiselle, L. (2012) Pathologizing behavior: meanings of behaviors in dementia care, *Journal of Aging Studies*, 26: 162–173.

Dworkin, G., Frey, R.G. and Bok, S. (1998) *Euthanasia and Physician-Assisted Suicide (For and Against)*. Cambridge: Cambridge University Press.

Dworkin, R. (1993) *Life's Dominion: An Argument About Abortion and Euthanasia*. London: Harper Collins.

Ebell, M.H., Becker, L.A., Barryt, H.C. and Hagen, M. (1998) Survival after in-hospital cardiopulmonary resuscitation. A meta-analysis. *Journal of General Internal Medicine*, 13: 805–816.

Ellis, C., Hunt, M. R., and Chambers-Evans, J. (2011). Relational autonomy as an essential component of patient-centred care, *International Journal of Feminist Approaches to Bioethics*, 4: 79–101.

Elvish, R., James, I. and Milne, D. (2010) Lying in dementia care: an example of a culture that deceives in people's best interests, *Aging & Mental Health*, 14: 255–262.

Elwyn, G., Coulter, A., Laitner, S., et al. (2010) Implementing shared decision making in the NHS. *British Medical Journal*, 341: 971–973.

Elwyn, G., Frosch, D., Thomson, R., et al. (2012) Shared decision making: a model for clinical practice, *Journal of General Internal Medicine*, 27: 1361–1367.

Emanuel, E.J., Grady, C., Crouch, R.A., Lie, R.K., Miller, F.G. and Wendler, D. (2008a) *The Oxford Textbook of Clinical Research Ethics*. Oxford: Oxford University Press.

Emanuel, E.J., Wendler, D. and Grady, C. (2008b) An ethical framework for biomedical research, in E.J. Emanuel, C. Grady, R.A. Crouch, R.K. Lie, F.G. Miller and D. Wendler (eds) *The Oxford Textbook of Clinical Research Ethics*. Oxford: Oxford University Press.

Emanuel, L.L., Emanuel, E.J., Stoeckle, J.D., et al. (1994) Advance directives. Stability of patients' treatment choices. *Archives of Internal Medicine*, 154: 209–217.

Emmett, C. and Hughes, J.C. (2019) Best interests, in *Mental Capacity Legislation: Principles and Practice*, 2nd edn. Cambridge: Cambridge University Press.

Emmett, C. and Hughes, J.C. (2021) Mental capacity and decision-making, in T. Dening, A. Thomas, R. Stewart and J-P. Taylor (eds) *Oxford Textbook of Old Age Psychiatry*, 3rd edn. Oxford: Oxford University Press.

Emmett, C., Poole, M., Bond, J. and Hughes, J.C. (2013) Homeward bound or bound for a home? Assessing the capacity of dementia patients to make decisions about hospital discharge: comparing practice with legal standards, *International Journal of Law and Psychiatry*, 36: 73–82.

European Parliament and European Council. (2001) *Directive 2001/20/Ec of the European Parliament and of the Council of 4 April 2001*. The European Parliament and The Council of the European Union. Available at: https://ec.europa.eu/health/system/files/2016-11/dir_2001_20_en_0.pdf (accessed 7 March 2022).

Evans, J., Brown, M., Coughlan, T., et al. (2015) A systematic review of dementia focused assistive technology, in M. Kurosu (ed.) *Human-Computer Interaction: Interaction Technologies. Lecture Notes in Computer Science*, vol 9170. Cham, Switzerland: Springer. Available at: https://doi.org/10.1007/978-3-319-20916-6_38 (accessed 31 March 2022).

Fabiszewski, K.J., Volicer, B. and Volicer, L. (1990) Effect of antibiotic treatment on outcome of fevers in institutionalized Alzheimer patients, *Journal of the American Medical Association*, 263: 3168–3172.

Faggioni, M.P., González-Melado, F.J. and Di Pietro, M.L. (2021) National health system cuts and triage decisions during the COVID-19 pandemic in Italy and Spain: ethical implications, *Journal of Medical Ethics*, 47: 300–307.

Fallon, A. and O'Neill, D. (2017) Driving and dementia, in D. Ames, J.T. O'Brien and A. Burns (eds) *Dementia*, 5th edn. Boca Raton, FL: CRC Press, Taylor & Francis Group.

Feil, N. and Altman, R. (2004) Validation theory and the myth of the therapeutic lie, *American Journal of Alzheimer's Disease and Other Dementias*, 19: 77–78.

Feinberg, L.F. and Whitlatch, C.J. (2001) Are persons with cognitive impairment able to state consistent choices? *The Gerontologist*, 41: 374–382.

Fellows, L.K. (1998) Competency and consent in dementia, *Journal of the American Geriatrics Society*, 46: 922–926.

Fetherstonhaugh, D., McAuliffe, L., Bauer, M. and Shanley, C. (2017) Decision-making on behalf of people living with dementia: how do surrogate decision-makers decide? *Journal of Medical Ethics*, 43: 35–40.

Finnis, J. (2011) *Natural Law and Natural Rights*, 2nd edn. Oxford: Oxford University Press.

Finucane, T.E., Christmas, C. and Travis, K. (1999) Tube feeding in patients with advanced dementia: a review of the evidence, *Journal of the American Medical Association*, 282: 1365–1370.

Flynn, E. (2018) Legal capacity for people with dementia: a human rights approach, in S. Cahill *Dementia and Human Rights*. Bristol and Chicago: Policy Press.

Foot, P. (1977) Euthanasia, *Philosophy and Public Affairs*, 6: 85–112.

Foot, P. (2001) *Natural Goodness*. Oxford: Clarendon Press.

Fossey, J., Ballard, C., Juszczak, E., et al. (2006) Effect of enhanced psychosocial care on antipsychotic use in nursing home residents with severe dementia: cluster randomised trial, *British Medical Journal*, 332: 756–761.

Foster, C., Herring, J. and Doron, I. (eds) (2014) *The Law and Ethics of Dementia*. Oxford and Portland, Oregon: Hart Publishing.

Freedman, B. (1987) Equipoise and the ethics of clinical research. *New England Journal of Medicine*, 317: 141–145.

Freedman, M.L. and Freedman, D.L. (1996) Should Alzheimer's disease patients be allowed to drive? A medical, legal, and ethical dilemma, *Journal of the American Geriatrics Society*, 44: 876–877.

Friedman, L.M., Furberg, C.D., DeMets, D.L., Reboussin, D.M. and Granger, C.B. (2015) *Fundamentals of Clinical Trials*, 5th edn. Cham, Switzerland: Springer.

Frisoni, G.B. (2004) Breaking the diagnosis of dementia, *The Lancet Neurology*, 3: 125–126.

Fulford, K.W.M. (Bill). (2004) Facts/values: ten principles of values-based medicine, in J. Radden (ed.) *The Philosophy of Psychiatry: A Companion*. Oxford: Oxford University Press.

Fulford, K.W.M. (Bill)., Peile, E., Carroll, H. (2012) *Essential Values-Based Practice: Clinical Stories Linking Science with People*. Cambridge: Cambridge University Press.

Fullbrook, S. (2007) Best interest. A review of the legal principles involved: Part 2(a). *British Journal of Nursing*, 16: 682–683.

Furberg, E. (2012) Advance directives and personal identity: what is the problem? *Journal of Medicine and Philosophy*, 37: 60–73.

Gaines, A.D. and Whitehouse, P.J. (2006) Building a mystery: Alzheimer's disease, mild cognitive impairment, and beyond, *Philosophy, Psychiatry, & Psychology*, 13: 61–74.

Gastmans, C. and de Lepeleire, J. (2010) Living to the bitter end? A personalist approach to euthanasia in persons with severe dementia, *Bioethics*, 24: 78–86.

Gauthier, S., Leuzy, A., Racince, E. and Rosa-Neto, P. (2013) Diagnosis and management of Alzheimer's disease: past, present and future ethical issues, *Progress in Neurobiology*, 110: 102–113.

Gedge, E.B. (2004) Collective moral imagination: making decisions for persons with dementia, *Journal of Medicine and Philosophy*, 29: 435–450.

Gendler, T.S. (2008) Alief and belief, *Journal of Philosophy*, 105: 634–663.

General Medical Council. (2017) Confidentiality: Patients' Fitness to Drive and Reporting Concerns to the DVLA or DVA. London: General Medical Council. Available at: https://www.gmc-uk.org/ethical-guidance/ethical-guidance-for-doctors/confidentiality-patients-fitness-to-drive-and-reporting-concerns-to-the-dvla-or-dva (accessed 29 March 2022).

Giebel, C., Lion, K., Mackowiak, M., et al. (2022) A qualitative 5-country comparison of the perceived impacts of COVID-19 on people living with dementia and unpaid carers, *BMC Geriatrics*, 22: 116. Available at: https://doi.org/10.1186/s12877-022-02821-1 (accessed 14 May 2022).

Giebel, C., Lord, K., Cooper, C., et al. (2021) A UK survey of COVID 19 related social support closures and their effects on older people, people with dementia, and carers, *International Journal of Geriatric Psychiatry*, 36: 393–402.

Gilbert, F., Viaña, J.N.M., Bittlinger, M., et al. (2022) Invasive experimental brain surgery for dementia: ethical shifts in clinical research practices? *Bioethics*, 36: 25–41.

Gillett, G. (2019) Advance decisions in dementia: when the past conflicts with the present, *Journal of Medica Ethics*, 45: 204–208.

Gilliard, J. and Gwilliam, C. (1996) Sharing the diagnosis: a survey of memory disorders clinics, their policies of informing people with dementia and their families, and the support they offer, *International Journal of Geriatric Psychiatry*, 11: 1001–1003.

Gillick, M.R. (2000) Rethinking the role of tube feeding in patients with advanced dementia, *New England Journal of Medicine*, 342: 206–210.

Gillick, M.R. (2001) Artificial nutrition and hydration in the patient with advanced dementia: is withholding treatment compatible with traditional Judaism? *Journal of Medical Ethics*, 27: 12–15.

Gilligan, C. (1982) *In a Different Voice: Psychological Theory and Women's Moral Development*. Cambridge MA: Harvard University Press.

Gillon, R. (1986) *Philosophical Medical Ethics*. Chichester: John Wiley & Sons.

Gillon, R. (1994) Medical ethics: four principles plus attention to scope, *British Medical Journal*, 309: 184–188.

Gilmour, J.A. and Brannelly, T. (2010) Representations of people with dementia – subaltern, person, citizen, *Nursing Inquiry*, 17: 240–247.

Gjellestad, A., Oksholm, T. and Bruvik, F. (2021) Forced treatment and care in home-dwelling persons with dementia, *Nursing Ethics*, 28: 372–386.

Glover, J. (1977) *Causing Death and Saving Lives*. Harmondsworth: Penguin.

Goffman, E. (1963) *Stigma: notes on the management of spoiled identity*. New York: Simon and Schuster.

Goldsteen, M. (2008) Empirical ethics in action in practices of dementia care, in G. Widdershoven, J. McMillan, T. Hope and L. van der Scheer (eds) *Empirical Ethics in Psychiatry*. Oxford: Oxford University Press.

Gómez-Vírseda, C. and Gastmans, C. (2021) Euthanasia in persons with advanced dementia: a dignity-enhancing care approach, *Journal of Medical Ethics*, online. Available at: https://doi.org/10.1136/medethics-2021-107308 (accessed 2 June 2022).

Gordon, M. (2006) Ethical and clinical issues in cardiopulmonary resuscitation (CPR) in the frail elderly with dementia: a Jewish perspective, *Journal of Ethics in Mental Health*, 1: 1–4. Available at: https://jemh.ca/issues/v1n1/documents/JEMH_V1N1_article_EthicalClinicalIssuesinCPR.pdf (accessed 6 May 2022).

Götzelmann, T.G., Strech, D. and Kahrass, H. (2021) The full spectrum of ethical issues in dementia research: findings of a systematic qualitative review, *BMC Medical Ethics*, 22: 32. Available at: https://doi.org/10.1186/s12910-020-00572-5 (accessed 28 October 2022).

Gove, D., Beatty, A., Capstick, A., et al. (2021) *2021 Alzheimer Europe Report: Sex, Gender and Sexuality in the Context of Dementia: A Discussion Paper*. Luxembourg: Alzheimer Europe. Available at: https://www.alzheimer-europe.org/reports-publication/2021-alzheimer-europe-report-sex-gender-and-sexuality-context-dementia (accessed 22 April 2022).

Gove, D., Downs, M., Vernooij-Dassen, M. et al. (2016) Stigma and GPs' perceptions of dementia, *Aging & Mental Health*, 20: 391–400.

Graham, J.E. and Ritchie, K. (2006) Mild cognitive impairment: ethical considerations for nosological flexibility in human kinds, *Philosophy, Psychiatry, & Psychology*, 13: 31–43.

Graham, P. and Hughes, J.C. (2014). Assisted dying – the debate: *Videtur … sed contra*, *Advances in Psychiatric Treatment*, 20: 250–257.

Greener, H., Poole, M., Emmett, C., et al. (2012) Value judgements and conceptual tensions: decision-making in relation to hospital discharge for people with dementia. *Clinical Ethics*, 7: 166–174.

Gregory, G. (2022) Poetry and crafting for people living with dementia, in I. Parker, R. Coaten and M. Hopfenbeck (eds) *The Practical Handbook of Living with Dementia*. Monmouth: PCCS Books.

Griffin, J. (1986) *Well-Being: Its Meaning, Measurement, and Moral Importance*. Oxford: Clarendon Press.

Grigorovich, A., Kontos, P. and Kontos, A.P. (2019) The 'violent resident': a critical exploration of the ethics of resident-to-resident aggression, *Bioethical Inquiry*, 16: 173–183.

Grisso, T. and Appelbaum, P.A. (1998) *The Assessment of Decision-Making Capacity: A Guide for Physicians and Other Health Professionals*. Oxford: Oxford University Press.

Grotius, H. (1925) *On the Law of War and Peace* (translated by F W Kelsey; first published 1625). Indianapolis: Bobbs-Merrill.

Guidry-Grimes, L., Dean, M. and Victor, E.K. (2021) Covert administration of medication in food: a worthwhile moral gamble? *Journal of Medical Ethics*, 47: 389–393.

Habermas, J. (1990) *Moral Consciousness and Communicative Action* (translated by C. Lenhardt and S. Weber Nicholsen). Cambridge MA: Massachusetts Institute of Technology Press. (First published in German in 1983 as *Moralbewußtsein und kommunikatives Handeln*. Frankfurt am Main: Suhrkamp Verlag.)

Hachinski, V. (2008) Shifts in thinking about dementia. *Journal of the American Medical Association*, 300: 2172–2173.

Hagan, R.J. and Campbell, S. (2021) Doing their damnedest to seek change: how group identity helps people with dementia confront public stigma and maintain purpose, *Dementia*, 20: 2362–2379.

Hallich, O. (2015) Tom Buller on the principle of precedent autonomy and the relation between critical and experiential interests, *Journal of Medical Ethics*, 41: 709–711.

Hamet, P. and Tremblay, J. (2017) Artificial intelligence in medicine, *Metabolism: Clinical and Experimental*, 69: S36–S40.

Hanna, K., Giebel, C., Tetlow, H., et al. (2022) Emotional and mental wellbeing following COVID-19 public health measures on people living with dementia and carers, *Journal of Geriatric Psychiatry and Neurology*, 35: 344–352.

Hariyanto, T.I., Putri, C., Arisa, J., et al. (2021) Dementia and outcomes from coronavirus disease 2019 (COVID-19) pneumonia: a systematic review and meta-analysis, *Archives of Gerontology and Geriatrics*, 93: 104299. Available at: https://doi.org/ 10.1016/j.archger.2020.104299 (accessed 18 May 2022).

Harper, L., Dobbs, B.M., Stites, S.D., et al. (2019) Stigma in dementia: It's time to talk about it: There's much you can do to address stigmatizing attitudes, beliefs, and behaviors, *Current Psychiatry*, 18: 16–24.

Harrefors, C., Axelsson, K. and Sävenstedt, S. (2010) Using assistive technology services at differing levels of care: healthy elder couples' perceptions, *Journal of Advanced Nursing*, 66: 1523–1532.

Harris, J. (1987) QALYfying the value of life. *Journal of Medical Ethics*, 13: 117–123.

Harrison, C. (1993) Personhood, dementia and the integrity of a life, *Canadian Journal on Aging / La Revue Canadienne do vieillissement*, 12: 428–440.

Harrison, C., Molloy, D.W., Darzins, P. and Bédard, M. (1995) Should people do unto others as they would want done unto themselves? *Journal of Clinical Ethics*, 6: 14–19.

Harwood, R.H. (2014) Feeding decisions in advanced dementia, *Journal of the Royal College of Physicians of Edinburgh*, 44: 232–237.

Haw, C. and Stubbs, J. (2010) Covert administration of medication to older adults: a review of the literature and published studies, *Journal of Psychiatric and Mental Health Nursing*, 17: 761–768.

Heersmink, R. (2022) Preserving narrative identity for dementia patients: embodiment, active environments, and distributed memory, *Neuroethics*, 15: 8. Available at: https://doi.org/10.1007/s12152-022-09479-x (accessed 25 February 2022).

Heidegger, M. (1962) *Being and Time* (trans. J. Macquarrie and E. Robinson), Malden MA, Oxford, and Carlton (Australia): Blackwell. (*Sein und Zeit* was first published in 1927.)

Her Majesty's Stationery Office (HMSO) (2005) *The Mental Capacity Act 2005*. London: HMSO. Available at: https://www.legislation.gov.uk/ukpga/2005/9/pdfs/ukpga_20050009_en.pdf (accessed 7 March 2022).

Herskovits, E. (1995) Struggling over subjectivity: debates about the 'self' and Alzheimer's disease, *Medical Anthropology Quarterly*, 9: 146–164.

Hertogh, C.M.P.M., de Boer, M.E., Dröes, R-M. and Eefsting, J.A. (2007) Would we rather lose our life than lose our self? Lessons from the Dutch debate on euthanasia for patients with dementia, *The American Journal of Bioethics*, 7: 48–56.

Hertogh, C.M.P.M., The, B.A.M., Miesen, B.M.L. and Eefsting, J.A. (2004) Truth telling and truthfulness in the care for patients with advanced dementia: an ethnographic study in Dutch nursing homes, *Social Science & Medicine*, 59: 1685–1693.

Higgs, P. and Gilleard, C. (2016) Interrogating personhood and dementia, *Aging & Mental Health*, 20: 773–780.

Hillman, A. (2017) Diagnosing dementia: ethnography, interactional ethics and everyday moral reasoning, *Social Theory & Health*, 15: 44–65.

Hinchliff, S. and Fileborn, B. (2021) Sexuality in old age, in T. Dening, A. Thomas, R. Stewart and J-P. Taylor (eds) *Oxford Textbook of Old Age Psychiatry*, 3rd edn. Oxford: Oxford University Press.

Hodge, G. (2021) Where are the children? An autoethnography of deception in dementia in an acute hospital, *Bioethics*, 35: 864–869.

Hoerl, C. (2013) Jaspers on explaining and understanding in psychiatry, in G. Stanghellini and T. Fuchs (eds) *One Century of Karl Jaspers' General Psychopathology*. Oxford: Oxford University Press.

Hoffer, L.J. (2006) Tube feeding in advanced dementia: the metabolic perspective, *British Medical Journal*, 333: 1214–1215.

Holder, J.M. and Jolley, D. (2012) Forced relocation between nursing homes: residents' health outcomes and potential moderators, *Reviews in Clinical Gerontology*, 22: 301–319.

Holm, S. (2001) Autonomy, authenticity, or best interest: everyday decision-making and persons with dementia, *Medicine, Health Care and Philosophy*, 4: 153–159.

Holton, R. (2016) Memory, persons and dementia, *Studies in Christian Ethics*, 29: 256–260.

Home Office (1998) *Human Rights Act 1998*. The Stationery Office: London.

Hope, R.A. and Fairburn, C.G. (1990) The nature of wandering in dementia: a community-based study, *International Journal of Geriatric Psychiatry*, 5: 239–245.

Hope, T. (1995) Personal identity and psychiatric illness, in A.P. Griffiths (ed.) *Philosophy, Psychology and Psychiatry*. Cambridge: Cambridge University Press.

Hope, T., Savulescu, J. and Hendrick, J. (2003) *Medical Ethics and Law: The Core Curriculum*. Edinburgh: Churchill Livingstone.

Hope, T., Slowther, A. and Eccles, J. (2009) Best interests, dementia and the Mental Capacity Act (2005), *Journal of Medical Ethics*, 35: 733–738.

Hotopf, M., Lee, W. and Price, A. (2011a) Assisted suicide: why psychiatrists should engage in the debate, *British Journal of Psychiatry*, 198: 83–84.

Hotopf, M., Price, A. and Lee, W. (2011b) Assisted suicide: two sides to the debate. Authors' reply, *British Journal of Psychiatry*, 198: 493.

House of Lords. (2014) *Mental Capacity Act 2005: Post- Legislative Scrutiny*. HMSO: London. Available at: https://publications.parliament.uk/pa/ld201314/ldselect/ldmentalcap/139/139.pdf (accessed 7 February 2022).

Howard, R., Gathercole, R., Bradley, R., et al. (2021) The effectiveness and cost-effectiveness of assistive technology and telecare for independent living in dementia: a randomised controlled trial, *Age and Ageing*, 50: 882–890.

Howarth, A., Crooks, M. and Sells, D. (2017) The use of physical restraint to deliver essential personal care to incapacitated older adults with dementia: can it be person-centred? in I.A. James and L. Jackman (eds) *Understanding Behaviour in Dementia that Challenges: A Guide to Assessment and Treatment*, 2nd edn. London and Philadelphia: Jessica Kingsley.

Howarth, A., Sells, D., Mackenzie, L. and Hope, A. (2014) Are we forcing people with dementia to receive care? *International Journal of Geriatric Psychiatry*, 29: 768–770.

Hudson, W.D. (1969) *The Is/Ought Question: A Collection of Papers on the Central Problem in Moral Philosophy*. London: Macmillan.

Hughes, J.A. (2021) Advance euthanasia directives and the Dutch prosecution, *Journal of Medical Ethics*, 47: 253–256.

Hughes, J.C. (2000) Ethics and the anti-dementia drugs, *International Journal of Geriatric Psychiatry*, 15: 538–543.

Hughes, J.C. (2001) Views of the person with dementia, *Journal of Medical Ethics*, 27: 86–91.

Hughes, J.C. (2003) Quality of life in dementia: an ethical and philosophical perspective, *Expert Review of Pharmacoeconomics and Outcomes Research*, 3: 525–534.

Hughes, J.C. (2006) Patterns of practice: a useful notion in medical ethics? *Journal of Ethics in Mental Health*, 1: 1–5. Available via www.jemh.ca (accessed 14 January 2022).

Hughes, J.C. (2009) Ethical issues and patterns of practice, in M.F. Weiner and A.M. Lipton (eds) *The American Psychiatric Publishing Textbook of Alzheimer Disease and Other Dementias*. Washington DC and London, England: American Psychiatric Publishing.

Hughes, J.C. (2011a) *Alzheimer's and Other Dementias: The Facts*. Oxford: Oxford University Press.

Hughes, J.C. (2011b) *Thinking Through Dementia*. Oxford: Oxford University Press.

Hughes, J.C. (2012) Justice, guidelines, and virtues, in H. Lesser (ed.) *Justice for Older People*. Amsterdam and New York: Ropodi.

Hughes, J.C. (2014a) Maintaining wellbeing through the end of life, in T.B.L. Kirkwood and C.L. Cooper (eds) *Wellbeing in Later Life. Volume IV of Wellbeing: A Complete Reference Guide*. Chichester: Wiley Blackwell.

Hughes, J.C. (2014b) The use of new technologies in managing dementia patients, in C. Foster, J. Herring, and I. Doron (eds) *The Law and Ethics of Dementia*. Oxford and Portland, Oregon: Hart Publishing.

Hughes, J.C. (2014c) The aesthetic approach to people with dementia. *International Psychogeriatrics*, 26: 1407–1413.

Hughes, J.C. (2019) Dementia as a psychiatric category, in: T. Kitwood (edited by D. Brooker) *Dementia Reconsidered, Revisited*, 2nd edn. London: Open University Press.

Hughes, J.C. (2020a) 'Dementia: ethical issues' – over ten years on, *Nuffield Council on Bioethics Blog*. Available at: https://www.nuffieldbioethics.org/blog/dementia-ethical-issues-over-ten-years-on (accessed on 22 March 2022).

Hughes, J.C. (2020b) What the virtues have to offer in the midst of COVID-19, *Journal of Medical Ethics blog*. Available at: https://blogs.bmj.com/medical-ethics/2020/04/19/what-the-virtues-have-to-offer-in-the-midst-of-covid-19/ (accessed 20 May 2020).

Hughes, J.C. (2021) Truthfulness and the person living with dementia: embedded intentions, speech acts and conforming to the reality, *Bioethics*, 35: 842–849.

Hughes, J.C. (forthcoming) The aesthetics of dementia, in M. Poltrum, M. Musalek, H. Fox, et al. (eds) *The Oxford Handbook of Mental Health and Contemporary Western Aesthetics*. Oxford: Oxford University Press.

Hughes, J.C. and Baldwin, C. (2006) *Ethical Issues in Dementia Care: Making Difficult Decisions*. London and Philadelphia: Jessica Kingsley.

Hughes, J.C. and Beatty, A. (2013) Understanding the person with dementia: a clinicophilosophical case discussion, *Advances in Psychiatric Treatment*, 19: 337–343.

Hughes, J.C. and Heginbotham, C. (2013) Mental capacity and decision-making, in T. Dening and A. Thomas (eds) *Oxford Textbook of Old Age Psychiatry*, 2nd edn. Oxford: Oxford University Press.

Hughes, J.C. and Louw, S.J. (2002a) Confidentiality and cognitive impairment: professional and philosophical ethics, *Age and Ageing*, 31: 147–150.

Hughes, J.C. and Louw, S.J. (2002b) Electronic tagging of people with dementia who wander, *British Medical Journal*, 325: 847–848.

Hughes, J.C. and Ramplin, S. (2012) Clinical and ethical judgement, in C. Cowley (ed.) *Reconceiving Medical Ethics*. London and New York: Continuum.

Hughes, J.C. and Sabat, S.R. (2008) The advance directive conjuring trick and the person with dementia, in G. Widdershoven, J. McMillan, T. Hope and L. van der Scheer (eds) *Empirical Ethics in Psychiatry*. Oxford: Oxford University Press.

Hughes, J.C. and Strech, D. (2017) Ethical issues, in D. Ames, J.T. O'Brien and A. Burns (eds) *Dementia*, 5th edn. Boca Raton, FL: CRC Press, Taylor & Francis Group.

Hughes, J.C. and Williamson, T. (2019) *The Dementia Manifesto: Putting Values-Based Practice to Work*. Cambridge: Cambridge University Press.

Hughes, J.C., Bamford, C. and May, C. (2008) Types of centredness in health care: themes and concepts, *Medicine, Health Care and Philosophy*, 11: 455–463.

Hughes, J.C., Beatty, A. and Emmett, C. (2021a) *Dementia, Law and Ethics: A Practical Guide for Nurses and Other Healthcare Professionals*. London and Philadelphia: Jessica Kingsley.

Hughes, J.C., Beatty, A. and Shippen, J. (2014) Sexuality in dementia, in C. Foster, J. Herring, and I. Doron (eds) *The Law and Ethics of Dementia*. Oxford and Portland, Oregon: Hart Publishing.

Hughes, J.C., Louw, S.J. and Sabat, S.R. (2006) *Dementia: Mind, Meaning, and the Person*. Oxford: Oxford University Press.

Hughes, J.C., Crepaz-Keay, D., Emmett, C. and Fulford, K.W.M. (2018) The Montgomery ruling, individual values and shared decision-making in psychiatry, *BJPsych Advances*, 24: 93–100.

Hughes, J.C., Hope, T., Reader, S. and Rice, D. (2002a) Dementia and ethics: the views of informal carers, *Journal of the Royal Society of Medicine*, 95: 242–246.

Hughes, J.C., Hope, T., Savulescu, J. and Ziebland, S. (2002b) Carers, ethics and dementia: a survey and review of the literature, *International Journal of Geriatric Psychiatry*, 17: 35–40.

Hughes, J.C., Jolley, D., Jordan, A. and Sampson, E.L. (2020) Palliative care in dementia: issues and evidence, in P. Lilford and J.C. Hughes (eds) *Clinical Topics in Old Age Psychiatry*. Cambridge: Cambridge University Press.

Hughes, J.C., Baseman, J., Hearne, C., et al. (2021b) Art, authenticity and citizenship for people living with dementia in a care home. *Ageing & Society*, 1–21. Available at: https://doi.org/10.1017/S0144686X21000271 (accessed on 5 April 2022).

Hughes, J.C., Haimes, E., Summerville, L., et al. (2009) Consenting older adults: research as a virtuous relationship, in O. Corrigan, J. McMillan, K. Liddell, K., et al. (eds) *The Limits of Consent – A Socio-Ethical Approach to Human Subject Research in Medicine*. Oxford: Oxford University Press.

Hughes, J.C., Ingram, T.A., Jarvis, A., et al. (2017) Consent for the diagnosis of preclinical dementia states: a review, *Maturitas*, 98: 30–34.

Hughes, J.C., Newby, J., Louw, S. J., et al. (2008) Ethical issues and tagging in dementia: a survey. *Journal of Ethics in Mental Health*, 3: 1–6. Available at: https://jemh.ca/issues/v3n1/documents/JEMH_V3N1_Ethical_Issues_and_Tagging_in_Dementia.pdf (accessed 2 April 2022).

Hughes, J.C., Poole, M., Louw, S.J., et al. (2015). Residence capacity: its nature and assessment, *BJPsych Advances*, 21: 307–312.

Humbert, I.A., McLaren, D.G. and Kosmatka, K. (2010) Early deficits in cortical control of swallowing in Alzheimer's disease, *Journal of Alzheimer's Disease*, 19: 1185–1197.

Hume, D. (1962) *A Treatise of Human Nature*, edited by D.G.C. Macnabb. Glasgow: Fontana/Collins. First published in 1739.

Hursthouse, R. (1999) *On Virtue Ethics*. Oxford: Oxford University Press.

Husband, H.J. (2000) Diagnostic disclosure in dementia: an opportunity for intervention? *International Journal of Geriatric Psychiatry*, 15: 544–547.

Hydén, L-C. (2013) Storytelling in dementia: embodiment as a resource, *Dementia*, 12: 359–367.

Hye, A. and Velayudhan, L. (2021) Molecular genetics and biology of dementia, in T. Dening, A. Thomas, R. Stewart and J-P. Taylor (eds) *Oxford Textbook of Old Age Psychiatry*, 3rd edn. Oxford: Oxford University Press.

Israel, M. (2015) *Research Ethics and Integrity for Social Scientists: Beyond Regulatory Compliance*, 2nd edn. London: Sage.

Jackman, L. and Emmett, C. (2014) Two important legal events that may radically shape the future delivery of dementia care in England and Wales, *International Journal of Geriatric Psychiatry*, 30: 105.

Jackman, L., Emmett, C., Sharp, T. and Marshall, J. (2014) Legal implications of restrictive physical interventions in people with dementia, *Nursing Older People*, 26: 24–29.

Jacobson, H. (2004) How the search for a little joy in this miserable world can kill you, *The Independent* (30 October 2004). Available at: https://www.independent.co.uk/voices/commentators/howard-jacobson/how-the-search-for-a-little-joy-in-this-miserable-world-can-kill-you-31091.html (accessed on 22 April 2022).

James, I.A. and Jackman, L. (2017) *Understanding Behaviour in Dementia that Challenges: A Guide to Assessment and Treatment*, 2nd edn. London and Philadelphia: Jessica Kingsley.

James, I.A., Reichelt, K., Moniz-Cook, E. and Lee, K. (2020) Challenging behaviour in dementia care: a novel framework for translating knowledge to practice, *The Cognitive Behaviour Therapist*, 13: e43. Available at: https://doi.org/10.1017/S1754470X20000434 (accessed 6 April 2022).

James, I.A., Wood-Mitchell, A., Waterworth, A.M., et al. (2006) Lying to people with dementia: developing ethical guidelines for care settings, *International Journal of Geriatric Psychiatry*, 21: 800–801.

Jaspers, K. (1963) *General Psychopathology* (translated by J. Hoenig and M.W. Hamilton). Manchester: Manchester University Press. Originally published in 1923 as *Allgemeine Psycholpathologie*, Berlin: Springer Verlag.

Jaworska, A. (1999) Respecting the margins of agency: Alzheimer's patients and the capacity to value, *Philosophy and Public Affairs*, 28: 105–138.

Jennings, L. (ed.) (2014) *Welcome to Our World: A Collection of Life Writing by People Living with Dementia*. Canterbury: Forget-Me-Nots.

Jha, A., Tabet, N. and Orrell, M. (2001) To tell or not to tell – comparison of older patients' reaction to their diagnosis of dementia and depression, *International Journal of Geriatric Psychiatry*, 16: 879–885.

John, S.D. (2007) Ordinary and extraordinary means, in R.E. Ashcroft, A. Dawson, H. Draper and J.R. McMillan (eds) *Principles of Health Care Ethics*, 2nd edn. Chichester: John Wiley & Sons.

Johnson, R.A. and Karlawish, J. (2015) A review of ethical issues in dementia, *International Psychogeriatrics*, 27: 1635–1647.

Johnston, B., Lawton, S., McCaw, C. et al. (2016) Living well with dementia: enhancing dignity and quality of life, using a novel intervention, Dignity Therapy, *International Journal of Older People Nursing*, 11: 107–120.

Johnston, B. and Narayanasamy, M. (2016) Exploring psychosocial interventions for people with dementia that enhance personhood and relate to legacy – an integrative review, *BMC Geriatrics*, 16: 77. Available at: https://bmcgeriatr.biomedcentral.com/articles/10.1186/s12877-016-0250-1 (accessed 24 February 2022).

Johnstone, M-J. (2011) Metaphors, stigma and the 'Alzheimerization' of the euthanasia debate, *Dementia*, 12: 377–393.

Jolley, D., Jefferys, P., Katona, C. and Lennon, S. (2011) Enforced relocation of older people when Care Homes close: a question of life and death? *Age and Ageing*, 40: 534–537.

Jones, D.A. (2022) Euthanasia, assisted suicide, and suicide rates in Europe, *Journal of Ethics in Mental Health*, 11: online. Available at: https://jemh.ca/issues/open/documents/JEMH%20article%20EAS%20and%20suicide%20rates%20in%20Europe%20-%20copy-edited%20final.pdf (accessed on 3 June 2022).

Jones, R.G. (1997) Ethical and legal issues in the care of demented people, *Reviews in Clinical Gerontology*, 7: 147–162.

Jongsma, K.R. and van der Vathorst, S. (2015) Dementia research and advance consent: it is not about critical interests, *Journal of Medical Ethics*, 41: 708–709.

Jongsma, K.R., Kars, M.C. and van Delden, J.J.M. (2019) Dementia and advance directives: some empirical and normative concerns, *Journal of Medical Ethics*, 45: 92–94.

Jonsen, A.R. and Toulmin, S. (1988) *The Abuse of Casuistry: A History of Moral Reasoning*. Berkeley, Los Angeles and London: University of California Press.

Jox, R.J., Denke, E., Hamann, J., et al. (2012) Surrogate decision making for patients with end-stage dementia, *International Journal of Geriatric Psychiatry*, 27: 1045–1052.

Kant, I. (1993) *Grounding for the Metaphysics of Morals with On a Supposed Right to Lie Because of Philanthropic Concerns*, 3rd edn. (translated by James W. Ellington; first published 1785). Indianapolis and Cambridge: Hackett Publishing Company.

Karlawish, J. (2011) Addressing the ethical, policy, and social challenges of preclinical Alzheimer disease, *Neurology*, 77: 1487–1493.

Kartalova-O'Doherty, Y., Morgan, K., Willetts, A. and Williamson, T. (2014) *Dementia – What is Truth? Exploring the Real Experience of People Living with More Severe Dementia. A Mental Health Foundation National Inquiry: A Rapid Literature Review*. London: Mental Health Foundation. Available at: https://www.mentalhealth.org.uk/sites/default/files/Dementia%20truth%20inquiry%20lit%20review%20FINAL%20%283%29.pdf (accessed 16 April 2022).

Kellogg, F.R., Crain, M., Corwin, J. and Brickner, P.W. (1992) Life-sustaining interventions in frail elderly persons, *Archives of Internal Medicine*, 152: 2317–2320.

Kelly, F. and Innes, A. (2013) Human rights, citizenship and dementia care nursing, *International Journal of Older People Nursing*, 8: 61–70.

Keogh, F., Carney, P. and O'Shea, E. (2021) Innovative methods for involving people with dementia and carers in the policymaking process *Health Expectations*, 24: 800–809.

Keown, J. (ed.) (1995) *Euthanasia Examined: Ethical, Clinical and Legal Perspectives*. Cambridge: Cambridge University Press.

Keown, J. (2002) *Euthanasia, Ethics and Public Policy: An Argument Against Legalisation*. Cambridge: Cambridge University Press.

Killick, J. (2013) *Dementia Positive: A Handbook Based on Lived Experiences*, Edinburgh: Luath Press.

Killick, J. (2017) *The Story of Dementia*. Edinburgh: Luath Press.

Killick, J. and Cordonnier, C. (2000) *Openings: Dementia Poems & Photographs*. London: Hawker Publications.

Kim, S., Richardson, A., Werner, P., et al. (2021a) Dementia stigma reduction (DESeRvE) through education and virtual contact in the general public: A multi-arm factorial randomised controlled trial, *Dementia*, 20: 2152–2169.

Kim, S.Y.H., Kane, N.B., Ruck Keene, A., Owen, G.S. (2021b) Broad concepts and messy realities: optimising the application of mental capacity criteria, *Journal of Medical Ethics*, Published Online First: 02 August 2021. doi: 10.1136/medethics-2021-107571.

Kim, S.Y.H., Mangino, D. and Nicolini, M. (2021c) Is this person with dementia (currently) competent to request euthanasia? A complicated and underexplored question, Journal of Medical Ethics, 47: e41. Available at: https://jme.bmj.com/content/47/12/e41 (accessed 3 June 2022).

Kim, S.Y.H., Miller, D.G. and Dresser, R. (2019) Response to: 'Dementia and advance directives: some empirical and normative concerns' by Jongsma et al., *Journal of Medical Ethics*, 45: 95–96.

King, L. and Series, H. (2014) Assessing capacity, in C. Foster, J. Herring, and I. Doron (eds) *The Law and Ethics of Dementia*. Oxford and Portland, Oregon: Hart Publishing.

Kissane, D.W. (1999) Euthanasia, dementia and ageing, *Current Opinion in Psychiatry*, 12: 457–461.

Kitwood, T. (1990) The dialectics of dementia: with particular reference to Alzheimer's disease, *Ageing and Society*, 10: 177–196.

Kitwood, T. (1995) Exploring the ethics of dementia research: a response to Berghmans and ter Meulen: a psychosocial perspective, *International Journal of Geriatric Psychiatry*, 10: 655–657.

Kitwood, T. (1997a) *Dementia Reconsidered: The Person Comes First*. Buckingham and Philadelphia: Open University Press.

Kitwood, T. (1997b) Personhood, dementia and dementia care, in S. Hunter (ed.) *Research Highlights in Social Work*. London: Jessica Kingsley.

Kitwood, T. (1998) Toward a theory of dementia care: ethics and interaction, *The Journal of Clinical Ethics*, 9: 23–34.

Kitwood, T. (2019) *Dementia Reconsidered, Revisited: The Person Still Comes First*, 2nd edn. (D. Brooker (ed.)). London: Open University Press.

Kitwood, T. and Bredin, K (1992) Towards a theory of dementia care: personhood and well-being, *Ageing and Society*, 12: 269–287.

Knüppel, H., Mertz, M., Schmidhuber, M., et al. (2013) Inclusion of ethical issues in dementia guidelines: a thematic text analysis, *PLoS Medicine*, 10: e1001498. Avaialable at: https://journals.plos.org/plosmedicine/article?id=10.1371/journal.pmed. 1001498 (accessed 21 March 2022).

Koh, W.Q., Ang, F.X.H. and Casey, D. (2021) Impacts of low-cost robotic pets for older adults and people with dementia: scoping review, *JMIR Rehabilitation and Assistive Technologies*, 8: e25340. Available at: https://doi.org/10.2196/25340 (accessed 1 April 2022).

Kontos, P.C. (2004) Ethnographic reflections on selfhood, embodiment and Alzheimer's disease, *Ageing and Society*, 24: 829–849.

Kontos, P.C. (2005) Embodied selfhood in Alzheimer's disease: rethinking person-centred care, *Dementia*, 4: 553–570.

Kontos, P. and Grigorovich, A. (2018) Integrating citizenship, embodiment, and relationality: towards a reconceptualization of dance and dementia in long-term care, *Journal of Law and Medical Ethics*, 46: 717–723.

Kontos, P., Miller, K.-L. and Kontos, A.P. (2017) Relational citizenship: supporting embodied selfhood and relationality in dementia care, *Sociology of Health and Illness*, 39: 182–198.

Kontos, P., Radnofsky, M.L., Fehr, P., et al. (2021a) Separate and unequal: a time to reimagine dementia, *Journal of Alzheimer's Disease*, 80: 1395–1399.

Kontos, P., Grigorovich, A., Kosurko, A., et al. (2021b) Dancing with dementia: exploring the embodied dimensions of creativity and social engagement, *Gerontologist*, 61: 714–723.

Koppelman, E.R. (2002) Dementia and dignity: towards a new method of surrogate decision making, *Journal of Medicine and Philosophy*, 27: 65–85.

Kouwenhoven, P.S.C., Raijmakers, N.J.H., van Delden, J.J.M. et al. (2015) Opinions about euthanasia and advanced dementia: a qualitative study among Dutch physicians and members of the general public, *BMC Medical Ethics*, 16: 7. Available at: http://www.biomedcentral.com/1472-6939/16/7 (accessed 2 June 2022).

Kruse, A. (2016) Benefactors or burdens? The social role of the old, in G. Scarre (ed.) *The Palgrave Handbook of the Philosophy of Aging*. London: Palgrave Macmillan.

Kruse, C.S., Fohn, J., Umunnakwe, G., et al. (2020) Evaluating the facilitators, barriers, and medical outcomes commensurate with the use of assistive technology to support people with dementia: a systematic review literature, *Healthcare*, 8: 278. Available at: https://doi.org/10.3390/healthcare8030278 (accessed 31 March 2022).

Laakkonen, M.-L., Raivio, M.M., Eloniemi-Sulkava, U., et al. (2008) How do elderly spouse care givers of people with Alzheimer disease experience the disclosure of dementia diagnosis and subsequent care? *Journal of Medical Ethics*, 34: 427–430.

Lamberg, J.L., Person, C.J., Kiely, D.K. and Mitchell, S.L. (2005) Decisions to hospitalize nursing home residents dying with advanced dementia, *Journal of the American Geriatrics Society*, 53: 1396–1401.

Lariviere, M., Poland, F., Woolham, J., et al. (2021) Placing assistive technology and telecare in everyday practices of people with dementia and their caregivers: findings from an embedded ethnography of a national dementia trial, *BMC Geriatrics*, 21: 121. Available at: https://doi.org/10.1186/s12877-020-01896-y (accessed 2 April 2022).

Laurance, J. (2004) Does an elderly man in a home have a right to pay for sex? *The Independent* (Saturday 23 October 2004). Available at: https://www.independent.co.uk/life-style/health-and-families/health-news/does-an-elderly-man-in-a-home-have-a-right-to-pay-for-sex-544740.html (accessed 22 April 2022).

Le Couteur, D.G., Doust, J., Creasey, H. and Brayne, C. (2013) Political drive to screen for pre-dementia: not evidence based and ignores the harms of diagnosis, *British Medical Journal*, 347: f5125. Available at: https://doi.org/10.1136/bmj.f5125 (accessed on 28 March 2022).

Lesser, A.H. (ed.) (1999) *Ageing, Autonomy and Resources*. Aldershot: Ashgate.

Lesser, A.H. (2006) Dementia and personal identity, in J.C. Hughes, S.J. Louw and S.R. Sabat (eds) *Dementia: Mind, Meaning, and the Person*. Oxford: Oxford University Press.

Lesser, H. (ed.) (2012a) *Justice for Older People*. Amsterdam and New York: Rodopi.

Lesser, H. (2012b) Triage and older patients, in H. Lesser (ed.) *Justice for Older People*. Amsterdam and New York: Ropodi.

Levinson, A-J.R. (1981) Termination of life support systems in the elderly: ethical issues, in *Journal of Geriatric Psychiatry*, 14: 71–85.

Lichtenberg, P.A. and Strzepek, D.M. (1990) Assessments of institutionalized dementia patients' competencies to participate in intimate relationships, *The Gerontologist*, 30: 117–120.

Lifton, R.J. (1986). *The Nazi Doctors*. New York: Basic Books.

Lightbody, E. (2014) Sexuality and dementia: for better or worse? *Old Age Psychiatrist*, 59: 15–23. Available at: https://catalogues.rcpsych.ac.uk/FILES/Spring%202014%20 Number%2059.pdf (accessed 20 April 2022).

Lilford, P. and Hughes, J.C. (2018) Biomarkers and the diagnosis of preclinical dementia, *BJPsych Advances*, 24: 422–430.

Lilford, P. and Hughes, J.C. (2020) Epidemiology and mental health in old age, *BJPsych Advances*, 26: 92–103.

Lindemann, H. (2009) Holding one another (well, wrongly, clumsily) in a time of dementia, *Metaphilosophy*, 40: 416–424.

Link, B.G. and Phelan, J.C. (2001) Conceptualizing stigma, *Annual Review of Sociology*, 27: 363–385.

Link, B.G. and Phelan, J.C. (2006). Stigma and its public health implications, *The Lancet*, 367: 528–529.

Locke, J. (1964) *An Essay Concerning Human Understanding*, edited by A.D. Woozley. Glasgow: William Collins/Fount. First published 1690.

Lohmeyer, J.L., Alpinar-Sencan, Z. and Schicktanz, S. (2021) Attitudes towards prediction and early diagnosis of late-onset dementia: a comparison of tested persons and family caregivers, *Aging & Mental Health*, 25: 832–843.

Lord Walton of Detchant (1994) *Medical Ethics: Select Committee Report*. House of Lords: *Hansard* 9 May: vol. 554, cc1344–412.

Louw, S.J. and Hughes, J.C. (2005) Moral reasoning – the unrealized place of casuistry in medical ethics, *International Psychogeriatrics*, 17: 149–54.

Low, L-F. and Purwaningrum, F. (2020) Negative stereotypes, fear and social distance: a systematic review of depictions of dementia in popular culture in the context of stigma, *BMC Geriatrics*, 20: 477. Available at: https://doi.org/10.1186/s12877-020-01754-x (accessed 22 January 2022).

Lustbader, W. (1999) Thoughts on the meaning of frailty, *Generations*, 23: 21-24.

Lyman, K.A. (1998) Living without Alzheimer's disease: the creation of meaning among persons with dementia, *The Journal of Clinical Ethics*, 9: 49–57.

Lynn, J.D., Rondón-Sulbarán, J., Quinn, E., et al. (2019) A systematic review of electronic assistive technology within supporting living environments for people with dementia, *Dementia*, 18: 2371–2435.

MacCormick, F.M.A., Emmett, C., Paes, P. and Hughes, J.C. (2018) Resuscitation decisions at the end of life: medical views and the juridification of practice. *Journal of Medical Ethics*, 44: 376–383.

MacIntyre, A. (1985) *After Virtue: A Study in Moral Theory*, 2nd edn. London: Duckworth.

MacIntyre, A. (2009) *Dependent Rational Animals: Why Human Beings Need the Virtues*. London: Duckworth (first published 1999).

Mackenzie, C. and Stoljar, N. (eds) (2000) *Relational Autonomy: Feminist Essays on Autonomy, Agency and the Social Self.* New York: Oxford University Press.

MacKenzie, J. (2021) Caring by lying, *Bioethics*, 35: 877–883.

Macklin, R. (2003) Dignity is a useless concept, *British Medical Journal*, 327: 1419–1420.

Macmillan, M.S. (1994) Hospital staff's perceptions of risk associated with the discharge of elderly people from acute hospital care, *Journal of Advanced Nursing*, 19: 249–256.

Maguire, P. (1999) Improving communication with cancer patients, *European Journal of Cancer*, 35: 1415–1422.

Mahieu, L. and Gastmans, C. (2012) Sexuality in institutionalized elderly persons: a systematic review of argument-based ethics literature, *International Psychogeriatrics*, 24: 346–357.

Mahieu, L., Anckaert, L. and Gastmans, C. (2014) Eternal sunshine of the spotless mind? An anthropological-ethical framework for understanding and dealing with sexuality in dementia care, *Medicine, Health Care and Philosophy*, 17: 377–387.

Mahieu, L., Anckaert, L. and Gastmans, C. (2017) Intimacy and sexuality in institutionalized dementia care: clinical-ethical considerations, *Health Care Analysis*, 25: 52–71.

Manthorpe, J., Iliffe, J.S., Samsi, K. et al. (2010) Dementia, dignity and quality of life: nursing practice and its dilemmas, *International Journal of Older People Nursing*, 5: 235–244.

Martens, R. and Hildebrand, C. (2021) Dementia care, robot pets, and aliefs, *Bioethics*, 35: 870–876.

Marzanski, M. (2000) Would you like to know what is wrong with you? On telling the truth to patients with dementia, *Journal of Medical Ethics*, 26: 108–113.

May, W.F. (1994) The virtues in a professional setting, in K.W.M. Fulford, G. Gillett and J.M. Soskice (eds) *Medicine and Moral Reasoning*. Cambridge: Cambridge University Press.

May, W.F. (2012) Testing the medical covenant: caring for patients with advanced dementia, *Journal of Law, Medicine & Ethics*, 40: 45–50.

McCullough, L.B., Coverdale, J.H. and Chervenak, F.A. (2007) Constructing a systematic review for argument-based clinical ethics literature: the example of concealed medications, *Journal of Medicine and Philosophy*, 32: 65–76.

McGettrick, G. and Williamson, T. (2015) *Dementia, rights, and the social model of disability. A new direction for policy and practice?* London: Mental Health Foundation.

McKenzie, K., Taylor, S., Murray, G. and James, I. (2020) The use of therapeutic untruths by learning disability nursing students, *Nursing Ethics*, 27: 1607–1617.

McKillop, J. (2016) Driving and dementia – my experiences. Glasgow: Life Change Trust. Available at: https://www.lifechangestrust.org.uk/publications/driving-and-dementia-my-experiences-james-mckillop (accessed 26 November 2022).

McMillan, J. (2006) Identity, self, and dementia, in J.C. Hughes, S.J. Louw and S.R. Sabat (eds) *Dementia: Mind, Meaning, and the Person.* Oxford: Oxford University Press.

McMillan, J. and Hope, T. (2008) The possibility of empirical psychiatric ethics, in G. Widdershoven, J. McMillan, T. Hope and L. van der Scheer (eds) *Empirical Ethics in Psychiatry.* Oxford: Oxford University Press.

Mental Health Foundation (2016) *What is Truth? An Inquiry about Truth and Lying in Dementia Care.* London: Mental Health Foundation. Available at: https://www.mentalhealth.org.uk/publications/what-truth-inquiry-about-truth-and-lying-dementia-care (accessed on 14 April 2022).

Menzel, P.T. (2019) AEDs are problematic, but Mrs A is a misleading case, *Journal of Medical Ethics*, 45: 90–91.

Merl, H., Doherty, K.V., Alty, J. and Salmon, K. (2022) Truth, hope and the disclosure of a dementia diagnosis: a scoping review of the ethical considerations from the perspective of the person, carer and clinician, *Dementia*, available at: https://doi.org/10.1177/14713012211067882 (accessed 28 March 2022).

Merleau-Ponty, M. (2002) *Phenomenology of Perception*. London and New York: Routledge (first published as *Phénomènologie de la Perception*, Paris: Gallimard (1945); translated by C. Smith).

Mill, J.S. (1859) On Liberty in M. Warnock (ed.)(1962) *Utilitarianism, On Liberty, Essay on Bentham, together with selected writings of Jeremy Bentham and John Austin*. Glasgow: William Collins, Fount.

Mill, J.S. (1861) *Utilitarianism* in M. Warnock (ed.)(1962) *Utilitarianism, On Liberty, Essay on Bentham, together with selected writings of Jeremy Bentham and John Austin*. Glasgow: William Collins, Fount.

Miller, D.G., Dresser, R. and Kim, S.Y.H. (2019) Advance euthanasia directives: a controversial case and its ethical implications, *Journal of Medical Ethics*, 45: 84–89.

Millett, S. (2011) Self and embodiment: a bio-phenomenological approach to dementia, *Dementia*, 10: 509–522.

Moe, C. and Schroll, M. (1997) What degree of medical treatment do nursing home residents want in case of life-threatening disease? *Age and Ageing*, 26: 133–137.

Montgomery, J. and Montgomery, E. (2016) Montgomery on informed consent: an inexpert decision? *Journal of Medical Ethics*, 42: 89–94.

Moody, H.R. (1992a) *Ethics in an Aging Society*. Baltimore: Johns Hopkins University Press.

Moody, H.R. (1992b) A critical view of ethical dilemmas in dementia, in R.H. Binstock, S.G. Post, and P.J. Whitehouse (eds) *Dementia and Aging: Ethics, Values and Policy Choices*. Baltimore: The Johns Hopkins University Press.

Moyle, W., Venturto, L., Griffiths, S., et al. (2011) Factors influencing quality of life for people with dementia: a qualitative perspective, *Aging & Mental Health*, 15: 970–979.

Mtande, T.K., Weijer, C., Hosseinipour, M.C., et al. (2019) Ethical issues raised by cluster randomised trials conducted in low-resource settings: identifying gaps in the *Ottawa Statement* through an analysis of the PURE Malawi trial, *Journal of Medical Ethics*, 45: 388–393.

Mugumbate, J.R. and Chereni, A. (2020) Now, the theory of ubuntu has its space in social work, *African Journal of Social Work*, 10: v–xvii.

Munden, L.M. (2017) The covert administration of medications: legal and ethical complexities for health care professionals, *Journal of Law, Medicine & Ethics*, 45: 182–192.

Muramoto, O. (2011) Socially and temporally extended end-of-life decision-making process for dementia patients, *Journal of Medical Ethics*, 37: 339–343.

Murdoch, I. (1970) *The Sovereignty of Good*. London and Henley: Routledge & Kegan Paul.

Murphy, D.J., Murray, A.M., Robinson, B.E. and Campion, E.W. (1989) Outcomes of cardiopulmonary resuscitation in the elderly, *Annals of Internal Medicine*, 111: 199–205.

Murphy, E. (1984) Ethical dilemmas of brain failure in the elderly, *British Medical Journal*, 288: 61–62.

Murphy, E. (1988) Psychiatric implications, in S.R. Hirsch and J. Harris (eds) *Consent and the Incompetent Patient: Ethics, Law and Medicine*. London: Gaskell.

Murphy, G.H. and O'Callaghan, A. (2004) Capacity of adults with intellectual disabilities to consent to sexual relationships, *Psychological Medicine*, 34: 1347–1357.

Murray, T.H. (1994) Medical ethics, moral philosophy and moral tradition, in K.W.M. Fulford, G. Gillett and J.M. Soskice (eds) *Medicine and Moral Reasoning*. Cambridge: Cambridge University Press.

Naue, U. (2008) 'Self-care without a self': Alzheimer's disease and the concept of personal responsibility for health, *Medicine, Health Care and Philosophy*, 11: 315–324.

Nedlund, A.-C. and Larsson, A.T. (2016) To protect and to support: how citizenship and self-determination are legally constructed and managed in practice for people living with dementia in Sweden, *Dementia*, 15: 343–357.

Nelson, J.L. (1995) Critical interests and sources of familial decision-making authority for incapacitated patients, *Journal of Law, Medicine & Ethics*, 23: 143–148.

Nelson, T. (2004) *Ageism: Stereotyping and Prejudice Against Older Persons*. Cambridge, MA: MIT Press.

Nestor, S., O'Tuathaigh, C. and Tony O'Brien, T. (2021) Assessing the impact of COVID-19 on healthcare staff at a combined elderly care and specialist palliative care facility: a cross-sectional study, *Palliative Medicine*, 35: 1492–1501.

Nguyen, T. and Li, X. (2020) Understanding public-stigma and self-stigma in the context of dementia: A systematic review of the global literature, *Dementia*, 19: 148–181.

NICE (2018) *Dementia: assessment, management and support for people living with dementia and their carers*. NICE guideline [NG97]. Available at: https://www.nice.org.uk/guidance/ng97/chapter/Recommendations#managing-non-cognitive-symptoms (accessed 7 April 2022).

Niemeijer, A.R., Frederiks, B.J.M., Depla, M.F.I.A., et al. (2011) The ideal application of surveillance technology in residential care for people with dementia, *Journal of Medical Ethics*, 37: 303–310.

Nilsson, M-L., Gershater, M.A. and Bengtsson, M. (2022) Registered Nurses' experiences of caring for persons with dementia expressing their sexuality, *Nursing Open*, 00: 1–8. Available at: https://doi.org/10.1002/nop2.1197 (accessed on 22 April 2022).

Noddings, N. (1984) *Caring: A Feminine Approach to Ethics and Moral Education*. Berkeley: University of California Press.

Nolan, M., Keady, J. and Aveyard, B. (2001) Relationship-centred care is the next logical step, *British Journal of Nursing*, 10: 757.

Noone, S. and Jenkins, N. (2018) Digging for dementia: exploring the experience of community gardening from the perspectives of people with dementia, *Aging and Mental Health*, 22: 881–888.

Norris, C. (1995) Hermeneutic circle, in T. Honderich (ed.) *The Oxford Companion to Philosophy*. Oxford: Oxford University Press.

Nuffield Council on Bioethics. (2009) *Dementia: Ethical Issues*. London: Nuffield Council on Bioethics. Available at: https://www.nuffieldbioethics.org/publications/dementia (accessed on 21 March 2022).

Oakley, J. (2007) Virtue theory, in in R.E. Ashcroft, A. Dawson, H. Draper and J.R. McMillan (eds) *Principles of Health Care Ethics*, 2nd edn. Chichester: John Wiley & Sons.

O'Connor, D., Phinney, A., Smith, A., et al. (2007) Personhood in dementia care: developing a research agenda for broadening the vision, *Dementia*, 6: 121–142.

O'Keefe, S.T. (2001) Autonomy vs welfare? Anatomy of a risky discharge. *Irish Medical Journal*, 94: 234–236.

Oliver, K. (2022) The me in dementia, in I. Parker, R. Coaten and M. Hopfenbeck (eds) *The Practical Handbook of Living with Dementia*. Monmouth: PCCS Books.

Osler, W. (1892) *Principles and Practice of Medicine Designed for the Use of Practitioners and Students of Medicine*. New York: D. Appleton and Company.

Oyebode, J. and Parveen, S. (2021) Carers and dementia, in T. Dening, A. Thomas, R. Stewart and J-P. Taylor (eds) *Oxford Textbook of Old Age Psychiatry*, 3rd edn. Oxford: Oxford University Press.

Pappadà, A., Chattat, R., Chirico, I., et al. (2021) Assistive technologies in dementia care: an updated analysis of the literature, *Frontiers in Psychology*, 12: 644587. Available at: https://www.frontiersin.org/articles/10.3389/fpsyg.2021.644587/full (accessed 31 March 2022).

Parfit, D. (1984) *Reasons and Persons*. Oxford: Oxford University Press.

Parker, I., Coaten, R. and Hopfenbeck, M. (2022) *The Practical Handbook of Living with Dementia*. Monmouth: PCCS Books.

Parsons, C. and van der Steen, J.T. (2017) Antimicrobial use in patients with dementia: current concerns and future recommendations, *CNS Drugs*, 31: 433–438.

Peisah, C., Ayalon, L., Verbeek, H., et al. (2021) Sexuality and the human rights of persons with dementia, *American Journal of Geriatric Psychiatry*, 29: 1021–1026.

Peisah, C., Byrnes, A., Doron, I., et al. (2020) Advocacy for the human rights of older people in the COVID pandemic and beyond: a call to mental health professionals, *International Psychogeriatrics*, 32: 1199–1204.

Pellegrino, E.D. and Thomasma, D.C. (1993) *The Virtues in Medical Practice*. New York and Oxford: Oxford University Press.

Penn, D., Lanceley, A., Petrie, A., et al. (2021) Mental capacity assessment: a descriptive, cross-sectional study of what doctors think, know and do, *Journal of Medical Ethics*, 47: e6. Available at: http://dx.doi.org/10.1136/medethics-2019-105819 (accessed on 7 February 2022).

Persad, G. (2019) Authority without identity: defending advanced directives via posthumous rights over one's body, *Journal of Medical Ethics*, 45: 249–256.

Pettit, P. (1980) *Judging Justice: An Introduction to Contemporary Political Philosophy*. London, Boston and Henley-on-Thames: Routledge and Kegan Paul.

Phillips, C.R. (2018) Quality of life in the contemporary politics of healthcare: … but what is a life? *Journal of Aging Studies*, 44: 9–14.

Phillipson, L. and Hammond, A. (2018) More than talking: a scoping review of innovative approaches to qualitative research involving people with dementia, *International Journal of Qualitative Methods*, 17: 1–13.

Phinney, A. and Chesla, C.A. (2003) The lived body in dementia, *Journal of Aging Studies*, 17: 283–299.

Pickering, N.J. (2021) Covert medication and patient identity: placing the ethical analysis in a worldwide context, *Journal of Medical Ethics*, 47: e59. Available at: http://dx.doi.org/10.1136/medethics-2020-106695 (accessed 11 April 2022).

Pinner, G. (2000) Truth-telling and the diagnosis of dementia, *British Journal of Psychiatry*, 176: 514–515.

Pinner, G. and Bouman, P. (2002) To tell or not to tell: on disclosing the diagnosis of dementia, *International Psychogeriatrics*, 14: 127–137.

Plato (1970) Apology, in B. Jowett (translator) *The Dialogues of Plato* Volume 1. London: Sphere Books.

Polden, E.R. (1989) Social work and people with dementia: putting principles into practice, *International Journal of Geriatric Psychiatry*, 4: 173–181.

Poole, M., Bond, J., Emmett, C., et al. (2014) Going home? An ethnographic study of assessment of capacity and best interests in people with dementia being discharged from hospital, *BMC Geriatrics*, 14: 56. Available at: http://www.biomedcentral.com/1471-2318/14/56 (accessed on 7 February 2022).

Pope, A. (2017) A psychological history of ageism and its implications for elder suicide, in R.E. McCue and M. Balasubramaniam (eds) *Rational Suicide in the Elderly: Clinical, Ethical, and Sociocultural Aspects*. Cham, Switzerland: Springer.

Pope John Paul II. (1995) *Evangelium Vitae – Encyclical Letter by the Supreme Pontiff John Paul II on the Value and Inviolability of Human Life*. Vatican City: Libreria Editrice Vaticana.

Post, S. (2004) Breaking the diagnosis of dementia, *The Lancet Neurology*, 3: 126–127.

Post, S.G. (1990) Severely demented elderly people: a case against senicide, *Journal of the American Geriatrics Society*, 38: 715–718.

Post, S.G. (1994a) Genetics, ethics, and Alzheimer disease, *Journal of the American Geriatrics Society*, 42: 782–786.

Post, S.G. (1994b) Alzheimer's disease: ethics and the progression of dementia, *Clinics in Geriatric Medicine*, 10: 379–394.

Post, S.G. (1995) *The Moral Challenge of Alzheimer Disease*, 1st edn. Baltimore and London: The Johns Hopkins University Press.

Post, S.G. (1997) Physician-assisted suicide in Alzheimer's disease, *Journal of the American Geriatrics Society*, 45: 647–651.

Post, S.G. (2000) *The Moral Challenge of Alzheimer Disease: Ethical Issues from Diagnosis to Dying*, 2nd edn. Baltimore and London: The Johns Hopkins University Press.

Post, S.G. (2006) *Respectare:* moral respect for the lives of the deeply forgetful, in J.C. Hughes, S.J. Louw and S.R. Sabat (eds) *Dementia: Mind, Meaning, and the Person.* Oxford: Oxford University Press.

Post, S.G., Whitehouse, P.J., Binstock, R.H., et al. (1997) The clinical introduction of genetic testing for Alzheimer disease: an ethical perspective, *Journal of the American Medical Association*, 277: 832–836.

Powell, R. (2014) Is preventive suicide a rational response to a presymptomatic diagnosis of dementia? *Journal of Medical Ethics*, 40: 511–512.

Prainsack, B. and Buyx, A. (2011) *Solidarity: Reflections on an Emerging Concept in Bioethics.* London: Nuffield Council on Bioethics.

Priefer, B.A. and Robbins, J. (1997) Eating changes in mild-stage Alzheimer's disease: a pilot study, *Dysphagia*, 12: 212–221.

Pucci, E., Belardinelli, N., Borsetti, G., et al. (2001) Information and competency for consent to pharmacologic clinical trials in Alzheimer disease: an empirical analysis in patients and family caregivers. *Alzheimer Disease and Associated Disorders*, 15: 146–154.

Purandare, N., Oude Voshaar, R.C., Rodway, C., et al. (2009) Suicide in dementia: 9-year national clinical survey in England and Wales, *British Journal of Psychiatry*, 194: 175–180.

Purtilo, R.B. and ten Have, H.A.M.J. (eds) (2004) *Ethical Foundations of Palliative Care for Alzheimer Disease.* Baltimore and London: The Johns Hopkins University Press.

Quinn, C., Hart, N., Henderson, C., et al. (2021) Developing supportive local communities: perspectives from people with dementia and caregivers participating in the IDEAL programme, *Journal of Aging & Social Policy.* Available at: https://doi.org/10.1080/08959420.2021.1973341 (accessed 22 January 2022).

Radden, J. and Fordyce, J.M. (2006) Into the darkness: losing identity with dementia, in J.C. Hughes, S.J. Louw and S.R. Sabat (eds) *Dementia: Mind, Meaning, and the Person.* Oxford: Oxford University Press.

Radden, J. and Sadler, J.Z. (2010) *The Virtuous Psychiatrist: Character Ethics in Psychiatric Practice.* New York: Oxford University Press.

Raphael, D.D. (1981) *Moral Philosophy*, 1st edn. Oxford: Oxford University Press.

Rapley, T. (2007) Distributed decision making: the anatomy of decisions-in-action, *Sociology of Health & Illness*, 30: 429–444.

Rawls, J. (1971) *A Theory of Justice.* Cambridge, Mass. and London England: Belknap Press of Harvard University Press.

Redley, M., Hughes, J.C. and Holland, A. (2010) Voting and mental capacity, *British Medical Journal*, 341: 466–467.

Regnard, C., Leslie, P., Crawford, H., et al. (2010) Gastrostomies in dementia: bad practice or bad evidence? *Age and Ageing*, 39: 282–284.

Reilly, S.T., Harding, A.J.E., Morbey, H., et al. (2020) What is important to people with dementia living at home? A set of core outcome items for use in the evaluation of non-pharmacological community-based health and social care interventions, *Age and Ageing*, 49: 664–671.

Rice, K. and Warner, N. (1994) Breaking the bad news: what do psychiatrists tell patients with dementia about their illness? *International Journal of Geriatric Psychiatry*, 9: 467–471.

Rivlin, M. (2012) Setting limits fairly: a critique of some of Daniel Callahan's views, in H. Lesser (ed.) *Justice for Older People*. Amsterdam and New York: Ropodi.

Robertson, G.S. (1983) Ethical dilemmas of brain failure in the elderly, *British Medical Journal*, 287: 1775–1777.

Rosenbaum, L. (2015) The paternalism preference – choosing unshared decision making, *New England Journal of Medicine*, 373: 589–592.

Roy, N., Stemple, J., Merrill, R.M. and Thomas, L. (2007) Dysphagia in the elderly: preliminary evidence of prevalence, risk factors, and socioemotional effects, *Annals of Otology, Rhinology & Laryngology*, 116: 858–865.

Royal College of Psychiatrists (2014). *Good Psychiatric Practice. Code of Ethics* College Report CR186. London: Royal College of Psychiatrists. Available at: https://www.rcpsych.ac.uk/docs/default-source/improving-care/better-mh-policy/college-reports/college-report-cr186.pdf?sfvrsn=15f49e84_2 (accessed 3 January 2022).

Russell, B. (1912) *The Problems of Philosophy*. Oxford: Oxford University Press (Paperback version published 1967).

Ryan, E.B., Bannister, K.A., Anas, A.P. (2009) The dementia narrative: writing to reclaim social identity, *Journal of Aging Studies*, 23: 145–157.

Sabat, S.R. (2001) *The Experience of Alzheimer's Disease: Life Through a Tangled Veil*. Oxford: Blackwell.

Sabat, S.R. (2005) Capacity for decision-making in Alzheimer's disease: selfhood, positioning and semiotic people, *Australian and New Zealand Journal of Psychiatry*, 39: 1030–1035.

Sabat, S.R. and Harré, R. (1992) The construction and deconstruction of self in Alzheimer's disease, *Ageing and Society*, 12: 443–461.

Sabat, S.R. and Harré, R. (1994) The Alzheimer's disease sufferer as a semiotic subject, *Philosophy, Psychiatry, & Psychology*, 1: 145–160.

Sabat, S.R., Johnson, A., Swarbrick, C. and Keady, J. (2011) The 'demented other' or simply 'a person'? Extending the philosophical discourse of Naue and Kroll through the situated self, *Nursing Philosophy*, 12: 282–292.

Saint Isaac (1997) *The Wisdom of Saint Isaac the Syrian* (translated by S. Brock). Oxford: SLG Press.

Sampson, E.L. (2010) Hospital admissions in dementia, in J.C. Hughes, M. Lloyd-Williams, G.A. Sachs (eds) *Supportive Care for the Person with Dementia*. Oxford: Oxford University Press.

Sampson, E.L. Blanchard, M.R., Jones, L., et al. (2009) Dementia in the acute hospital: prospective cohort study of prevalence and mortality, *British Journal of Psychiatry*, 195: 61–66.

Sanders, D. and Scott, P. (2020) Literature review: technological interventions and their impact on quality of life for people living with dementia, *BMJ Health Care Informatics*, 27: e100064. Available at: https://doi.org/10.1136/bmjhci-2019-100064 (accessed on 1 April 2022).

Schermer, M. (2007) Nothing but the truth? On truth and deception in dementia care, *Bioethics*, 21: 13–22.

Schmutte, T., Olfson, M., Maust, D.T., Xie, M. and Marcus, S.C. (2021) Suicide risk in first year after dementia diagnosis in older adults, *Alzheimer's and Dementia*, 1–10. Available via: https://doi.org/10.1002/alz.12390 (accessed on 9 March 2022).

Schneewind, J.B. (1991) Book Review: *Sources of the Self*, Charles Taylor. *The Journal of Philosophy*, 88: 422–426.

Scholten, M. and Jakov Gather, J. (2018) Adverse consequences of article 12 of the UN Convention on the Rights of Persons with Disabilities for persons with mental disabilities and an alternative way forward, *Journal of Medical Ethics*, 44: 226–233.

Schou-Juul, F., Nørgaard, S. and Lauridsen, S.M.R. (2022) Ethical issues in dementia guidelines for people with dementia and informal caregivers in Denmark: a qualitative thematic synthesis, *Dementia*, 0: 1–18 (online).

Schouten, V., Henrickson, M., Cook, C. M. et al. (2021) Intimacy for older adults in long-term care: a need, a right, a privilege – or a kind of care? *Journal of Medical Ethics*, 0: 1–5. Available at: http://dx.doi.org/10.1136/medethics-2020-107171 (accessed on 22 April 2022).

Secinaro, S., Calandra, D., Secinaro, A., et al. (2021) The role of artificial intelligence in healthcare: a structured literature review, *BMC Medical Informatics and Decision Making*, 21: 125. Available at: https://doi.org/10.1186/s12911-021-01488-9 (accessed 3 May 2022).

Seckler, A.B., Meier, D.E., Mulvihill, M. and Paris, B.E. (1991) Substituted judgment: how accurate are proxy predictions? *Annals of Internal Medicine*, 115: 92–98.

Sells, D. and Howarth, A. (2014) The Forced Care Framework: guidance for staff, *Journal of Dementia Care*, 22: 30–34.

Shakespeare, T. (2014). *Disability Rights and Wrongs Revisited* 2nd edn. London: Routledge.

Shakespeare, T., Zeilig, H. and Mittler, P. (2019) Rights in mind: thinking differently about dementia and disability, *Dementia*, 18: 1075–1088.

Shalowitz, D.I., Garrett-Mayer, E. and Wendler, D. (2006) The accuracy of surrogate decision makers: a systematic review, *Archives of Internal Medicine*, 166: 493–497.

Sharp, R. (2012) The dangers of euthanasia and dementia: how Kantian thinking might be used to support non-voluntary euthanasia in cases of extreme dementia, *Bioethics*, 26: 231–235.

Shaw, D. (2012) A direct advance on advance directives, *Bioethics*, 26: 267–274.

Shelton, C., El-Boghdadly, K. and Appleby, J.B. (2021) The 'haves' and 'have-nots' of personal protective equipment during the COVID-19 pandemic: the ethics of emerging inequalities amongst healthcare workers, *Journal of Medical Ethics*, Published Online First: 17 December 2021. Available at: https://doi.org/10.1136/medethics-2021-107501 (accessed 20 May 2022).

Shepherd, V., Griffith, R., Sheehan, M., et al. (2018) Healthcare professionals' understanding of the legislation governing research involving adults lacking capacity in England and Wales: a national survey, *Journal of Medical Ethics*, 44: 632–637.

Shepherd, V., Sheehan, M., Hood, K., et al. (2021) Constructing authentic decisions: proxy decision making for research involving adults who lack capacity to consent, *Journal of Medical Ethics*, 47: e42. Available at: https://jme.bmj.com/content/medethics/47/12/e42.full.pdf (accessed 10 March 2022).

Sherwin, S. (2007) Feminist approaches to health care ethics, in R.E. Ashcroft, A. Dawson, H. Draper and J.R. McMillan (eds) *Principles of Health Care Ethics*, 2nd edn. Chichester: John Wiley & Sons.

Shua-Haim, J.R. and Gross, J.S. (1996) The 'co-pilot' driver syndrome, *Journal of the American Geriatrics Society*, 44: 815–817.

Sinoff, G. and Blaja-Lisnic, N. (2014). Advance decisions and proxy decision-making in the elderly: a medical perspective, in C. Foster, J. Herring, and I. Doron (eds) *The Law and Ethics of Dementia*. Oxford and Portland, Oregon: Hart Publishing.

Slors, M. (1998) Two conceptions of psychological continuity, *Philosophical Explorations*, 1: 61–80.

Smart, J.J.C. and Bernard Williams, B. (1973) *Utilitarianism: For and Against*. Cambridge: Cambridge University Press.

Smith, A., King, E., Hindley, N., et al. (1998) The experience of research participation and the value of diagnosis in dementia: implications for practice, *Journal of Mental Health*, 7: 309–321.

Smith, M. (2017) Genetics of Alzheimer's disease, in D. Ames, J.T. O'Brien and A. Burns (eds) *Dementia*, 5th edn. Boca Raton, FL: CRC Press, Taylor & Francis Group.

sm-Rahman, A., Lo, C.H. and Jahan, Y. (2021) Dementia in Media Coverage: A Comparative Analysis of Two Online Newspapers across Time. *International Journal of Environmental Research and Public Health*, 18: 10539. Available at: https://doi.org/10.3390/ijerph181910539 (accessed 22 January 2022).

Social Care Institute for Excellence (2022) Dementia at a Glance: Key UK Statistics. Available at: https://www.scie.org.uk/dementia/about/ (accessed 25 January 2022).

Sonnicksen, J. (2016) Dementia and representative democracy: Exploring challenges and implications for democratic citizenship, *Dementia*, 15: 330–342.

Spencer, B. and Hotopf, M. (2019) The assessment of mental capacity, in R. Jacob, M. Gunn and A Holland (eds) *Mental Capacity Legislation: Principles and Practice*, 2nd edn. Cambridge: Cambridge University Press.

Srinivasan, T.N. and Thara, R. (2002) At issue: management of medication noncompliance in schizophrenia by families in India, *Schizophrenia Bulletin*, 28: 531–535.

Sriram, V., Jenkinson, C. and Peters, M. (2019) Informal carers' experience of assistive technology use in dementia care at home: a systematic review, *BMC Geriatrics*, 19: 160. Available at: https://doi.org/10.1186/s12877-019-1169-0 (accessed 31 March 2022).

Steele, L., Swaffer, K., Carr, R., Phillipson, L., and Fleming, R. (2021) Ending confinement and segregation: barriers to realising human rights in the everyday lives of people living with dementia in residential aged care. *Australian Journal of Human Rights*, 26: 308–328.

Steele, L., Swaffer, K., Phillipson, L. and Fleming, R. (2019) Questioning segregation of people living with dementia in Australia: an international human rights approach to care homes, *Laws*, 8: 18. Available at https://doi.org/10.3390/laws8030018 (accessed 20 May 2022).

Stein-Parbury, J., Chenoweth, L., Jeon, Y.H., et al. (2012) Implementing person-centred care in residential dementia care, *Clinical Gerontology*, 35: 404–424.

Strang, D.G., Molloy, D.W. and Harrison, C. (1998) Capacity to choose place of residence: autonomy vs beneficence? *Journal of Palliative Care*, 14: 25–29.

Stratford, J. (2017) Sexuality and dementia, in D. Ames, J.T. O'Brien and A. Burns (eds) *Dementia*, 5th edn. Boca Raton, FL: CRC Press, Taylor & Francis Group.

Strawson, G. (2004) Against narrativity, *Ratio*, 17: 428–452.

Strech, D., Mertz, M., Knüppel, H. et al. (2013) The full spectrum of ethical issues in dementia care: systematic qualitative review, *The British Journal of Psychiatry*, 202: 400–406.

Sugarman, J., Cain, C., Wallace, R. and Welsh-Bohmer, K.A. (2001) How proxies make decisions about research for patients with Alzheimer's disease, *Journal of the American Geriatric Society*, 49: 1110–1119.

Sulmasy, D.P. (2013) The varieties of human dignity: a logical and conceptual analysis, *Medicine Health Care and Philosophy*, 16: 937–944.

Swaffer, K. (2014) Dementia: stigma, language, and dementia-friendly, *Dementia*, 13: 709–716.

Swidler, R.N., Seastrum, T. and Shelton, W. (2007) Difficult hospital inpatient discharge decisions: ethical, legal and clinical practice issues, *American Journal of Bioethics*, 7: 23–28.

Swinnen, A. and Schweda, M. (2015) Popularizing dementia: public expressions and representations of forgetfulness, in A. Swinnen and M. Schweda (eds) *Popularizing Dementia: Public Expressions and Representations of Forgetfulness*. Bielefeld: transcript Verlag.

Tarzia, L., Fetherstonhaugh, D. and Bauer, M. (2012) Dementia, sexuality and consent in residential aged care facilities, *Journal of Medical Ethics*, 38: 609–613.

Taylor, C. (1985) *Human Agency and Language: Philosophical Papers I*. Cambridge: Cambridge University Press.

Taylor, C. (1989) *Sources of the Self: The Making of the Modern Identity*. Cambridge: Cambridge University Press.

Taylor, C. (1995) *Philosophical Arguments*. Cambridge, MA: Harvard University Press.

Teles Sarmento, J., Lírio Pedrosa, C. and Carvalho, A.S. (2021) What is common and what is different: recommendations from European scientific societies for triage in the first outbreak of COVID-19, *Journal of Medical Ethics*, Epub ahead of print. Available at: https://doi.org/10.1136/medethics-2020-10696 (accessed 20 May 2022).

ter Meulen, R. and Wright, K. (2012) Family solidarity and informal care: the case of care for people with dementia, *Bioethics*, 26: 361–368.

Thornton, T. (2006) The discursive turn, social constructionism, and dementia, in J.C. Hughes, S.J. Louw and S.R. Sabat (eds) *Dementia: Mind, Meaning, and the Person*. Oxford: Oxford University Press.

Thornton, T. (2007) *Essential Philosophy of Psychiatry*. Oxford: Oxford University Press.

Tieu, M. (2021) Truth and diversion: self and other regarding lies in dementia care, *Bioethics*, 35: 857–863.

Tieu, M. and Matthews, S. (forthcoming) The relational care framework: promoting continuity or maintenance of selfhood in person-centred care, *Journal of Medicine and Philosophy*.

Tooley, M. (2009) Personhood, in H. Kuhse and P. Singer (eds) *A Companion to Bioethics*, 2nd edn. Chichester: Wiley-Blackwell.

Torke, A.M., Alexander, G.C. and Lantos, J. (2008) Substituted judgment: the limitations of autonomy in surrogate decision making, *Journal of General Internal Medicine*, 23: 1514–1517.

Trachtenberg, D.I. and Trojanowski, J.Q. (2008) Dementia: a word to be forgotten. *Archives of Neurology*, 65: 593–595.

Train, G.H., Nurock, S.A., Manela, M., et al. (2005) A qualitative study of the experiences of long-term care for residents with dementia, their relatives and staff, *Aging & Mental Health*, 9: 119–128.

Treloar, A., Beats, B. and Philpot, M. (2000) A pill in the sandwich: covert medication in food and drink, *Journal of the Royal Society of Medicine*, 93: 408–411.

Treloar, A., Philpot, M. and Beats, B. (2001) Concealing medication in patients' food, *Lancet*, 357: 62–64.

Treloar, A., Crugel, M. and Prasanna, A., et al. (2010) Ethical dilemmas: should antipsychotics ever be prescribed for people with dementia? *British Journal of Psychiatry*, 197: 88–90.

Tuckett, A.G. (2004) Truth-telling in clinical practice and the arguments for and against: a review of the literature, *Nursing Ethics*, 11: 500–513.

Tuckett, A.G. (2012) The experience of lying in dementia care: a qualitative study, *Nursing Ethics*, 19: 7–20.

Tuijt, R., Rait, G., Frost, R., et al. (2021) Remote primary care consultations for people living with dementia during the COVID-19 pandemic: experiences of people living with dementia and their carers, *British Journal of General Practice*, August 2021, e574–e582. Available at: https://doi.org/10.3399/BJGP.2020.1094 (accessed 14 May 2022).

Tulloch, G. (2005) *Euthanasia – Choice and Death*. Edinburgh: Edinburgh Press.

Turner, A., Eccles, F., Keady, J., et al. (2017) The use of the truth and deception in dementia care amongst general hospital staff, *Aging and Mental Health*, 21: 862–869.

Uniacke, S. (2007) The doctrine of double effect, in R.E. Ashcroft, A. Dawson, H. Draper and J.R. McMillan (eds) *Principles of Health Care Ethics*, 2nd edn. Chichester: John Wiley & Sons.

United Nations General Assembly (1948) *Universal Declaration of Human Rights*. Available at: https://www.un.org/sites/un2.un.org/files/udhr.pdf (accessed 7 April 2022).

United Nations General Assembly (2006) *Convention on the Rights of Persons with Disabilities*, 13 December 2006, A/RES/61/106, Annex I. Available at: https://legal.un.org/avl/ha/crpd/crpd.html (accessed 29 January 2022).

United Nations General Assembly (2014) *Convention on the Rights of Persons with Disabilities: General Comment No. 1 (19th May 2014)*, Article 12: Equal recognition before the law. Available at: https://www.ohchr.org/en/hrbodies/crpd/pages/gc.aspx (last accessed 10 February 2022).

van Delden, J.J.M. (2004) The unfeasibility of requests for euthanasia in advance directives, *Journal of Medical Ethics*, 30: 447–452.

van der Maaden, T., van der Steen, J.T., de Vet, H.C.W., et al. (2016) Prospective observations of discomfort, pain, and dyspnea in nursing home residents with dementia and pneumonia, *Journal of the American Medical Directors Association*, 17: 128–135.

van der Steen, J.T., Helton, M.R. and Ribbe, M.W. (2009b) Prognosis is important in decision making in Dutch nursing home patients with dementia and pneumonia, *International Journal of Geriatric Psychiatry*, 24: 933–936.

van der Steen, J.T., Ooms, M.E., van der Wal, G. and Ribbe, M.W. (2002a) Pneumonia: the demented patient's best friend? Discomfort after starting or withholding antibiotic treatment, *Journal of the American Geriatric Society*, 50: 1681–1688.

van der Steen, J.T., Lane, P., Kowall, N.W., et al. (2012) Antibiotics and mortality in patients with lower respiratory infection and advanced dementia, *Journal of the American Medical Directors Association*, 13: 156–161.

van der Steen, J.T., Ooms, M.E., Ader, H.J., et al. (2002b) Withholding antibiotic treatment in pneumonia patients with dementia: a quantitative observational study, *Archives of Internal Medicine*, 162: 1753–1760.

van der Steen, J.T., Pasman, H.R.W., Ribbe, M.W. et al. (2009a) Discomfort in dementia patients dying from pneumonia and its relief by antibiotics, *Scandinavian Journal of Infectious Diseases*, 41: 143–151.

van der Steen, J.T., Radbruch, L., Hertogh, C.M.P.M., et al. (2014) White paper defining optimal palliative care in older people with dementia: a Delphi study and recommendations from the European Association for Palliative Care, *Palliative Medicine*, 28: 197–209.

Volicer, L., Rheaume, Y., Brown, J., et al. (1986) Hospice approach to the treatment of patients with advanced dementia of the Alzheimer type. *Journal of the American Medical Association*, 256: 2210–2213.

Wagland, R. (2012a) Social injustice: distributive egalitarianism, the complete-life view, and age discrimination, in H. Lesser (ed.) *Justice for Older People*. Amsterdam and New York: Ropodi.

Wagland, R. (2012b) A fair innings or a complete life: another attempt at an egalitarian justification of ageism, in H. Lesser (ed.) *Justice for Older People*. Amsterdam and New York: Ropodi.

Wall, J. (2019) 'Mrs A': a controversial or extreme case? *Journal of Medical Ethics*, 45: 77–78.

Walsh, S., Merrick, R., Milne, R. and Brayne, C. (2021) Aducanumab for Alzheimer's disease? Patients and families need hope, not false hope, *British Medical Journal*, 374: n1682.

Walsh, S.C., Murph, E., Devane, D., et al. (2021) Palliative care interventions in advanced dementia, *Cochrane Database of Systematic Reviews 2021*, Issue 9. Art. No.: CD011513. Available at: https://www.cochranelibrary.com/cdsr/doi/10.1002/14651858. CD011513.pub3/full (accessed on 3 June 2022).

Wang, Q., Davis, P.B., Gurney, M.E. and Xu, R. (2021) COVID-19 and dementia: analyses of risk, disparity, and outcomes from electronic health records in the US, *Alzheimer's & Dementia*, 17: 1297–1306.

Ward, R., Campbell, S. and Keady, J. (2016) 'Gonna make yer gorgeous': everyday transformation, resistance and belonging in the care-based hair salon, *Dementia*, 15: 395–413.

Weil, S. (2002) *The Need for Roots: Prelude to a Declaration of Duties towards Mankind*, (trans. A. Wills). London: Routledge. (Originally published as *L'Enracinement* in 1949; Paris: Editions Gallimard.)

Weiss, G.B. (1985) Paternalism modernised, *Journal of Medical Ethics*, 11: 184–187.

Weissman, J.S., Haas, J.S., Fowler, F.J. Jr., et al. (1999) The stability of preferences for life-sustaining care among persons with AIDS in the Boston Health Study, *Medical Decision Making*, 19: 16–26.

Welie, S. (2008) Patient incompetence in the practice of old age psychiatry: the significance of empirical research for the law, in G. Widdershoven, J. McMillan, T. Hope and L. van der Scheer (eds) *Empirical Ethics in Psychiatry*. Oxford: Oxford University Press.

Welie, S.P.K. (2001) Criteria for patient decision making (in)competence: a review of and commentary on some empirical approaches, *Medicine, Health Care and Philosophy*, 4: 139–151.

Wells, L.A. (1974) 'Why not try the experiment?' The scientific education of Edward Jenner, *Proceedings of the American Philosophical Society*, 118: 135–145.

Welsh, S. and Deahl, M. (2002) Cover medication – ever ethically justifiable? *Psychiatric Bulletin*, 26: 123–126.

Werner, P. (2006) Lay perceptions regarding the competence of persons with Alzheimer's disease, *International Journal of Geriatric Psychiatry* 21: 674–680.

Whitehouse, P. (2004) Breaking the diagnosis of dementia, *The Lancet Neurology*, 3: 124.

Whitehouse, P.J. (1996) Future prospects for Alzheimer's disease therapy: ethical and policy issues for the international community, *Acta Neurologica Scandinavica*, 165: 145–149.

Whitehouse, P.J. (2000) Quality of life: future directions, in S.M. Albert and R.G. Logsdon (eds) *Assessing Quality of Life in Alzheimer's Disease*. New York: Springer Publishing Company.

Whitehouse, P.J. and George, D. (2008) *The Myth of Alzheimer's: What You Aren't Being Told About Today's Most Dreaded Diagnosis*. New York: St. Martin's Press.

Widdershoven, G. and van der Scheer, L. (2008) Theory and methodology of empirical ethics: a pragmatic hermeneutic perspective, in G. Widdershoven, J. McMillan, T. Hope and L. van der Scheer (eds) *Empirical Ethics in Psychiatry*. Oxford: Oxford University Press.

Widdershoven, G.A.M. and Abma, T.A. (2007) Hermeneutic ethics between practice and theory, in R.E. Ashcroft, A. Dawson, H. Draper and J.R. McMillan (eds) *Principles of Health Care Ethics*, 2nd edn. Chichester: John Wiley & Sons.

Widdershoven, G.A.M. and Berghmans, R.L.P. (2001) Advance directives in dementia care: from instructions to instruments, *Patient Education and Counseling*, 44: 179–186.

Widdershoven, G.A.M. and Berghmans, R.L.P. (2006) Meaning-making in dementia: a hermeneutic perspective, in J.C. Hughes, S.J. Louw, and S.R. Sabat (eds) *Dementia: Mind, Meaning, and the Person*. Oxford: Oxford University Press.

Widdershoven, G.A.M. and Widdershoven-Heerding, I. (2003) Understanding dementia: a hermeneutic perspective, in K.W.M. Fulford, K. Morris, J.Z. Sadler, and G. Stanghellini (eds) *Nature and Narrative: An Introduction to the New Philosophy of Psychiatry*. Oxford: Oxford University Press.

Williams, B. (1972) *Morality: An Introduction to Ethics*. Cambridge: Cambridge University Press.

Wilson, S. and Pinner, G. (2020) Driving in dementia: a clinician's guide, in P. Lilford and J.C. Hughes (eds) *Clinical Topics in Old Age Psychiatry*. Cambridge: Cambridge University Press.

Winner, S. (1999) Practical problems with the discharge of old people from hospital – a physician's perspective, in A.H. Lesser (ed.) *Ageing, Autonomy and Resources*. Aldershot, England and Brookfield, Vermont: Ashgate.

Wittgenstein, L. (1967) *Philosophical Investigations* (G.E.M. Anscombe and R. Rhees (eds); G.E.M. Anscombe (trans)). Oxford: Blackwell. (First published 1953.)

Wittgenstein, L. (1981) *Zettel* (G.E.M. Anscombe and G.H. von Wright (eds); G.E.M. Anscombe (trans)). Oxford: Blackwell.

Wolff, J. (2012) Dementia, death and advance directives, *Health Economics, Policy and Law*, 7: 499–506.

Wolverson, E., Dunn, R., Moniz-Cook, E., et al. (2021) The language of behaviour changes in dementia: a mixed methods survey exploring the perspectives of people with dementia, *Journal of Advanced Nursing*, 77: 1992–2001.

Woodford, H. (2010) *Essential Geriatrics*, 2nd edn. Oxford, New York: Radcliffe Publishing.

Wood-Mitchell, A., Waterworth, A., Stephenson, M., et al. (2006) Lying to people with dementia: sparking the debate. *Journal of Dementia Care*, 14: 30–31.

Woodruff, R. (2016) Aging and the maintenance of dignity, in G. Scarre (ed.) *The Palgrave Handbook of the Philosophy of Aging*. London: Palgrave Macmillan.

Woods, S. (2007) *Death's Dominion: Ethics at the End of Life*. Maidenhead: Open University Press.

World Health Organization (2004) *Ageing and Health Technical Report, Volume 5: A Glossary of Terms for Community Health Care and Services for Older Persons*. Kobe: World Health Organization Centre for Health Development.

World Medical Association (WMA) (2013) World Medical Association Declaration of Helsinki: Ethical principles for medical research involving human subjects, *Journal of the American Medical Association*, 310: 2191–2194.

Zeilig, H. (2013) Dementia as a cultural metaphor, *The Gerontologist*, 54: 258–267.

Zeilig, H., West, J., and van der Byl Williams, M. (2018) Co-creativity: possibilities for using the arts with people with a dementia, *Quality in Ageing and Older Adults*, 19: 135–14.

Zeilig, H., Poland, F., Fox, C. and Killick, J. (2015) The arts in dementia care education: a developmental study, *Journal of Public Mental Health*, 14: 18–23.

Zeilig, H., Tischler V., van der Byl Williams, M., et al. (2019) Co-creativity, well-being and agency: a case study analysis of a co-creative arts group for people with dementia, *Journal of Aging Studies*, 49: 16–24.

Zuckerman, C. (1987) Conclusions and guidelines for practice, *Generations*, 11: 67–73.

Zwijsen, S.A., Niemeijer, A.R. and Hertogh, C.M.P.M. (2011) Ethics of using assistive technology in the care for community-dwelling elderly people: an overview of the literature, *Aging & Mental Health*, 15: 419–427.

Subject Index

Name Index